CIRCULATION

CIRCULATION

Björn Folkow

Professor of Physiology
The University of Göteborg
Sweden

Eric Neil

John Astor Professor of Physiology
in the University of London
at the Middlesex Hospital Medical School
London

New York

OXFORD UNIVERSITY PRESS

London   Toronto

1971

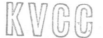

Second printing, 1973

Copyright © 1971 by Oxford University Press, Inc.
Library of Congress Catalogue Card Number: 70-83036
Printed in the United States of America

*This book
is dedicated to Anglo-Swedish friendship,
which barely survived it*

Preface

Charles Dickens (1843) prefaced *A Christmas Carol* thus:

"I have endeavoured in this Ghostly little book to raise the Ghost of an Idea, which shall not put my readers out of humour with themselves, with each other, with the season, or with me. May it haunt their houses pleasantly and no one wish to lay it."

We have had the same end in view—to raise the Ghost of an Idea. If the reader substitutes "reason" for "the season" and adds the word "down" to the end of the last sentence of Dickens's Preface we will be content to leave it at that. Whether he changes the word "ghostly" to "ghastly" is up to him.

We acknowledge the help of our colleagues and friends—both of them. We thank, fervently, our Secretaries, Grania Fetherstonhaugh, Kerstin Andréasson, and Helena Öberg for services beyond the bounds of duty.

The Publishers—well, after all they *did* publish the book.

Björn Folkow
Eric Neil

Göteborg and London
November 1970

Contents

CIRCULATION

I

General Principles

Introduction

The greatest discovery in medical science was made by William Harvey, who showed in 1628 that the heart pumped blood around the circulatory system. He had a clear grasp of the general principles of cardiovascular function and understood that the circulation provided nourishment for the tissues. Harvey had no direct knowledge about the capillaries, which were not described until 1661 by Malpighi, but he understood what happened when blood passed from the arteries over to the veins in the tissues. In Chapter 14 of *De Motu Cordis* Harvey wrote of blood which "forcibly ejected to all parts of the body, therein steals into the veins and porosities of the flesh, flows back everywhere through those very veins ... to the auricle of the heart" (Harvey, 1628). Three and a half centuries have elapsed since this introduction to modern experimental medicine, and a vast number of contributions have been made in cardiovascular physiology.

The Heart

No pump yet devised has the long-term performance of the heart. This little organ, the "size of a clenched fist" and weighing 300 g, supplies blood for the "ideal man" of 70 kg weight for 70 years. In resting man

3

each ventricle of the heart ejects 5 to 5.5 l/min—in 70 years the output of the two ventricles is about 400 million litres, even if the man remains in the resting state. The heart beats 65 to 75/min in resting man. Each cardiac cycle therefore lasts some 0.8 sec, and of that cycle 0.3 sec is spent in contraction of the ventricles and 0.5 sec in their relaxation. In the latter period the ventricles are refilled by venous return.

The heart is in essence two pumps—a *right heart* (atrium and ventricle) and a *left heart* (atrium and ventricle). In the contraction phase (*systole*) the left heart ejects 70 to 80 ml/beat into the aorta, and blood received from the systemic veins (venae cavae) is pumped out by the right ventricle into the pulmonary circuit.

The metabolic requirements of the body vary according to the state of activity. The heart may service the body at rest by providing about 5 to 5.5 l/min, but during strenuous exercise it may pump 25 l/min or more by increasing its force of contraction and by accelerating its rate of beat. Some of these changes in cardiac performance are due to nervous influences on the cardiac muscle fibres; some are a simple physical consequence of the effect of the "distending force" of venous return on the diastolic length and hence the contractile force of the cardiac muscle fibres.

Every pump has to be "primed", or filled, before it can perform. The heart receives blood via the veins at a pressure which only slightly exceeds zero during its filling, or relaxation, phase—*diastole*. The contraction, and consequent downward displacement, of the heart ventricles causes a passive expansion of the atria and hence exerts some suction on blood in the central veins which contributes to the forces responsible for venous filling ("priming of the pump").

The Vessels

General Organization

During systole the intraventricular pressure changes from near zero to 120 mm Hg in the left ventricle and to 25 mm Hg in the right. The systolic pressures in the aorta and the pulmonary artery consequently rise to 120 mm Hg and to 25 mm Hg, respectively. At the end of the contraction phase the heart muscle relaxes, the semilunar valves close off the aorta and the pulmonary artery, and intraventricular pressures fall steeply to near zero.

Owing to the elasticity of the large arteries and the resistance to flow in the peripheral vessels, arterial pressure varies far less than that in the ventricles, resulting in a diastolic pressure of approximately 80 mm Hg in the systemic vascular bed. Therefore the phasic pressure cycle of the left ventricle—120 to 0 mm Hg—is changed into an arterial pulse pressure of $120/80 = 40$ mm Hg. For the pulmonary circuit the corresponding pressures are approximately 25/10, with a pulse pressure of about 15 mm Hg.

The two ventricles thus phasically provide the energy for circulation in the pulmonary and systemic circuits, respectively, furnishing the *pressure head* which drives the flow. The analogy of Ohm's law enables an understanding of the factors involved:

$$I = E/R \text{ (Ohm)}$$

E is the pressure head for flow and is equal to the mean pressure difference between the arterial and venous ends of the circuits. R is the total resistance offered by the vessels of the systemic and pulmonary circuits, respectively, where the arterioles make the biggest contribution to resistance. The quotient between the pressure head (E) and the regional flow resistance (R) determines the blood flow (I) to any one circuit.

The *left* ventricle thus pumps blood out into the systemic vascular bed, which consists of many regional circuits—liver, kidney, brain, muscle, etc.—specialized in design and control and arranged in parallel. Each such circuit supplies the metabolic requirements of the relevant region: solutes for nutrition and oxygen for the combustion of such substrates by the tissue cells. To secure this the arteries branch repeatedly, first into arterioles (which control resistance to flow) and then into capillaries. The thin-walled capillaries, by virtue of their dense distribution and enormous surface area, form the key point of the circulation. Across their walls (total surface area about 1000 m^2 in the whole body) occurs the all-important exchange between cells and bloodstream. Metabolites and CO_2 produced by cellular metabolism diffuse into and are removed by the blood leaving the tissues. The capillary network is collected by the venules leading to the veins which serve as adjustable conduits to the heart.

The *right* ventricle pumps blood out into the pulmonary vascular bed, which is uniform in design and where exchange of oxygen and carbon

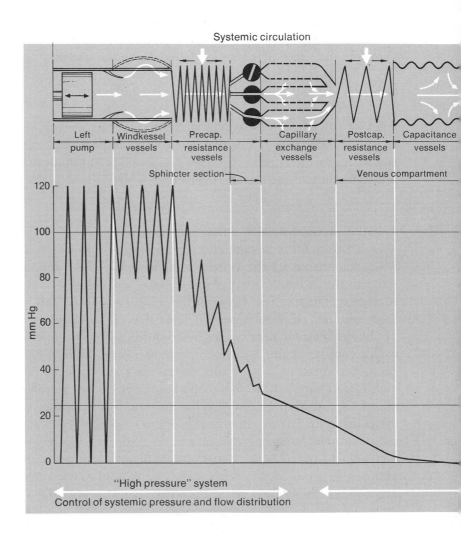

Fig. 1-1. Diagrammatic illustration of the functionally specialized series-coupl
sections of the cardiovascular system as related to the pressure levels.

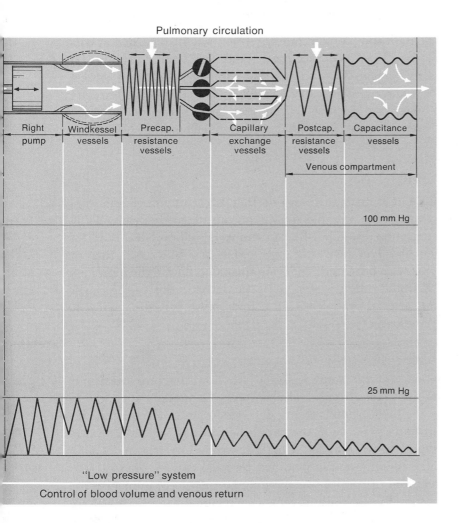

dioxide takes place with the alveolar air across the walls of the capillaries (total surface area in the lungs about 90 m²).

Vascular Differentiation

Each vascular circuit, pulmonary and systemic, may be regarded as containing the following *series-coupled* sections: Windkessel vessels, precapillary resistance vessels, precapillary sphincters, capillary exchange vessels, postcapillary resistance vessels, capacitance vessels and, in some circuits, shunt vessels (Fig. 1-1). These subdivisions are made on *functional* grounds and are of great importance for understanding circulatory phenomena.

Windkessel Vessels

These offer little resistance to flow but they are distensible and consequently they damp the pulsatile systolic output of the ventricle. Thus, left ventricular ejection distends the aorta and its large branches. With the closure of the aortic valves the elastic aorta and its branches recoil, thereby sustaining the pressure head and rendering the blood flow to the periphery steadier than it would otherwise be. Geriatric deterioration of the elastic elements of the arterial wall leads to a high pulse pressure owing to reduction of Windkessel function.

Precapillary Resistance Vessels

These furnish most of the total resistance to flow and are essentially represented by the small arteries and arterioles. Changes in their radius mainly decide the blood supply of any one region and, moreover, determine the hydrostatic pressure in the capillaries of that region. The precapillary resistance vessels manifest a high degree of intrinsic (myogenic) basal tone which is continuously modified by local factors, physical and chemical. Alterations of basal myogenic tone by such local influences are almost solely responsible for the adjustments of regional vascular resistance in the all important circuits that supply the heart and brain. Elsewhere the resistance vessels of the regional circuits are subjected also to the influence of extrinsic sympathetic nerves. The effects of such a nervous supply are relatively trivial in the circumstances of resting equilibrium, but they may become profound in conditions of stress.

Precapillary Sphincters

These, though part of the precapillary resistance vessels, determine in particular the size of the capillary exchange area by modifying the number of capillaries perfused at any one moment. Again, their control is predominantly local—that of an intrinsic myogenic activity continuously modified by local vasodilator metabolites.

The Capillary Exchange Vessels

These vessels—the key point of the cardiovascular system—are tubes formed by a single layer of endothelial cells. Across their walls solutes pass to and fro; lipid-soluble substances utilizing the entire surface, and water-soluble molecules traversing only the capillary "pores". The capillaries themselves exert no "active" influence on either flow rate or the all-important exchange mechanisms of diffusion and filtration-absorption.

Postcapillary Resistance Vessels

The venules and small veins contribute little to *total* peripheral resistance. Nevertheless they are important, for the *ratio* of the precapillary to postcapillary resistance determines the hydrostatic pressure in the capillaries themselves and this pressure itself chiefly decides the net fluid transfer between blood and interstitial fluid. Thus, while changes in the *sum* of the pre- and post-capillary resistances affect blood *flow*, changes in the pre/postcapillary *ratio* affect blood *volume*.

Capacitance Vessels

These vessels—the whole of the venous compartment—add very little to *total* resistance but notably affect vascular capacity by changes in their luminal configuration and diameter. Cardiac output is dependent upon venous return; correspondingly, changes of venous capacity, due essentially to extrinsic sympathetic constrictor activity, can profoundly influence the priming of the cardiac pump. The venous compartment may be regarded as the adjustable "forechamber" of the pump.

Shunt Vessels

These are the exception rather than the rule in most circuits. They constitute direct connections between small arteries and veins, bypassing the capillary bed. As a consequence they subserve no metabolic function and, appropriately, are found in abundance in parts of the skin (fingers, toes,

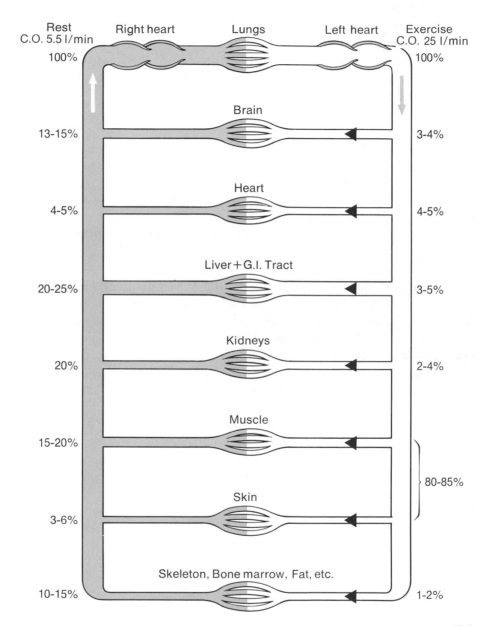

Fig. 1-2. Diagram illustrating the flow distribution among the various parallel-coupled vascular circuits in man during rest and during heavy exercise.

ears, etc.) which fulfill a purely thermoregulatory function. Their tone is greatly dependent upon the influence of sympathetic constrictor nerves.

Dimensions

The heart pumps about 5 to 5.5 l/min round the body in an average sized man at rest (3.25 l/m² body surface area, which best describes the relationship between cardiac output and body size). The blood volume is only 5 to 6 litres, so this implies a complete circulation of the total blood volume in one minute. During intense exercise the cardiac output can increase up to 25 l/min in a healthy man, extreme values in outstanding athletes being 35 to 40 l/min.

Regional flow measurements *at rest* reveal that the brain receives 750 ml/min, the liver 1300 ml/min, the kidneys 1200 ml/min, the muscles 1000 ml/min, and the heart itself 250 ml/min. These total nearly 4.5 l/min—and no account has been made for skin, fat, and bone flow. At exercise the flow pattern changes markedly (Fig. 1-2). Clearly the husbandry of the cardiovascular system is careful. As the blood flow to any one regional circuit depends on its pressure head and its local vascular resistance and as the pressure head is virtually the same for each, the separate blood flows of these circuits is determined by their respective vascular resistances.

Resistance can only be expressed quantitatively from a knowledge of flow and pressure. For this calculation, flow must be expressed in unit of quantitatively comparable weights of tissue. It is conventional to express flow in terms of ml/min/100 g. Occasionally such expressions yield information which borders on the ludicrous: for example, the blood flow for the carotid body is then 2000 ml/min/100 g, while that of resting skeletal muscle is about 3 ml/min/100 g. The carotid body weighs 2 mg and its actual flow is 40 μl (0.040 ml/min), while skeletal muscles weigh some 35 kg and receive some 1000 ml during rest. Nevertheless, the bulk flow information thus expressed has its uses, giving as it does a vivid impression of the tremendous differences in blood supply that different tissues enjoy.

Table 1-1 provides some quantitative data in cardiovascular physiology in resting man, giving in approximative terms an idea of both the regional *oxygen consumption* and the *dimensions* of the various regional circuits during normal "resting" tone of their resistance vessels. As a contrast, the approximate figures for regional blood flow at maximal dilatation at a pressure head of about 100 mm Hg are also given. Clearly, the heart would not be

Table 1-1.

ORGAN	Weight kg	Blood flow during rest (Max. vasodil. = [1])			Oxygen usage during rest			
		ml/min	ml/min/100 g	% total card. output	A-V O₂ difference, ml/100 ml blood	ml/min	ml/min/100 g	% total O₂ usage
Brain	1.4	750 [1500]	55	14	6	45	3	18
Heart	0.3	250 [1200]	80	5	10	25	8	10
Liver G.I. tract	1.5 / 2.5	1300 [5000] / 1000 [4000]	85 } / 40	23	6	75	2	30
Kidneys	0.3	1200 [1800]	400	22	1.3	15	5	6
Muscle	35	1000 [20,000]	3	18	5	50	0.15	20
Skin	2	200 [3000]	10	4	2.5	5	0.2	2
Remainder (skeleton, bone marrow, fat, connective tissue, etc.)	27	800 [4000]	3	14	5	35	0.15	14
TOTAL	70 kg	5500 ml/min		100		250		100

The values in the table are "rounded" figures and roughly describe the situation in average man during rest. Figures within [1] give in very approximate terms organ blood flows at maximal vasodilatation of the respective circuits.

able to provide all tissues simultaneously with a maximal blood supply; nor does this ever occur normally. Thus, exercise hyperaemia (Fig. 1-2), which constitutes the largest work load for the heart, is combined with flow restrictions in areas outside the muscle circuit.

References

Harvey, William (1628). "Movement of the heart and blood in animals. An anatomical essay." Trans. by Kenneth J. Franklin (1957). Oxford: Blackwell.

2

Poiseuille's Law

Historical Background

Although since prehistoric times moving water must have fascinated man
—while fishing, wading, or swimming in calm and turbulent streams—
Newton (1713) was responsible for the first theoretical considerations
concerning the laws that govern fluids in motion. He outlined in *Principia
Mathematica* how gentle movement, imparted to a fluid relative to a surface, created laminae moving at velocities which increased with the
distance from the surface. A velocity gradient perpendicular to the surface,
the *rate of shear*, thus characterized this laminar flow.

No further experimental studies of fluid movements were published until
1813, when Girard described the flow of water in brass pipes. He correctly
defined the relationship between flow, pressure, and tube length. However, he concluded that flow varied with the *third* power of the radius—
possibly because some turbulence had disturbed the laminar flow conditions—and it remained for Hagen and Poiseuille to provide the final
experimental solution.

Experimental Evidence

In 1839, the engineer Hagen studied the water flow through brass tubes.
Using tubes 47.2 to 108.7 cm long and 12.7 to 29.4 mm radius, he found

the flow varied as the pressure to a power of the radius and was inversely proportional to the tube length. The exponent of the radius was found experimentally to be 4.12, and Hagen concluded that it should theoretically be 4.

Hagen was thus the first to suggest the importance of r^4 in the flow through any given tube. A more complete analysis, published in an abstract in 1842 and in full in 1846, was provided by Poiseuille. It is worth noting that Poiseuille (1799–1869) first studied physics and mathematics at the École Polytechnique in Paris, but transferred to medical school, taking his M.D. degree with a thesis on the study of the strength of the aortic beat. On qualifying he became free teacher of medical physics. The experiments that stimulated him to study the flow of water in glass capillary tubes arose from his previous studies of blood flow in animal capillaries, conducted in 1835 and 1840–41, in which he had proved that the movement of corpuscles in capillaries was solely due to the action of the heart and was not due to attraction of these corpuscles to one another. He also observed (as had Malpighi) that the velocity of the blood cells was greatest in the centre of the minute vessels and, moreover, described the transparent cell-free layer at the periphery of the smallest vessels.

Poiscuille used five capillary tubes, each smaller than the last, with diameters from 140 μ down to 30 μ. Using compressed air, he forced a constant water volume through them, measuring the time taken to do so. He found that, provided the length of the tube exceeded a certain minimum, the volume discharged in unit time Q was proportional to the pressure head P, to the fourth power of the radius r and inversely proportional to the tube length L.

Hence
$$Q = K \cdot \frac{Pr^4}{L}$$

where K is a constant characteristic of the liquid and is temperature dependent; i.e. K represents the viscosity of the liquid which is nowadays denoted by the Greek letter η (eta).

Mathematical Derivation

Wiedemann (1856) and Hagenbach (1860) independently calculated the equation for flow in these circumstances, each using Newton's hypothesis—

without, however, giving any credit to Newton. Hagenbach's solution is given here.

Consider a length AB of a cylindrical tube of radius R (Fig. 2-1). Let a pressure head P be maintained along the length L causing liquid to flow from A to B. The flow is assumed to be such that each particle of liquid moves parallel to the axis with a constant velocity. This velocity is the same for all points lying on the same circle, so the liquid may be regarded as being composed of cylindrical laminae moving at velocities v which are functions of their radii.

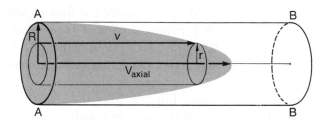

Fig. 2-1. The velocity profile in a tube AB in steady laminar flow. This profile forms a parabola. The *average* velocity (V) is half the axial velocity (V_{axial}).

The force F exerted by the pressure P on a cylindrical unit of radius r is

$$F_P = \pi r^2 P \tag{1}$$

The viscous force (F_{visc}) retarding the motion of the liquid is given by the product: area × viscosity × velocity gradient

$$F_{visc} = 2\pi r L \eta (dv/dr) \tag{2}$$

If v is to remain constant the forces acting on the cylinder must be equal and opposite.

$$F_P = -F_{visc}$$

Therefore
$$rP = -2L\eta(dv/dr) \tag{3}$$

Hence the velocity gradient is

$$dv/dr = -\frac{rP}{2L\eta} \tag{4}$$

On integration,

$$v = -\frac{r^2 P}{4L\eta} + C \qquad (5)$$

If we assume that the lamina in contact with the wall of the tube is stationary, then here $v = 0$ and $r = R$, and

$$C = \frac{R^2 P}{4L\eta} \qquad (6)$$

Combining (5) and (6),

$$v = \frac{P}{4L\eta}(R^2 - r^2) \qquad (7)$$

This is the equation of a parabola whose axis is the axis of AB while the axis of r is at the distance $R^2 P/4L\eta$ from the apex of the curve. v has its maximum when $r = 0$, i.e. along the axis of AB. As v is the distance traversed in unit time, all liquid particles which lie on the plane AA at zero time will be on the surface of this paraboloid after unit time. Hence the volume of the paraboloid is the volume of fluid Q which flows in unit time.

The volume of this solid of revolution is

$$Q = 2\pi \int_0^R vr \cdot dr \qquad (8)$$

Combining (7) and (8) and substituting for v,

$$Q = \frac{2\pi P}{4L\eta} \int_0^R (R^2 - r^2)r \cdot dr$$

$$Q = \frac{\pi P R^4}{8L\eta}$$

Applicability

Poiseuille's law—sometimes called the Hagen-Poiseuille law—is strictly valid *only* for streamline flow and when flow is nonpulsatile with uniform viscosity for the fluid (see McDonald, 1960). Even if these prerequisites are not met in the circulation, this fundamental law, with due approximations, is largely valid for haemodynamics. In Chapters 3 through 6 the type of fluid movement within the cardiovascular system is discussed, together with the different factors in the formula, with particular emphasis on the magnitude, range of variation, etc., of the pressure head, the radius and the length of the tube, and the viscosity of blood in the situation *in vivo*.

When the Poiseuille formula is used in haemodynamics, the pressure head is written as $P_1 - P_2$, thereby denoting the difference between the pressures at the two ends of the system. The radius is usually written as r, since R has come to stand for *flow resistance*. The formula is nowadays usually written thus:

$$Q = \frac{\pi r^4 (P_1 - P_2)}{8L\eta}$$

The Poiseuille formula can also be written in a simplified form, as a direct analogue to Ohm's first law for the relationship between electric current, voltage, and resistance:

$$Q = \frac{P_1 - P_2}{R}; \quad \text{where} \quad R = \frac{8L\eta}{\pi r^4}$$

In some situations it is more convenient to use the flow *conductance*, C, instead of the flow *resistance*, R; C being equal to $1/R$.

R is sometimes expressed in *peripheral resistance units* (*PRU*), being equal to the pressure gradient (mm Hg) divided by the flow (ml/min) (see Green *et al.*, 1963). However, to give the proper relationship to the perfused tissue mass, the unit PRU_{100}—expressing flow resistance per 100 g tissue—is more convenient in studies of *regional* haemodynamics:

$$PRU_{100} = \frac{P_1 - P_2 (\text{mm Hg})}{Q (\text{ml/min/100 g})}$$

The proper physical unit for calculations of *total systemic* (or *pulmonary*) *resistance* (*TPR*) is dyne sec/cm^5, where cardiac output is given as flow/sec (e.g. 90 ml) and the pressure head in mm Hg (e.g. 100 mm Hg):

$$TPR = \frac{100 \times 13.6 \times 980}{90} = 14{,}810 \text{ dynes} \times \text{sec/cm}^5$$

In the cardiovascular system Q is, of course, the important factor in the Poiseuille formula, and the radius r is the main determinant of Q in any individual tissue. This is so mainly because flow is proportional to the *fourth* power of r, but also because the other factors, $P_1 - P_2$, L, and η, do not vary extensively under ordinary circumstances.

References

Girard, P. S. (1813–15). "Mémoire sur le mouvement des fluides dans les tubes capillaires et l'influence de la temperature sur ce mouvement," *Mém. de l'Inst.* 249–380. (Paris.)

Green, H. D., C. E. Rapela, and M. C. Conrad (1963). "Resistance (conductance) and capacitance phenomena in terminal vascular beds," *Handbook of Physiology*, 2, Circulation **II**, 935–60.

Hagen, G. H. L. (1839). "Über die Bewegung des Wassers in engen cylindrischen Röhren," *Ann. d. Phys. u. Chem.* **46**, 423–42.

Hagenbach, E. (1860). "Über die Bestimming der Sähigkeit einer Flüssigkeit durch den Ausfluss aus Röhren," *Ann. der Physik.* **109**, 385–426.

McDonald, D. A. (1960). *Blood flow in arteries.* London: Arnold.

Newton, I. (1713). *Principia mathematica.* 2nd edition, lib. **II**, sect. IX, The circular motion of liquids, Proposition LI, Theorem **XXXIX**.

Poiseuille, J. L. M. (1846). "Recherches expérimentales sur le mouvement des liquides dans les tubes de très petits diamètres," *Mém. Savant Étrangers*, **9**, 433–544. (Paris.)

Wiedemann, G. (1856). *Ann. der Physik.* **99**, 221; Quoted by E. Hatschek (1928) in *The viscosity of liquids*, p. 239. London: Bell.

3

Streamline and Turbulent Flow

Poiseuille himself observed that the relationship between pressure and flow ceased to be linear at high rates of flow, but it was Osborne Reynolds (1883) who provided the first serious analysis of the problem (see Mc-Donald, 1960). Using a long cylindrical tube, he injected dye into the axial stream and showed that the flow of fluid was streamline, or laminar, until the rate of flow reached a critical value, whereupon the flow became turbulent with vortices. He derived the formula

$$Re = \frac{VD\sigma}{\eta}$$

in which V = average velocity, D = diameter of the tube, σ (sigma) = density, and η = viscosity. Re is the Reynolds number. When V is measured in cm/sec, D in cm, and viscosity in poise (see Chapter 4), turbulence appears when Re exceeds 2000. (Note that if the radius of the tube is used in the formula, as is sometimes the case, Re has a critical value of 1000.)

When turbulence develops, it does so gradually; when turbulence becomes conspicuous the fluid flow becomes largely proportional to the square root of the pressure drop along the tube (Fig. 3-1). In other words, there is a greater energy loss incurred in turbulent flow because more energy is wasted in creating the kinetic energy of the eddies (see Coulter and Pappenheimer, 1949). "Big whirls have little whirls which feed on their velocity. Little whirls have smaller whirls and so on to vorticity" (L.F. Richardson).

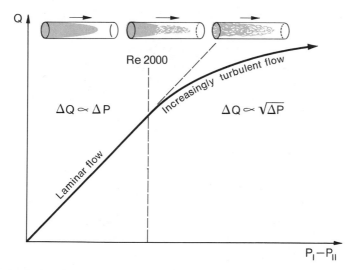

Fig. 3-1. Relationship between pressure head $(P_I\text{-}P_{II})$ and flow (Q) in a rigid tube during streamline flow and its transition to turbulent flow. (Modified from Coulter and Pappenheimer, 1949. By permission.)

Blood flow is streamline in all the smaller vessels which constitute the "resistance channels" and thus haemodynamic behaviour is largely dependent on this type of flow. Turbulence, however, occurs normally in the ventricles and to some extent in the atria, with the great benefit of mixing the blood thoroughly on both sides of the heart. For example, even if blood oxygenation is not equally efficient in all parts of the lung, the turbulence in the left ventricle ensures thorough mixing, so that all tissues are supplied with equally well-oxygenated blood.

The aorta too may exhibit turbulence: here the pulsatile flow might favour turbulence even at Reynolds numbers well below 2000 for *net forward* flow. With a resting cardiac output of 5.5 litres and a pulse rate of 65, about 85 ml of blood are pushed through the aorta per second and as the cross-sectional area is some 4 cm² $(D = 2.2$ cm) the *mean* velocity of blood flow is 85/4, or about 21 cm/sec. The viscosity of the blood when flowing in large-bore tubes at 37°C is about 0.03 poise, so calculating Re at *mean* flow (σ set at 1),

$$Re = \frac{21 \times 2.2}{0.03} = 1540$$

However, as the blood is ejected into the aorta only during systole the Reynolds number must during this phase be several times higher than the number calculated for mean flow. Some turbulence, then, might occur at systolic ejection into the aorta, even in resting man. The flow resistance of the aorta and its main branches is, however, almost negligible; hence such moderate phasic turbulence, if it occurs, has little effect on over-all flow resistance. In heavy exercise, with cardiac outputs perhaps exceeding 25 l/min the peak velocity of aortic ejection increases more than fivefold and turbulence would then appear to have greater chances to develop. If so, this may partly explain the substantial pressure drop that seems to occur along central parts of the arterial tree in heavy exercise (Åstrand *et al.*, 1965). On the other hand, the very intermittency of flow seems to "protect" against turbulence which takes some time to develop (Cotton 1960); thus aortic turbulence might after all be slight even at high instantaneous Reynolds numbers.

As each successive branching of the arterial tree entails an increase in the total cross-sectional vascular area (Chapter 5), the linear velocity of flow decreases proportionately. Moreover, each single branch has a smaller diameter than has the parent vessel, so both V and D decrease and the Reynolds number calculated has a progressively smaller value. Therefore, turbulent flow is *not* a normal feature of the peripheral arterial or venous circulation. However, pathological changes, such as plaques of atheroma, favour local turbulence, just beyond the site where the diameter of the vessel is decreased; moreover, where turbulence occurs, secondary aggregates of thrombocytes and organized blood clots follow more easily and further diminish the lumen.

Turbulent flow itself does not cause murmurs or bruits. However, when turbulence occurs in a region where wall resonance is prominent with distinct vibrations of the wall, murmurs can be heard. Vibrations of such nature occur especially easily where blood is rapidly pushed through a narrow segment into a wider lumen. Aortic or mitral stenosis, and patent ductus arteriosus, are all associated with murmurs of this type. The Korotkow sounds of sphygmomanometry have their origin in turbulence, as the systolic blood flow is rapidly pushed through the semicollapsed artery beyond the blood pressure cuff. The sounds usually disappear when the cuff pressure falls below diastolic pressure, for the artery then remains wide open with essentially streamline flow.

References

Åstrand, P. O., B. Ekblom, R. Messin, B. Saltin, and J. Svedberg (1965). "Intra-arterial blood pressure during exercise with different muscle groups," *J. Appl. Physiol.* **20,** 253–56.

Cotton, K. L. (1960). "The instantaneous measurement of blood flow and of vascular impedance," Ph.D. Thesis, London.

Coulter, N. A., Jr., and J. R. Pappenheimer (1949). "Development of turbulence in flowing blood," *Am. J. Physiol.*, **159,** 401–8.

McDonald, D. A. (1960). *Blood flow in arteries.* London: Arnold.

Reynolds, O. (1883). "An experimental investigation of the circumstances which determine whether the motion of water shall be direct or sinusoid, and of the law of resistance in parallel channels," *Phil. Trans.* **174,** 935–82.

4

The Viscosity Factor

Historical Background

It is common knowledge that if some part of a liquid bulk is kept moving, e.g. if one stirs a cup of coffee, the motion is gradually communicated to the rest of the liquid; conversely, if one ceases stirring, the liquid comes to rest. Newton analyzed this problem and ascribed the effects to a "lack of slipperiness" (*defectus lubricitatis*) between the liquid particles—a property resembling *attritus* (friction) seen between solid surfaces. In *Principia* (Lib. ii, Sect. ix) he formulated a hypothesis regarding the force required to overcome this lack of slipperiness:

> that the resistance which arises from the lack of slipperiness of the parts of the liquid, other things being equal, is proportional to the velocity with which the parts of the liquid are separated from one another.

The terms "internal friction" and "viscosity" have since supplanted *defectus lubricitatis*. How the word "viscosity" came to be used is not sure, but as Hatschek (1928) has pointed out, it comes from the word *viscum*—the mistletoe. This is indeed true—and is no help whatever of itself. However, the Romans used the same word, *viscum*, to signify bird-lime—a sticky substance made from mistletoe and holly, which they painted on tree branches to ensnare small birds. Hence the use of the word "viscous".

Characterisation of Fluids

Homogeneous fluids like water possess a viscosity which is independent of the rate of shear. They are called "Newtonian" fluids. Although blood plasma contains protein macromolecules and other solutes, it behaves rheologically very like a Newtonian fluid. "Non-Newtonian" fluids are heterogeneous. Emulsions (containing insoluble fluid droplets), suspensions (containing solid particles), and foams (containing gas bubbles) belong to this group. Such fluids show *anomalous viscosity*—their viscosity increases as the flow velocity falls.

Although blood is a suspension, the deformable erythrocytes can be squeezed through capillary lumina well below their normal diameter with remarkably little extra force. However, blood does exhibit anomalous viscosity, and, at very low shear rates, its viscosity measured *in vitro* far exceeds that seen in normal circulatory conditions (Fig. 4-1A). Erythrocytes tend to aggregate at very low shear rates, and this property presumably contributes to the anomalous viscosity that blood displays. Nevertheless blood does not exhibit true *plasticity*—a state in which a certain driving force has to be reached before the fluid begins to move. Thus, the pressure-flow curve for blood flowing through rigid tubes does not show an intercept at the positive pressure axis but actually converges towards the origin (Fig. 4-1B).

Excellent surveys of blood viscosity are available and should be consulted for details (Bayliss, 1952, 1962; Haynes, 1961; Whitmore, 1968).

Measurement of Viscosity

Two types of viscosimeter are commonly employed for measurements *in vitro* (see Whitmore, 1968). In one, the fluid passes through a calibrated tube system, and pressure and flow rate are measured in relationship to that of water. In the other, the fluid is kept in a container where it is exposed to two smooth surfaces that can be moved relative to each other at measured rates, and the force required to produce a given rate of shear is then recorded and is related to that for water.

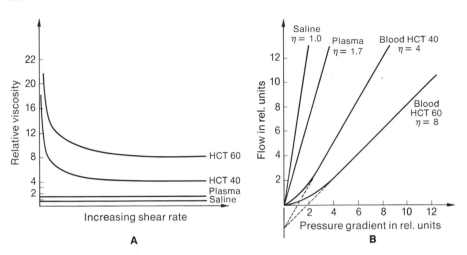

Fig. 4-1. A. Approximate relationship between shear rate and relative viscosity of plasma and blood of haematocrits 40 and 60. B. Approximate pressure-flow relationship in a rigid tube (diameter about 1 mm) for saline, plasma, and blood of haematocrits 40 and 60. (Modified from Haynes, 1961. By permission.)

The viscosity of blood can also be estimated *in vivo*, e.g. by comparing the flows of blood and plasma at equal pressure heads *and* transmural pressures in a maximally dilated vascular bed (Whittaker and Winton, 1933). Then the radius factor is kept constant, and plasma—the viscosity of which is the same *in vivo* and *in vitro*—is used as the reference fluid. For example, if at equal pressures 10 ml of plasma (viscosity of 1.2 *cP* at 37°C) passes per unit time, but only 5 ml of blood, then the viscosity of blood *in vivo* at that flow rate is 2.4 *cP*.

Although the unit for viscosity is the *poise* (*P*), the *centipoise* (*cP*) is more convenient. The viscosity of water is set at 1 *cP* at a temperature of 20.3°C. Temperature is very important: at 0°C water has a viscosity of 1.792 *cP*, while at 37°C it has a viscosity of 0.6947 *cP*. Blood viscosity may be even more affected by temperature.

Commonly, the term *relative viscosity* is used: the viscosity of a fluid is expressed relative to that of water. At 37°C the relative viscosity of plasma is usually 1.7 (so its viscosity is 1.7 × 0.6947 = 1.2 *cP*). Fibrinogen molecules have an especially important effect on plasma viscosity because their elongate molecular form greatly increases the internal friction of the solution. Hyperfibrinogenaemia markedly increases plasma viscosity.

Factors Influencing Blood Viscosity

Normal whole blood has a relative viscosity of 4 to 5 (Fig. 4-1) when measured *in vitro* at moderate or high shear rates in the conventional viscosimeters. However, in addition to the influence of shear rate, other factors—haematocrit, tube diameter, and temperature—are very important in influencing blood viscosity *in vivo* (Fåhraeus and Lindqvist, 1931).

The Influence of Shear Rate

When the shear rate is very low it causes a great increase of blood viscosity *in vitro*. The situation *in vivo* is different, however, owing to the complexity of the vascular bed. Thus, even during the most extensive reductions in flow rates which may occur in normal conditions, especially when this involves a narrowing of the vessels, the viscosity measured *in vivo* increases only a little, perhaps by a factor of only 30 to 50%, provided that the blood *composition* remains unaltered (Djojosugito *et al.*, 1970).

Although several factors contribute to the anomalous viscosity of blood, it is clear that the suspended erythrocytes confer this property, for plasma itself behaves largely like a Newtonian fluid.

Axial Streaming

It seems that the erythrocytes tend to rotate slowly in a regular direction (Fig. 4-2A) when exposed to the variable rates of shear that are inherent in the parabolic flow profile (Magnus effect). It is clear from the arrows

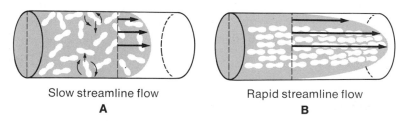

Slow streamline flow	Rapid streamline flow
A	**B**

Fig. 4-2. Orientation of the erythrocytes in small vessels during slow (*A*) and rapid (*B*) streamline flow, where the axial cell orientation is maximal.

in Fig. 4-2A that the rotation of the cells implies a relatively higher linear speed for their axial ends. This appears to create a minor pressure gradient transversely directed from the tube wall to the axis, tending to push the cells towards the axis.

As long as the shear rate is low, this axial tendency created for the cells is offset by their mutual collisions, but as shear rate increases the cells come to occupy the central part of the tube. Eventually they move with their long axes parallel to the direction of flow in that part of the stream where the linear flow rate is highest but where the intermolecular differences in shear rate are least (Fig. 4-2B). This last factor tends to minimize the friction between cell and plasma fractions (which is normally responsible for blood having a higher viscosity than plasma). This development of axial streaming of the cells as the flow rate increases is associated with a progressive decrease of viscosity as the shear rate rises, until the maximal axial orientation is reached. At still higher flow rates blood therefore behaves largely as a Newtonian fluid with almost constant viscosity, showing a linear pressure-flow relationship (Fig. 4-1A).

The extent of this axial displacement of the cells is limited in blood of normal haematocrit value. Thus, even if the cells were so closely packed as to be in direct contact with each other, but *without* deformation, they would largely fill the entire vascular lumen if the haematocrit value were slightly above 60 with the 35 to 40% plasma compartment trapped between them. Even at the normal haematocrit of 40 to 45 there is only a limited space available if the cells are not to be deformed, and it is an experimental finding that the relatively cell-free zone close to the wall is usually quite narrow.

The *dynamic haematocrit* is always smaller in narrow vessels than in the general vascular bed, as the cells then mainly travel in the rapidly moving axial parts. The higher the flow rate, the lower the dynamic haematocrit, as was clearly shown by Fåhraeus and Lindqvist (1931) in experiments on models. When, for example, the rapid renal circulation is arrested by clamping both artery and vein, the blood trapped within the kidney has a substantially lower haematocrit than does that in the general circulation.

Plasma Skimming

When the flow rates are high, this axial orientation of the cells presumably accounts for the phenomenon of *plasma skimming*. This may occur at sites where the angle of branching is large, with the result that the haematocrit value of the blood is lower in the side branch than in the main branch. Plasma skimming is of no importance where *large* vessels branch because of the very narrow limits of the marginal cell-free zone.

Anomalous Viscosity *in Vivo*

Usually blood flows in the body are sufficiently high to minimize the importance of the anomalous viscosity. However, marked decreases in flow rate, caused by asynchronous changes in local tone, normally occur intermittently in the interconnected vascular loops of the microvessels. On the other hand, these events generally occur in vessels so narrow that the cells usually traverse them in single file and the blood therefore behaves rheologically almost like plasma (see below).

It has generally been assumed that anomalous viscosity would become very important when the over-all flow rate is grossly reduced, as in shock. However, as has already been stated, viscosity *in vivo* increases relatively little at low flow rates, provided that the blood *composition* has not been simultaneously altered. One cannot draw too close parallels between the behaviour of blood *in vitro* and that of blood flowing naturally in the vascular bed. In any case, it is the viscosity of blood *in vivo* that is really important.

On the other hand, the linear flow rate is always less in small veins than in small arteries because of the dimensional difference in the size of the total cross-sectional area. In shock, the average velocity of flow may become so slow that the anomalous properties of blood raise its viscosity in the wide postcapillary compartment well above that of the blood passing through the precapillary vessels. For this reason the postcapillary resistance may increase relative to that of the precapillary compartment, even though the impact of such a regional increase of viscosity on *total* flow resistance is small. Nevertheless, such a "rheologically determined" reduction in the pre/postcapillary resistance ratio is serious, for it tends to raise the capillary pressure and thus tends to cause additional fluid loss from the capillaries (see Chapter 8). Also, the increased tendency of the cells to aggregate and sludge, particularly when sepsis and trauma are involved, further exacerbates this situation. Moreover, aggregation causes capillary plugging, which reduces the total surface area available for exchange and therefore minimizes the opportunity for diffusion of oxygen and other nutrients.

The Influence of Haematocrit

The viscosity of blood increases out of proportion to the increase of the cell fraction when the haematocrit exceeds 40 to 45, when flows are measured in tubes of diameter similar to those of the important "resistance" section of the vascular bed (Fig. 4-3). Curve A shows intercepts that give the viscosities for bloods of 20 and 60 compared with blood of haematocrit 40. It can be understood that at low haematocrits the oxygen capacity of the blood is decreased more than the gain in oxygen supply that results from

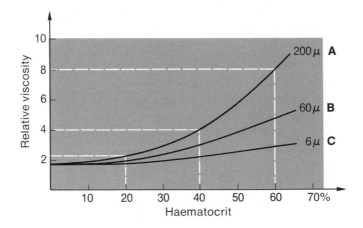

Fig. 4-3. Approximate relationship between haematocrit and relative viscosity when blood passes at high rates through tubes of various diameters: (A) 200μ, (B) 60μ, and (C) 6μ. (Modified from Haynes, 1961. By permission.)

the increased flow at the lower viscosity. Conversely, at haematocrit 60 the increase in oxygen capacity (50%) from the normal value is more than offset by the increase in viscosity, which largely halves the rate of oxygen supply. These are problems found in anaemia and polycythaemia.

Such effects of the haematocrit value on viscosity are of less moment in very small pre- and post-capillary vessels (Curve B) and are almost insignificant in tubes of capillary diameter (Curve C). This seems remarkable, as the systemic capillary diameter of 4 to 7 microns cause the cells to be deformed to be squeezed through the lumen in single file, thereby dividing the plasma stream into more or less separate compartments. Prothero and Burton (1962a, b) have shown, however, that the cells are very deformable and can be squeezed through pores of 3 to 4 microns with very little extra force; whether few or many erythrocytes traverse a capillary per second has little effect on the regional viscosity, which in the capillaries approaches that of plasma.

The Influence of Tube Diameter

Once the tube diameter is of the order of 200 microns the regional viscosity of the blood traversing the tube falls progressively as the tube diameter further decreases, providing that the shear rate is reasonably high (Fig. 4-4). This is the classical *Fåhraeus-Lindqvist effect* (1931); it is due to the presence of the red cells, though its exact explanation is still not certain. One hypothesis implies that the suspended cells, closely packed in the axial parts of the stream, move in such small vessels as parallel columns with largely "unsheared" fluid compartments trapped between cells

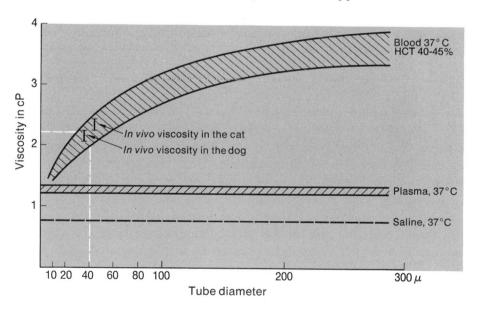

Fig. 4-4. Diagram illustrating approximate relationship between blood viscosity and tube diameter, varying from capillary up to resistance vessel dimensions, at "physiological" rates of flow. (Modified from Bayliss, 1952. By permission.)

belonging to the same column. Hence the main shear is limited essentially to the narrow plasma zones between the parallel cell columns. The narrower the vessel, the fewer such sheared plasma columns exist, and hence the smaller the total internal friction (the "Sigma" phenomenon).

Another hypothesis suggests that the width of the marginal cell-free zone is fairly constant and only little dependent on the tube diameter, thus occupying a greater fraction of the flow profile in smaller tubes. As this marginal zone is the site of the highest shear rates, but also comprises the low viscosity plasma compartment, it would follow that blood viscosity would be reduced in proportion to the narrowing of the lumen.

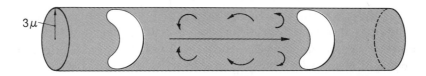

Fig. 4-5. "Bolus" flow in capillaries with some stirring of the plasma columns "trapped" between the erythrocytes, when these move like pistons in the capillary.

Either of these hypotheses would serve to explain the Fåhraeus-Lindqvist effect in vessels of arteriolar or venular dimensions, and both are probably of importance in such sites. Neither suffices as an explanation for capillary flow, which is not parabolic, where cells squeeze through in a single row with plasma "columns" trapped in between, and where there is presumably some stirring within the fluid columns between the cells traversing the capillaries (Prothero and Burton, 1962a, b) (Fig. 4-5). In this special vascular section the surface characteristics of the vascular endothelium, which seems to be covered by a thin muco-polysaccharide film (see Chapter 8), may be important, as the fluid closest to the capillary wall is hardly stagnant. It has been suggested (Copley, 1960) that the vascular endothelium may help here to lower the viscosity *in vivo*. Such a factor, together with the fact that very little force is needed to deform the erythrocytes, may explain why the viscosity of blood passing through the capillaries is almost as low as that of plasma (Fig. 4-3, Curve C).

A consequence of the Fåhraeus-Lindqvist phenomenon is that flow in an arteriole increases slightly *less* than in proportion to r^4 when the vessel dilates, because the increase in luminal diameter raises the regional viscosity. This is the case if we are dealing with flows of fairly *high* shear rate. However, if flow were initially *low* then the vasodilatation might have an opposite effect because of a reduction in the anomalous viscosity of the blood as flow increases, this effect being preponderant over the Fåhraeus-Lindqvist effect which itself is relatively small at low flow rates. These circumstances illustrate the complexities of describing the viscous properties of blood *in vivo*.

The Influence of Temperature

Even in homeothermic animals only the body core itself is maintained at 37°C. The peripheral parts of the body may be exposed to considerable cooling, which predictably increases the blood viscosity. In fingers cooled in ice water, regional viscosity may be increased three times or perhaps even more. In addition, cooling may reduce the suspension stability of the cells, producing a reversible aggregation which further increases blood viscosity.

Viscosity of Blood in Vivo

Measurements of blood viscosity *in vivo*, first performed by Whittaker and Winton in 1933, yield results which differ in some important respects from those obtained in most conditions *in vitro*. Hence the term *effective* or *apparent* viscosity is often used to denote the viscous properties of blood in the cardiovascular system. This apparent viscosity is decidedly lower than that measured *in vitro*, being in the dog only about twice that of plasma at high flow rates (Whittaker and Winton, 1933). Similarly, the viscosity of cat blood *in vivo*, being only about half of that *in vitro* at high shear (flow) rates, is 2.35 ± 0.04 *cP*, and even at quite low flow levels this *in vivo* value increases only moderately (Djojosugito *et al.*, 1970).

The Fåhraeus-Lindqvist effect is quite likely responsible for the fact that the apparent viscosity is lower than that measured *in vitro*. The majority of the normal hindrance to vascular flow probably occurs in arterial sections of 10 to 100 microns radius, where the Fåhraeus-Lindqvist effect is known to be most marked. *In vitro* measurements

(Bayliss, 1952) suggest that blood viscosity would be about 2.3 cP at 37°C when blood flows rapidly in tubes of some 20 to 25 μ radius (Fig. 4-4). Thus, the fact that the apparent blood viscosity shows approximately this same value may suggest that about half of the flow resistance is situated proximal to arterial vessels larger than 20 to 25 μ in radius, where regional blood viscosity is *higher* than 2.3 cP, while half of the resistance is placed distally to this point of the vascular bed, with regional blood viscosity reaching its lowest point—close to that of plasma—at the capillary level.

Effective or apparent viscosity thus represents a sort of approximate mean of regional viscosity values, perhaps ranging from about 3 to 3.5 cP in large vessels to slightly above 1.2 cP in capillaries. Further analysis of these problems is exceedingly complicated, however, and one must make a pragmatic approximation that proves sufficient for most biological situations. In any case, it should be realized that the flow resistance of each consecutive vascular section is the *product* of the hindrance inherent in its design and the regional blood viscosity, and *total* flow resistance is the *sum* of all these products.

References

Bayliss, L. E. (1952). "Rheology of blood and lymph," in *Deformation and flow in biological systems*, ed. A. Frey-Wyssling. Amsterdam: North Holland Publ. Co.

Bayliss, L. E. (1962). "The rheology of blood," *Handbook of Physiology*, 2, Circulation **I**, 137–50.

Copley, A. L. (1960). "Apparent viscosity and wall adherence of blood systems," in *Flow properties of blood and other biological systems*, eds. A. L. Copley and G. Stainsby, pp. 97–117. London: Pergamon.

Djojosugito, A. M., B. Folkow, B. Öberg, and S. White (1970). "A comparison of blood viscosity measured in vitro and in a vascular bed," *Acta Physiol. Scand.* **78**, 70–80.

Fåhraeus, R., and T. Lindqvist (1931). "The viscosity of the blood in narrow capillary tubes," *Am. J. Physiol.* **96**, 562–68.

Hatschek, E. (1928). *The viscosity of liquids*, p. 239. London: Bell.

Haynes, R. H. (1961). "The rheology of blood," *Trans. Soc. Rheol.* **5**, 85–101.

Prothero, J., and A. C. Burton (1962a). "The capillary resistance to flow," *Biophys. J.* **2,** 199–211.

Prothero, J., and A. C. Burton (1962b). "The pressure required to deform erythrocytes," *Biophys. J.* **2,** 213–22.

Whitmore, R. L. (1968). *Rheology of the circulation.* Oxford: Pergamon.

Whittaker, S. R. F., and F. R. Winton (1933). "The apparent viscosity of blood flowing in the isolated hind limb of the dog, and its variation with corpuscular concentration," *J. Physiol.,* **78,** 339–69.

5

Vascular Length and Radius

General Considerations

The length L and the internal radius r of the vessels, together with the viscosity η of the blood, determine the flow resistance R, and also the blood content, the total cross-sectional area, and the total wall surface area of each vascular section. L does not change much in most vessels and hence can be largely disregarded as a factor in haemodynamic *changes*, the more so since the vessels generally have a high longitudinal elasticity modulus *in vivo*, implying that only minor changes of L accompany alterations of vascular distension or vascular tone. At first sight it would appear that the vessels of hollow viscera (lungs, stomach, gut, bladder) might be stretched considerably by distension of the wall of the viscus, but when these visceral walls are *not* distended, the vessels usually present a coiled appearance, and distension only straightens these coils; it has little corresponding effect on vascular length. Only a few vascular sections, among them the portal vein and its mesenteric branches, have longitudinally oriented smooth muscles, which may moderately shorten these venous compartments.

In most vessels, especially those controlling flow resistance, the vascular smooth muscles are circular, with a slightly helical arrangement. They cause changes only of r, and this is the most important determinant of blood flow, which varies with r^4. Blood content, on the other hand, varies with r^2. However, even a major decrease of radius of a given vascular section adds little to the over-all resistance if the narrowed section is very

36

short. The importance of the length factor, L, is strikingly illustrated by tightening a ligature around the aorta. It is at first surprising to see how much the aorta has to be narrowed to produce any appreciable pressure drop downstream—until one understands that L for this added resistance is so short. Thus, for any calculation of resistance, capacity, or surface wall area of a particular vascular section, the *radius* of the tubes, the *number* of the tubes, and the *length* of the tubes must be known. Further, as blood viscosity also varies with the radius of the tube, this viscosity factor should be considered, too, in any calculation of regional flow resistance.

Architecture and Dimensions of the Capillary Bed

A dense network of narrow short tubes, arranged so that their total surface area and total cross-sectional area are large in relation to their length and volume, fulfills the requirements of the capillary section—i.e. that they offer an extensive exchange surface at a minimal distance for diffusion of gases and solutes to the tissues and a suitable time for this exchange.

The Systemic Capillaries

The *average* systemic capillary has a radius of about 3 μ and is some 750 μ long, though the range of variation is large. Each has, therefore, a wall surface area of $2\pi rL = 3.14 \times 6 \times 750 =$ about $15,000$ square microns and a cross-sectional area of $\pi r^2 = 30$ square microns. However, there is increasing evidence that considerable exchange takes place also in what are generally considered as the postcapillary venules (see Chapter 8). For such reasons it might be more appropriate for the deductions presented below to consider the *total* exchange surface of a systemic capillary as $25,000$ rather than $15,000$ square microns.

The volume flow through the capillary bed is the same as that through the aorta and is equal to the cross-sectional area times the velocity. In resting conditions about 85 ml of blood are ejected through the aorta per second (cross-sectional area $= 4$ cm^2) and the mean velocity is $85/4 = 21$ cm/sec. The *average* flow velocity through a systemic capillary may be of the order of 0.3 mm/sec in a resting tissue, so it would seem that the cross-sectional area of the *patent* capillary bed is $210/0.3 = 700$ times that of the

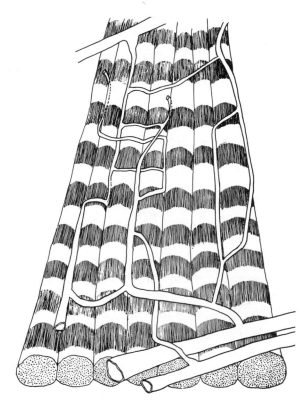

Fig. 5-1A. Capillary network in skeletal muscle. (From Wiedeman, 1963. By permission.)

aorta during rest. However, only some 25 to 35% of the capillaries seem to be patent in resting conditions, so that, if the whole of the capillary bed were to open, its cross-sectional area would then be at most 2800 times that of the aorta = 2800×400 million μ^2.

Such considerations imply that the total "capillary count" in a 70-kg man would be of the order of forty thousand million ($2800 \times 400{,}000{,}000/30$). The *total* capillary exchange surface would then be $40{,}000{,}000{,}000 \times 25{,}000$ square microns and thus be equivalent to some 1000 square metres. Their entire blood content is, however, only some 200 to 250 ml, i.e. at most 4 to 5% of the total blood volume. If the capillary density were uniform throughout the body of a 70-kg man (which it is not), there would be

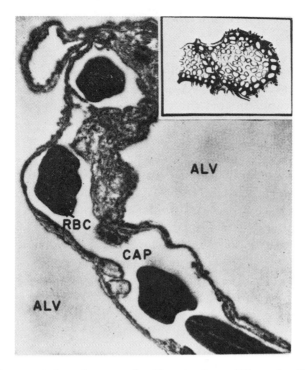

Fig. 5-1B. Electron microphotograph of human lung. The red cells (RBC) pass in single file through a pulmonary capillary (CAP) between adjacent alveoli (ALV). × 19,370. (From A. P. Fishman, 1963. By permission.)

nearly 1.5 m² of capillary wall surface per 100 g tissue, or 600 capillaries/mm³ tissue.

The muscle capillary bed has now been investigated both by anatomical methods (capillary counts) and by functional methods (see Chapter 8), and the capillary wall surface area proper in 100 g of "phasic" muscle seems to be about 0.7 m². Further, there seem to be 300 to 400 capillaries per cubic mm of phasic muscle, but the figure is perhaps 3 times higher than this in the slow "tonic" muscles. In a man of 70 kg with 30 to 35 kg of muscle mass, where perhaps 20% are "tonic", his muscles alone would contain a total of 275 to 325 m² of capillary wall surface. The principal arrangement of the capillary exchange section in skeletal muscle is shown in Fig. 5-1A, which should be compared with that of the lung (Fig. 5-1B).

Further, it varies also considerably in the different systemic circuits (see Wiedeman, 1963).

Other tissues, such as bone, fat, connective tissue, and smooth muscles, may have a somewhat lower capillary density. If the combined weight of such tissues is taken as 25 to 30 kg, we may postulate an average capillary density of 250 capillaries per cubic mm. This would give a total capillary surface area of about 200 m² for these tissues.

The heart, kidneys, brain, liver, red bone marrow, gastrointestinal and other exocrine and endocrine glands, together weighing some 7 to 9 kg, on the other hand, enjoy maximal blood flow rates per 100 g, which may be up to ten times that of phasic skeletal muscle. Anatomical and functional studies suggest that their total capillary surface area per unit weight is some 6 to 8 times that of skeletal muscle. If such tissues show an *average* capillary density of 2500–3000 capillaries/mm³, they would possess a *total* capillary surface area of about 500 m² (Fig. 5-2).

Of our total of forty thousand million capillaries, only 25 to 35% seem to be open at any one time in resting condition—with a combined ex-

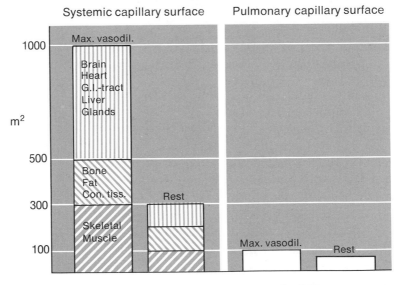

Fig. 5-2. Approximate size of capillary surface area in different *systemic* vascular beds as compared with the pulmonary circuit during "rest" and maximal vasodilatation.

change surface area of 250 to 350 m². In heavy exercise, the opening up of all the muscle and myocardial capillaries would raise the perfused wall surface for exchange in the body to perhaps 500 to 600 m², or to 50 to 60% of the possible total of about 1000 m². Such deductions and figures, though very approximate, nevertheless serve the purpose of providing semiquantitative information of the dimensions of the most important vascular section of all.

As stated, the *average* capillary flow rate in resting man with a 5.5 litre cardiac output seems to be about 0.3 mm/sec, but there are considerable differences in the individual tissues. Thus, in resting conditions, blood traverses muscle and skin capillaries in 1 to 2 sec, compared with a transit time of perhaps 3 to 4 seconds through fat depots. In heavy muscular exercise, with a fivefold increase of cardiac output, there may be a four-fold increase of patent "muscle" capillaries and up to a twentyfold increase in muscle blood flow; the blood then traverses the muscle capillaries in about 0.3 sec.

The Pulmonary Capillaries

In man at rest the pulmonary capillaries have an effective wall surface area of some 60 m²—only 20 to 25% of that available in the systemic circuit under the same conditions (see Fishman, 1963). This *entire* surface area is, however, available for gaseous exchange in the lungs, as O_2 and CO_2 are lipid soluble. In heavy exercise, the capillary surface area of the lungs increases to about 90 m²—i.e. by some 50% (Fig. 5-2).

Pulmonary capillaries are wider ($r = 4\ \mu$) and shorter than systemic capillaries. If their "effective" length should be half the alveolar circum-ference which they span, this would yield a value of 350 μ for length. However, the pulmonary capillaries form such a dense network around the alveoli that one can hardly speak of a specific capillary "length", and this expression is used only for approximate deductions of passage time (Fig. 5-1B).

This effective pulmonary wall surface area of 60 m² corresponds to some eight thousand million pulmonary capillaries (compared with about ten thousand million in the entire systemic circuit patent in resting con-ditions). As the cross-sectional area of each pulmonary capillary is $\pi r_p^2 = 3.14 \times 16$, and that of a systemic capillary is $\pi r_s^2 = 3.14 \times 9$, this means that each pulmonary capillary has a cross-sectional area that is 80%

higher than that of its systemic counterpart. Thus, the combined cross-sectional area of the pulmonary capillary bed may be bigger than that of the systemic capillary bed during rest, and the mean capillary flow rate would be correspondingly lower in the lung.

However, the effective length of the lung capillary is only about half that of its systemic counterpart, so the average passage time for pulmonary capillaries would be about 60% of the average passage time of those in the systemic circuit, or about 1 sec. With a pulmonary blood flow of 25 litres in heavy exercise, and the perfused capillary wall surface area increased to 90 m², the average pulmonary capillary transit time is about 0.3 sec. That is, the time available for gas exchange may be closely similar to that in the muscle capillaries in this situation.

Architecture and Dimensions of Precapillary Vessels

The precapillary vessels constitute the major fraction of the resistance section. With each arborization of the vessels the radius of the individual branches diminishes, but the combined cross-sectional area of the branches always *exceeds* that of the stem, usually by a factor of 1.2 to 1.3 when two branches are formed.

Let us suppose that a parent artery (volume flow Q_1, radius r_1, pressure drop P_1) divides into a number n of equal branches whose individual radius is r_2, pressure gradient P_2, and individual volume flow Q_2. For unit length L_1 equals L_2, and from Poiseuille's law:

$$Q_1 = \frac{P_1 r_1^4}{8\eta L_1} = nQ_2 = \frac{nP_2 r_2^4}{8\eta L_2}$$

$$\frac{P_1}{P_2} = \frac{nr_2^4}{r_1^4}$$

Let K be the factor of increase of the total cross-sectional area.

$$\frac{nr_2^2}{r_1^2} = K \qquad \text{and therefore} \qquad \frac{r_2^2}{r_1^2} = \frac{K}{n}$$

$$\frac{P_1}{P_2} = \frac{K^2}{n}$$

For steady flow then, the vascular resistance per unit length (or pressure drop) remains unaltered only if K equals $\sqrt{n}$. If there are only two branches, as $\sqrt{n}$ then equals 1.414, there will be a rise of resistance when the factor K is *lower* than 1.414.

In nearly all branchings of the arterial tree K is, indeed, *lower* than $\sqrt{n}$, so such arborizations do imply *increases* of regional resistance. However, since L meanwhile decreases with each consecutive arterial section, the progressive increase of resistance per section is only moderate, particularly as the regional viscosity tends to decrease as well (see Chapter 4). Hence, it is an oversimplification to identify the marked precapillary resistance solely with the "arterioles", for no precise morphological criteria can be defined by the resistance vessels. It is more correct to state that, though there is a gradual increase in resistance along the branching artery-arteriole-capillary system, the arteries themselves provide little of this and the small arteries (0.5 mm radius and below), arterioles, and metarterioles provide the most.

At maximal dilation, when the smallest precapillary vessels usually exhibit the largest percentage increase of radius, the *relative* importance of larger vessels for total resistance to flow increases accordingly. Then the sigmoid pressure drop curve along the circuit tends to flatten out, especially if turbulence in larger vessels adds to their regional resistance (see Chapter 6).

If any one precapillary section constricts, its contribution to the over-all resistance will increase correspondingly. Since the impact of local control mechanisms and extrinsic nerves are usually not equally pronounced within all the precapillary consecutive sections (Chapter 16), such more or less "selective" adjustments do occur *in vivo*.

Architecture and Dimensions of Postcapillary Vessels

The veins are usually described as the "capacitance" section of the vascular bed. The blood volume of a 70-kg man is about 5.5 l (7.5 to 8% of body weight), and when he is recumbent it is distributed roughly as follows (Fig. 5-3): pulmonary circuit about 550 to 650 ml (10 to 12%), heart 400 to 600 ml (8 to 11%), systemic capillaries 200 to 250 ml (4 to 5%), arteries 500 to 700 ml (10 to 12%), and veins 3500 to 4000 ml (60 to 70%).

Although the systemic venous content greatly exceeds that of the arterial compartment, the cross-sectional area of the *major* venous branches is not too dissimilar to that of the corresponding arteries, and the cross-sectional area of the two venae cavae together is only twice that of the aorta.

Clearly, then, it is the "small vein" compartment that mainly possesses the large dimensions and that predominantly justifies the designation of "*capacitance* section". Morphological measurements suggest that venules and veins of 10 to 15 μ up to 1 to 2 mm radius are most important in this context. Although the total cross-sectional area of such venules and small

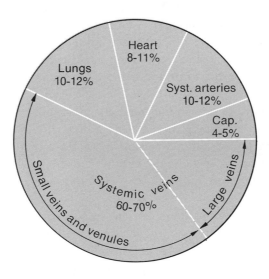

Fig. 5-3. Distribution of blood volume in resting man.

veins is much lower than that of the capillaries, their length is very much greater, so that their total volume or blood content is very large indeed.

As the radius of the veins is bigger than that of their arterial counterparts, their *resistance* is low, despite the fact that regional blood viscosity might be expected to be somewhat larger than in their arterial homologues (see Chapter 4). Indeed, the total postcapillary resistance is only 10 to 20% of that of the precapillary vessels, probably varying in the various regional circuits and certainly varying with the extent of smooth muscle activity in the two sections. Correspondingly, the total venous return of 5.5 l/min in resting man is achieved by a pressure gradient of only 10 to 20 mm Hg. The postcapillary resistance resides essentially in the smaller veins and venules; major veins are usually fairly unimportant in this respect. It must be admitted that the tendency of veins to assume a gradually more ellipsoidal shape when the transmural pressure falls below 6 to 9 mm Hg, complicates the measurement of venous resistance, for a vessel of elliptical cross-section offers greater flow resistance than does one whose profile is circular, of course. Thus, *in vivo*, postcapillary resistance and capacitance are passively affected far more by such changes in regional transmural pressure than are those of the precapillary side, where *active* luminal changes predominate.

Figure 5-4 shows the approximate relationship between the total cross-sectional area, linear flow velocity, and pressure drop (reflecting the regional resistances) at different parts of the systemic vascular circuit during rest.

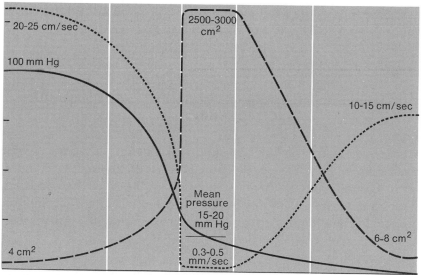

Fig. 5-4. Relationship between total cross-sectional area (– –), average linear flow velocity (. . .) and blood pressure level (   ) in the different consecutive sections of the systemic vascular bed during rest.

Series-coupled Flow Resistances

The relative flow resistances of the consecutive vascular sections may be calculated from the Poiseuille formula if the number of parallel-coupled vessels n, their radius r, length L, and the regional blood viscosity η are known. The flow Q through each consecutive section is of course the same, but the other factors vary considerably, even from moment to moment, with the possible exception of L in most cases.

$$\text{The regional pressure drop} = \frac{Q \cdot L \cdot \eta}{r^4 n}$$

Such calculations, though based on only approximate data, suggest that the capillary flow resistance is relatively small, because L is short, η is low, and n is quite large in comparison with the situation in the arterioles. The increase in n is so great as to overshadow the effect of the reduced r. Capillary resistance is, however, closely dependent upon the number of patent capillaries, and this in turn depends upon the tone of the precapillary sphincters. A widespread closure of the precapillary sphincters can no doubt cause a striking rise of the capillary flow resistance.

Wall/Lumen Relationship of Precapillary and Postcapillary Vessels

In a hollow circular structure (a cylindrical balloon, or a soap bubble) the tension in the wall, T, is given by the product of the pressure P and the radius r. This relationship $T = Pr$, though usually called Laplace's law, was first given by John Bernoulli in the seventeenth century. On the basis of "Laplace's" law, Frank (1920) defined the situation for a blood vessel where wall thickness, w, also has to be considered:

$$T = P(r/w)$$

Clearly, providing that the wall thickness diminishes in proportion to the reduction in r, the ability of the wall to withstand pressure is not reduced (see Burton, 1962). Thus, thin-walled blood vessels of *small* radius can withstand quite high pressures (a principle of design also used in

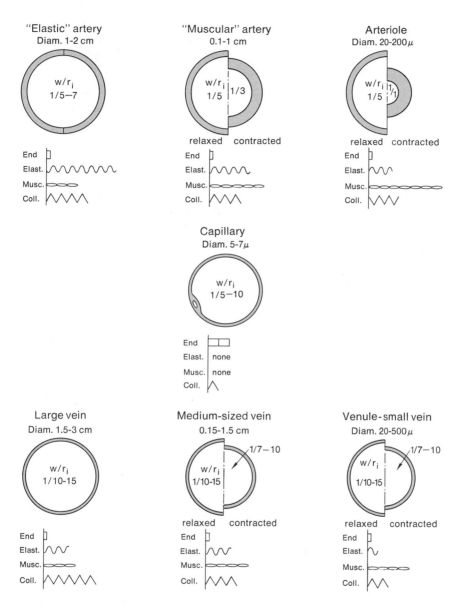

Fig. 5-5. Approximate wall composition and relationship between wall thickness and internal radius in different parts of the vascular bed. (Modified from Burton, 1962. By permission.)

engineering). Therefore, if one neglects the effect of hydrostatic pressure in dependent circuits, which is sporadically added as an extra load when the individual stands, the w/r ratio of the arterial system in recumbent man could decrease towards the capillary level, for the pressure head drops as the capillaries are approached and reached. However, the increased hydrostatic pressure in dependent circuits does seem to be partly compensated for by adaptive changes in vascular design: for example, the leg veins have thicker walls than those in e.g. the neck and arm (Svejcar *et al.*, 1962).

Small "muscular" arteries, and especially arterioles and metarterioles, show a larger w/r ratio than the "elastic" Windkessel arteries (Fig. 5-5). This morphological feature has two advantages. First, these resistance vessels, in which flow varies with the fourth power of the *internal* radius, are less distensible than the Windkessel arteries, and hence passive elastic effects cause less interference with "active" smooth muscle adjustments of vascular resistance.

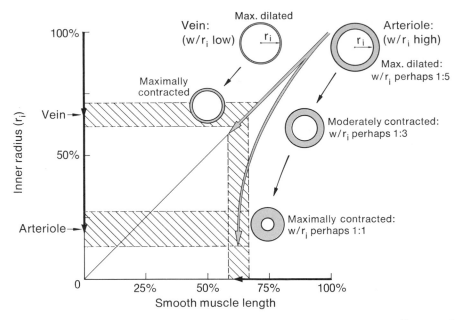

Fig. 5-6. Diagram illustrating in approximate terms how a difference in w/r_i ratio greatly affects the luminal reductions produced by a given smooth muscle contraction.

Second, and even more important, the high w/r ratio accentuates the reduction of the lumen produced by a given shortening of the vascular smooth muscle. Thus, as flow varies with r^4, where r is the *internal* radius, the high w/r ratio of resistance vessels allows them to alter flow dramatically even by only small changes in smooth muscle contraction (Fig. 5-6). The shortening of the external muscle layers (from which neurogenic constrictions are initiated) displaces the relatively large tissue mass situated inside their "line of force" in an inward direction and this accentuates the reduction in the lumen. The cutaneous A-V shunts which have a very high w/r ratio seem to close completely in response to the slightest neurogenic activation of their outermost smooth muscle layer (see Chapter 25).

Veins have a low transmural pressure and active adjustments of venous calibre do not require a high w/r ratio, which would further interfere with their ability to collapse—on the whole their w/r is quite low. Nevertheless, the w/r ratio in leg veins is, as mentioned, higher than that in veins not subjected to high hydrostatic pressures. Most veins also possess a stiff external jacket of collagen and often gain additional support from tight fasciae. Such arrangements are well developed in the leg veins of the giraffe, where transmural pressures may reach several hundred mm Hg.

In general, the w/r of veins is so small that the potentiating effect of wall thickness can be neglected in deductions of resistance and volume. Hence, the flow resistance in veins of circular profile varies largely with the fourth power of any "active" change in length of their smooth muscles, unlike the situation in the arterioles (Fig. 5-6). Likewise, the capacity of a vein is proportional to the second power of this length if the vein is circular, but, as is discussed in Chapter 10, veins are commonly semicollapsed and assume an ellipsoidal shape. Such an alteration greatly modifies both their resistance and capacitance.

To judge the true w/r ratio of vessels correctly, they should of course be examined in the state of *normal distension*. For example, the striking difference between stretched and unstretched arteries—with respect to thickness and structure of the wall—is obvious from Fig. 5-7. This figure shows identical wall segments of an "elastic" and a "muscular" artery, fixed when they are exposed to the normal stretch offered by the blood pressure and when completely undistended (see Bunce, 1964, 1965).

"Elastic" artery   "Muscular" artery

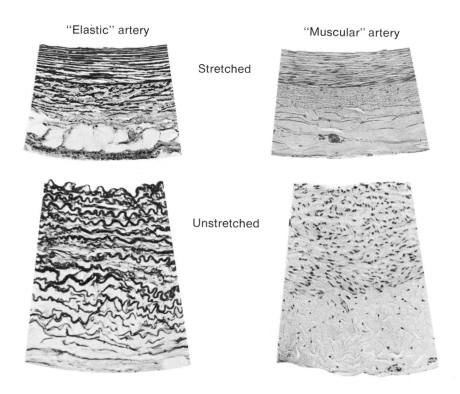

Stretched

Unstretched

Fig. 5-7. Wall appearance and thickness in an "elastic" and a "muscular" artery when exposed to the normal distension of the arterial blood pressure, as contrasted to the same wall when unstretched. (Courtesy of Dr. D. F. M. Bunce, Dept. of Human Physiology, Des Moines College of Medicine.)

Distensibility of Resistance and Capacitance Vessels

Generally, a change in distension of the precapillary vessels is mainly important in affecting flow *resistance*, which is inversely proportional to r^4, whereas a distension of the postcapillary vessels mainly affects *capacitance*, which is proportional to r^2. Capillaries in general appear to have very little distensibility, thanks to their delicate but stiff basal membranes (see Chapter 8).

Distensibility of Precapillary Vessels

It is not easy to define distensibility, for when the muscle layers are relaxed w/r is much smaller, and, as the relaxed muscle is largely "plastic", the load on the vessel wall is then borne mostly by the elastic fibres. Only when the transmural pressure is high enough to stretch the stiff collagen elements do these limit distensibility strikingly. Such a situation in a maximally relaxed vessel requires an arterial pressure of about 100 mm Hg or more.

The more the vascular muscles contract, the greater the w/r ratio and the smaller their distensibility. Hence the distensibility of precapillary vessels

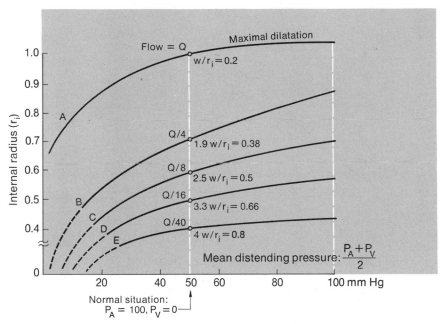

Fig. 5-8. Approximate relationship between internal radius (r_i) and mean vascular distending pressure $\left(\dfrac{P_A + P_V}{2}\right)$ of an "idealized" resistance vessel. *Curve A:* At maximal vascular relaxation; wall to radius ratio here denoted as w/r_i and blood flow as Q at 100 mm Hg pressure head. *Curves B–E:* At increasing levels of *stable* vasoconstriction, as defined by the changed values for w/r_i and Q. (From Folkow and Löfving, 1956; by permission; experimental data from cat muscle vascular bed.)

can only be expressed by a family of pressure-radius curves, as shown in
Fig. 5-8. In this figure the relative values of the average internal radius
and the *w/r* ratio of an "idealized" resistance vessel segment were derived
from measurements of the relationship between flow resistance and transmural pressure (i.e. the pressure difference across the wall). Recordings

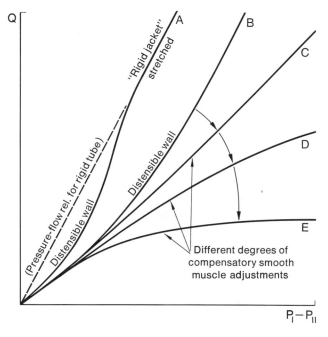

Fig. 5-9. Relationship between pressure head (P_I-P_{II}) and flow (Q) for the
vascular bed at:
A. Maximal dilatation. At lower transmural pressures the wall is quite distensible but gradually becomes more rigid when the collagen elements are
stretched. First, then, a linear pressure-flow relationship, pointing to origo, is
reached.
B. Moderate level of *stable* smooth muscle activity. *w/r* increased and resistance
to stretch now mainly offered by the activated smooth muscles. As these are
to some extent distensible (see Fig. 5-8), the pressure-flow curve is convex
towards the pressure axis.
C, D, E: These curves represent a more "physiological" situation than
B, as in most situations, where smooth muscle activity is present, the
smooth muscles tend to *counteract* the physical distensibility. This counteraction
is slight in C, apparently suggesting "rigid" vascular walls, moderate in D, and
so powerful in E as to establish a perfect "flow autoregulation".

were made first during maximal vasodilatation and subsequently during increasing vasoconstriction in cat skeletal muscle. The experiments were so arranged that very stable levels of smooth muscle activity could be maintained artificially. The figure shows the full range of distensibility of these particular resistance vessels at different levels of flow resistance, w/r ratio, and transmural pressure. Fully dilated vessels are quite distensible in the lower pressure range, but become less so as the intramural pressure rises and stretches the collagen fibrils. Vasoconstriction unloads the collagen fibrils, and in these circumstances the distensibility characteristics are mainly those of the contracted smooth muscle as modified by the w/r ratio. At low pressures luminal closure tends to occur, for reasons described below.

Note that, in normal conditions, the distensibility of resistance vessels is usually modified by active adjustments of smooth muscle tone ("autoregulation"; see Chapter 16). It should therefore be stressed that—except at maximal vasodilatation—there is almost always an interplay between the physical distensibility of the resistance vessels and the smooth muscle response evoked by such distensions. The situation—illustrated by the pressure-volume curve of Fig. 5-9—is indeed complex (see Folkow, 1962). Thus, any vascular bed can, depending on the circumstances, display a great variety of pressure-flow curves.

"Critical Closure" of Resistance Vessels

"Active" closure may occur in a vessel with a high w/r ratio even with a moderate shortening of its outer sheath of smooth muscle, because the lumen, narrowed out of proportion to the decrease in circumference, is finally obliterated.

Passive closure, on the other hand, may occur as a result of a fall in the transmural pressure, but even this presupposes the presence of some active tension in the outer sheath of smooth muscle. Such muscle activity, when intense, clearly unloads the bulky inner layers (see Van Citters *et al.*, 1962), with the result that the resistance of the vessel wall to distension is *mainly* furnished by the outer sheath of muscle. Even contracted smooth muscle is distensible, however (Fig. 5-8), and a fall in the transmural pressure therefore leads to some elastic recoil of the contracted outer muscle layer. This recoil, even when relatively slight, can obliterate the lumen by pushing the bulky inner layers inwards.

Even a moderate fall of transmural pressure may thus lead to an apparently abrupt shut-off of the vessel, as is illustrated in Fig. 5-10A. This is the probable explanation of the phenomenon sometimes referred to as "critical closure" (see Burton, 1962). This phenomenon occurs most readily in such vessels as the thick-walled cutaneous A-V shunts or in the ductus arteriosus Botalli (McIntyre, 1969), but is also seen in strongly

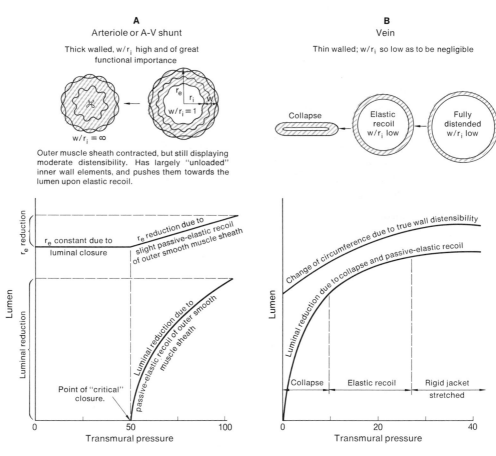

Fig. 5-10A. Schematic drawing of small pre-capillary vessel; outer muscle sheath contracted, but still displaying moderate distensibility. Has largely "unloaded" inner wall elements, and pushes them towards the lumen upon elastic recoil to produce luminal closure.

Fig. 5-10B. Schematic drawing of vein; thin-walled; w/r so low as to be negligible.

constricted arterioles-metarterioles-sphincters (Fig. 5-8). Most vessels, however, exhibit so-called "autoregulation" (see Chapter 16), where, for instance, the accumulation of metabolites surrounding them, which occurs when the vessel narrows and the flow decreases, exert a vasodilator action. This tends to offset the forces causing narrowing of the lumen and flow is thus usually re-established or stabilized. It is therefore only in vessels which exhibit little autoregulatory adjustments of their smooth muscles (e.g. arteriovenous shunts and arterioles of the skin) that may display a more prolonged closure in the physiological situation.

Distensibility of the Postcapillary Bed

Figure 5-10B shows the pressure-volume curve for veins. Venous distensibility at high pressures is quite small because of the stretching of stiff collagen elements. It has often been assumed that this curve reveals a high wall distensibility at low transmural pressures, but this is not the case at all. The initial phase of apparently high wall distensibility of veins simply reflects a change in the *geometry* of the vessel. A pressure of some 6 to 9 mm Hg is required to keep a vein fully rounded; at lower pressures it is ellipsoid. The cross-sectional area of an ellipse is less than that of a circle of the same perimeter. Hence, as the pressure rises from zero to, say, 6 mm Hg, the capacity of the venous segment alters greatly *only for this reason.* "True" distensibility of the venous wall, i.e. the increase in perimeter produced by a stretching force, is actually rather low in most veins, as indicated also by the change of circumference shown in Fig. 5-10B. Its physiological relevance is, however, restricted to circumstances in which the cross-sectional profile of the veins is circular—conditions which presuppose a transmural pressure sufficient to achieve this (as in the legs when the subject is standing). The "collapse" situation is dominant at pressures below 6 to 9 mm Hg and greatly affects both active and passive venous adjustments (see Öberg, 1967). Such considerations are of fundamental importance in the interpretation of venous function and control (see Chapter 10).

References

Bunce, D. F. M. (1964). "Formation of the intima in arteries," *Angéiologie*, **16,** 15–20.

Bunce, D. F. M. (1965). "Structural differences between distended and collapsed arteries," *Angiology*, **16,** 53–56.

Burton, A. C. (1962). "Physical principles of circulatory phenomena: the physical equilibria of the heart and blood vessels," *Handbook of Physiology*, 2, Circulation **I,** 85–106.

Fishman, A. P. (1963). "Dynamics of the pulmonary circulation," *Handbook of Physiology*, 2, Circulation, **II,** 1667–1743.

Folkow, B. (1962). "Transmural pressure and vascular tone, some aspects of an old controversy," *Arch. Int. Pharmacodyn.* **129,** 455–69.

Folkow, B., and B. Löfving (1956). "The distensibility of the systemic resistance blood vessels," *Acta Physiol. Scand.* **38,** 37–52.

Frank, O. (1920). "Die Elastizität der Blutgefässe," *Zeit. f. Biol.* **71,** 255–72.

McIntyre, T. W. (1969). "An analysis of critical closure in the isolated ductus arteriosus," *Biophys. J.* **9,** 685–99.

Öberg, B. (1967). "The relationship between active constriction and passive recoil of the veins at various distending pressures," *Acta Physiol. Scand.* **71,** 233–47.

Svejcar, J., I. Prerovsky, J. Linhart, and J. Kruml (1962). "Content of collagen, elastin and water in walls of the internal saphenous vein in man," *Circ. Res.* **11,** 296–300.

Van Citters, R. L., B. M. Wagner, and R. F. Rushmer (1962). "Architecture of small arteries during vasoconstriction," *Circ. Res.*, **10,** 668–75.

6

The Pressure

Mean Pressures

Central Arterial and Venous Pressures

In the Poiseuille formula, P denotes the pressure *head*, i.e. the pressure difference along the tube, $P_1 - P_2$. When applied to the vascular bed P_1 and P_2 are better labelled P_a and P_v, respectively. Thus, P_a corresponds to the mean aortic pressure (90 to 110 mm Hg) in the systemic circuit and P_v corresponds to the central venous pressure (sensibly zero). In the pulmonary circuit, P_a, the mean pulmonary arterial pressure, is 12 to 18 mm Hg, and P_v, the left atrial pressure, is at 3 to 5 mm Hg, slightly higher than its counterpart in the systemic circuit. P_v in the pulmonary circuit cannot be disregarded in calculations of resistance, because P_a is so low in this circuit.

In both circuits, $P_a - P_v$ is kept fairly constant. Even when the resting cardiac output of 5.5 l/min is increased to 25 l/min in heavy exercise, the average value for the systemic mean pressure head increases only by 15 to 20% (Holmberg, 1956). However, the *profile* of the pressure drop along the individual circuits alters depending on changes in their vascular tone. Thus, in the dilated muscle vessels the greatest reduction of resistance occurs in the small precapillary segments. Hence, other segments contribute relatively more to the resistance of the muscle circuits and the increased blood flow is associated with a larger pressure drop along the major arteries and veins. The muscle capillary pressure rises simultaneously. Therefore, the sigmoid pressure drop along the circuit, which characterises the situation at rest, now becomes more linear. The reverse occurs during precapillary constriction (Fig. 6-1).

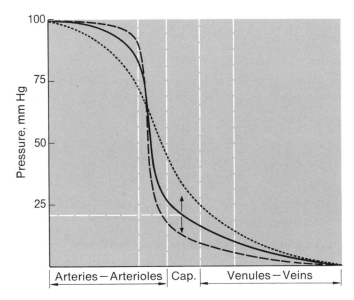

Fig. 6-1. Profile of pressure drop along a systemic vascular bed (muscle) during rest (—), vasodilation (. . . .), and vasoconstriction (- - -).

Capillary Pressure

Only from the capillaries can a net amount of fluid be lost or gained, and they therefore represent another key point of the pressure drop along the circuit. The opposing forces that determine net fluid movement to or from the capillary are those of the hydrostatic pressure and the colloid osmotic pressure. The transcapillary difference in colloid osmotic pressure and in hydrostatic pressure normally balance each other in the steady state (see Chapter 8).

Capillary hydrostatic pressure (Pc) is determined by the ratio of resistances in the precapillary region and in the postcapillary part of the circuit, respectively.

Let us consider the flow through a capillary, where Q is the volume of flow that passes the capillaries; R_a and R_v are the pre- and post-capillary resistances, respectively; P_a is the arterial pressure, say 100 mm Hg; and P_v is the central venous pressure, say 2 mm Hg. Then suppose that the *mean* capillary pressure is P_c.

$$Q = \frac{P_a - P_c}{R_a} = \frac{P_c - P_v}{R_v}$$

$\therefore$
$$P_a \cdot R_v - P_c \cdot R_v = P_c \cdot R_a - P_v \cdot R_a$$

$\therefore$
$$P_c(R_a + R_v) = P_a \cdot R_v + P_v \cdot R_a$$

Divide through by R_a:

$\therefore$
$$P_c[1 + (R_v/R_a)] = P_a \cdot (R_v/R_a) + P_v$$

$\therefore$
$$P_c = \frac{P_a \cdot (R_v/R_a) + P_v}{[1 + (R_v/R_a)]}$$

Let us suppose that the ratio R_v/R_a is $1/5$. Substituting:

$$P_c = \frac{100 \times (1/5) + 2}{1 + (1/5)} = \frac{22 \times 5}{6} = 18.3 \text{ mm Hg}$$

Roughly speaking, then, the resistance ratio of $5/1$ will provide a mean pressure of the capillary exchange section of nearly 20 mm Hg. (The consequences for the transcapillary fluid exchange will be dealt with in Chapter 8.) Thus, changes in the profile of the pressure drop along the vascular pathway can only be assessed by measuring the pressure at the relevant sites (e.g., see Wiederhielm, 1968).

The Piezometer

The apparatus in Fig. 6-2, often called a piezometer, serves to illustrate the situation. The left hand reservoir provides a mean pressure P_1 and represents a source of constant potential energy. Fluid passes through the rigid tube AB which represents the vascular bed, to reach the right hand reservoir, where P_2 represents the low, fairly constant pressure at the entrance of blood to the right heart.

This effective total pressure head, $P_1 - P_2$, is responsible for flow. During flow some of the potential energy is transformed into kinetic energy and

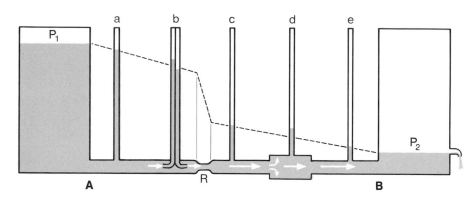

Fig. 6-2. Piezometer. The tube *AB* represents the vascular bed with a "precapillary" resistance, *R*; it is perfused at the pressure head P_1–P_2 and the pressure drop along AB is measured by the fluid levels in the side tubes *a–e*. The pressure levels in the double tube *b* illustrate the Pitot principle and the pressure level in *d*, as compared with those in *c* and *e*, illustrates the Bernoulli principle.

some into heat due to the frictional losses. Hence a gradual pressure drop occurs along the tube, being especially great between *b* and *c*, due to the high resistance at *R*.

If the radius is doubled at one point—at side tube *d* representing the capillary level—the mean flow velocity, *V*, is reduced to 1/4, being inversely proportional to the cross-sectional area. The kinetic energy, $mV^2/2$, which is proportional to the square of the velocity, thus is reduced to 1/16th of its value elsewhere in tube *AB*. As the fluid levels in side tubes a, c, d, and e reflect the regional lateral ("static") pressures—or total pressure *minus* local kinetic ("dynamic") pressures—it follows that the lateral pressure in the dilated segment d is clearly higher than it would have been if *AB* had not been widened at this site. This phenomenon is an expression of the *Bernoulli principle*, i.e. lateral ("static") pressure is higher where flow velocity is lower, and vice versa.

In the double tube *b* in Fig. 6-2 two lateral tubes project into the lumen, one facing the oncoming stream, the other facing downstream. The upstream tube records lateral pressure *plus* kinetic energy ("end pressure") and the downstream tube records lateral pressure *minus* kinetic energy ("downstream pressure"). The arrangement is that of a *Pitot tube*, which is widely used to measure velocity.

In such a tube system, then, the *total* pressure responsible for flow is equal to the difference between the static *plus* the dynamic pressures at the two ends of a tube system, *not* to the difference between the static (lateral) pressures alone. *In vivo*, however, most situations in the *systemic* circulation in resting man can be considered without taking kinetic energy into account, for it constitutes only a few per cent of the total energy. It becomes correspondingly more important in exercise, where the mean flow velocity increases perhaps fivefold. In the low-pressure *pulmonary* circuit the kinetic factor is important even in man at rest, and correspondingly more so during activity.

Transmural Pressure versus Pressure Head

Returning to Fig. 6-2, it is obvious that if both the end-reservoirs were raised by an equal amount above the level of the tube *AB* the pressure head and flow would remain the same, since the tube is rigid. However, the *transmural pressure* (i.e. the pressure difference across the wall) would be increased everywhere by an amount equal to the rise in height of the reservoirs. This is reflected by the proportionately higher levels in all the side tubes.

Similarly, nothing is added to the pressure head, $P_1 - P_2$, in immobile man when his position is changed from supine to upright; only the *transmural pressure* is affected. (Leg movements change this situation due to the venous valves; see below.) In upright man, blood is still pushed from the capillaries of the feet to the heart with a dissipation of pressure energy that remains as low as about 15 mm Hg. The addition of hydrostatic pressure thus puts an equal load on *both* limbs of a dependent circuit and is relevant *only* in circumstances in which the tubes are distensible and/or porous. However, the resistance vessels, and, more particularly, the capacitance vessels, are distensible and the capillaries are porous (see Chapter 8). Hence, important physical consequences of an increased transmural pressure are for such reasons induced *in vivo*, unless compensated by physiological adjustments (see Chapter 16).

Effects of Venous Valves

The leg and arm veins contain valves and the deep veins in these parts are surrounded by muscles. Even in quiet standing there are slight muscle movements that act like muscle pumps exerting external pressure on these veins and also to some extent on the subcutaneous ones. Because the valves permit only unidirectional flow, such movements squeeze the blood towards the heart (see Gauer and Thron, 1965). When a segment is thus "milked", the blood which remains therein is of less volume and the transmural pressure in the segment is lowered; therefore blood coming from the more peripheral parts flows more easily into the segment, and the "cycle" is then repeated (see Fig. 6-3).

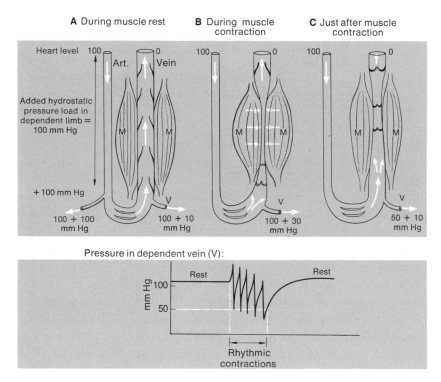

Fig. 6-3. A. Free flow at normal pressure head but at increased transmural pressure in the dependent limb.
B. Muscle contraction squeezes blood towards heart, the venous valves hinder backflow, but pressure in vein V increases phasically due to the contraction.
C. Muscles again relaxed but vein "milked empty," proximal valves therefore closed. Pressure in V therefore greatly lowered so that the effective pressure head is increased until the system is again filled up from the arterial side, restituting the situation in A.

Suppose now that the femoral artery is obstructed—a common patho-physiological situation. There is a consequent marked pressure drop in the arteries below this site. However, when the leg is kept dependent, both P_1 and P_2 increase proportionally, thereby distending the "low pressure" vessels, which improves flow for any given pressure head. Further, even slight rhythmic muscular movements squeeze blood towards the heart and intermittently lower P_2. This sporadically improves the effective pressure head, $P_1 - P_2$. Distension of the collateral arteries also helps to enhance the pressure head (Gaskell, 1969). Hence, ischaemic pain, a characteristic of a less than adequate circulatory supply to muscles, tends to vanish when the patient keeps his affected leg dependent and moves it intermittently. Patients so afflicted usually are well aware of these benefits, but sometimes their physicians insist on having the leg raised, not realizing the haemodynamics of the situation.

In the normal subject as well—even during heavy exercise, when the blood vessels are maximally dilated—a considerable extra gain in flow can be achieved by the rhythmic lowering of the local venous pressure, as caused, for instance, in rapid running, despite the very rapid refilling of the venous side in this situation (see Folkow *et al.*, 1970). For such reasons, flow in the lower limbs is considerably larger than would be expected from the levels of central arterial and venous pressures and the flow resistance in the maximally dilated muscle vessels of the legs. As an example, calf blood flow in man can be 50–60% larger when heavy rhythmic exercise is performed in the upright position as compared with the reclining position (Folkow *et al.*, 1971).

Pulsatile Pressures

The Windkessel Function

If fluid is suddenly forced into a rigid tube it emerges in essentially the same shape, and the pressure wave travels through the fluid at the speed of sound. But when the tube is distensible, as the blood vessels are, the speed of transmission of the pressure wave lessens in proportion to the decrease in the elasticity modulus (= increase of distensibility) and the wave is damped. Furthermore, much of a rhythmically injected fluid is now temporarily "stored" in the tube when the tube becomes distended by the pressure rise (Windkessel function). This temporary "storage" helps to transform an intermittent input to a more even outflow (Fig. 6-4). The aorta and the main arteries serve as Windkessel vessels, but their rhythmic changes in pressure and volume are very complex owing to the peculiar architecture of their walls (see Remington, 1963).

The aortic wall is composed of intricately interwoven elastic fibres (30%), collagen fibrils (30%), and smooth muscles (about 40%). Large "muscular" arteries have 20% elastic, 45% collagen, and 35% smooth

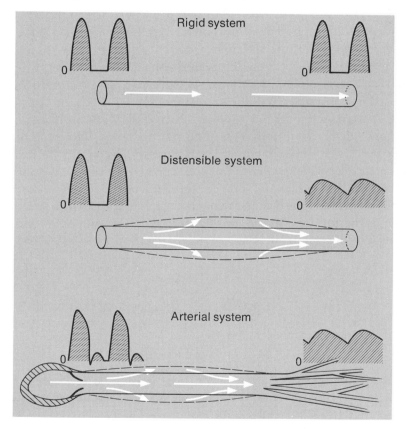

Fig. 6-4. Schematic illustration of the Windkessel effect of a distensible tube system: A rhythmic fluid ejection is transformed into a fairly uniform flow with reduced pressure oscillations.

musclc. In the Windkessel vessels, the muscle component by contraction causes increased wall stiffness in most situations but usually little change of their rather low w/r relationship (see Fig. 5-5), at least in the aorta (Bader, 1963). A rise of pressure in the arterial tree *in situ* increases the cross-sectional area, rather than its length, except perhaps in the aortic arch. The design of the larger arteries and their tissue connections together ensure that they are usually "prestretched", with a much higher longitudinal elasticity modulus (i.e. less stretchable) than that of the circumference. The opposite is the case for isolated segments of unstretched arteries.

According to Hooke's law, the deformation of a *perfectly* elastic material is proportional to the *size* but *not* to the *rate* of the applied force. However, once viscous properties are added ("visco-elastic" materials)—which is the case in blood vessels—such deformation will be somewhat *delayed* if the material is exposed to a rapid stretch, and its length then exhibits *creep*. The viscous properties of the material reveal themselves as a *stress relaxation*, or after-relaxation, with respect to its tension. Hence *hysteresis loops* are formed when a rapid stretch with some latency is followed by a rapid unloading. The visco-elastic properties of material can indeed be deduced from such loop characteristics (see Harding, 1962; Remington, 1963). The viscous properties imply that the more rapidly a given amount of blood is ejected into the Windkessel vessels, the larger the rise in pulse pressure, which occurs when the sympathetic influence on the heart increases (see Chapter 12). The rise in pulse pressure is still more increased if the walls of the Windkessel vessels are stiffened by smooth muscle contraction. Such factors explain why the pulse pressure increases far more than what can be accounted for by an increased stroke volume during heavy exercise.

Laplace's formula ($T = Pr/w$) shows that even if a tube wall were perfectly elastic—according to Hooke's law showing a linear relationship between wall deformation and applied force—the curve relating transmural pressure to wall tension would inevitably show a convexity towards the pressure axis. The wall tension thus increases out of proportion to the increase of pressure, for this rise of pressure itself causes an increase of radius and also a decrease of wall thickness. Hence a linear rise of pressure within distensible tubes brings them towards their breaking point at an accelerated rate.

This has important consequences also for the Windkessel vessels. Bursting at high pressure can only be avoided if a stiff and strong wall element exists, eventually protecting the wall from further distension. The collagen elements serve this purpose in normal vessels; they are usually slack but they prevent over-distension when the wall is excessively stretched. When they are damaged—as occurs in syphilis—aneurysmal sacs may result. Then the "yield point" of the vessel occurs even at normal transmural pressure and eventually, when $Pr/w > T$, such an aneurysm will burst.

At pressure levels below those which considerably involve its collagen elements, the thoracic aorta manifests the highest distensibility of all the systemic arteries—presumably due to its high proportion of elastic

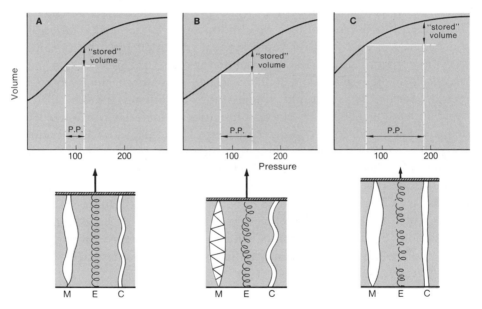

Fig. 6-5. Pressure-volume relationship of Windkessel vessels.
A. Smooth muscles relaxed and the elastic elements alone "damp" the rhythmic fluid ejection, which is temporarily "stored" at a comparatively small pressure rise (pulse pressure).
B. Smooth muscles contracted, stiffening the wall. The pressure rise for one and the same "stored" fluid volume is now somewhat bigger: pulse pressure is increased.
C. Elastic elements degenerated (old age), volume is increased, and resistance to distension is mainly offered by the stiff collagen elements. Therefore pulse pressure is greatly increased for a given "stored" volume.

fibres. Its diameter increases some 10% for a pulse pressure of 40 mm Hg (i.e. about 20% in volume, or more, as the length also increases), compared with that of abdominal aorta (5%) and that of large "muscular" arteries (3%). The thoracic aorta correspondingly displays the most pronounced Windkessel function *per unit volume*, although the *absolute* contribution of the other arteries to this property is greater because of their larger total volume.

The pressure-volume behaviour of Windkessel vessels is shown schematically in Fig. 6-5. Fig. 6-5A shows the situation when the smooth muscles are largely relaxed and the transmural pressure is initially low. The vessels are freely distensible owing to their elastic fibrils—their relaxed smooth muscle fibres are almost plastic and their collagen fibrils still slack. On further increases of pressure the collagen fibrils become stretched and henceforth the vessel is almost indistensible.

Figure 6-5B shows the result when contraction of the smooth muscles has added a "stiffer" element to the wall and has caused some decrease of circumference. In the lower range of transmural pressure the vessel is less distensible than in Fig. 6-5A. However, the "rigid jacket" of the collagen fibrils is not involved until the pressure level is higher than in Fig. 6-5A. However, smooth muscle contraction rarely causes more considerable decreases in the luminal diameter of large Windkessel vessels (unlike its effects on resistance vessels). It has been suggested that the muscle elements of the largest arteries are arranged in such a way as to change the distensibility of the wall rather than to exert a major effect on the w/r relationship (Bader, 1963).

Figure 6-5C illustrates the "geriatric" situation, with degeneration of the elastic fibrils—here the main load of pressure is placed on the collagen fibrils. Such a change in wall characteristics causes an increased volume and a lessened distensibility of the Windkessel arteries. The increased pulse pressure of age is largely due to this decreased distensibility. It should be remembered, however, that changes of *mean* arterial pressure are not attributable to reduction of Windkessel function alone; this only occurs when total peripheral resistance and/or cardiac output are changed.

The Nature of the Arterial Pulse Wave

The pulse pressure and the propagation of the pulse wave both are greatly influenced by the state of the elements of the arterial wall. Clearly, both are dependent on the stroke volume, and this has led to efforts to design a beat-by-beat measurement of the cardiac output. Unfortunately, unpredictable or inaccessible variables preclude this praiseworthy endeavour and the calculations made from the measurements have in the main proved unreliable when compared with results obtained from dye output or Fick methods (see Chapter 7). For example, an increased *rate* of blood expulsion into the aorta, or a smooth muscle contraction in the Windkessel vascular walls, will, for reasons discussed above, increase the pulse pressure even if stroke volume remains the same.

Recent studies of the pulse wave, notably by McDonald and Womersley (see McDonald, 1960; Harding, 1962; or Spencer and Denison, 1963), have helped to clarify some of the fundamental problems of the pulse wave. The more distensible the wall and the higher the fluid viscosity, the slower the propagation of the pulse wave and the more rapidly damped. The characteristics of the arterial wall and the architecture of tapering and arborization of the arterial tree both cause considerable damping. Thus, the dicrotic notch of the aortic pulse is already abolished at the lower end of the abdominal aorta (see Fig. 6-6).

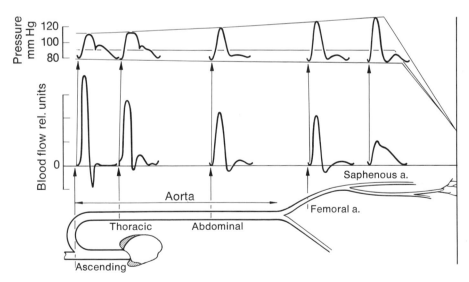

Fig. 6-6. Changes in mean and pulse pressures and in blood flow in different parts of the arterial tree. (Modified from McDonald, 1960. By permission.)

Wave reflection at various sites also occurs, and this complicates matters further. Although reflections occur at sites of major branches, the main site for positive wave reflection is at the precapillary resistance "barrier", which acts almost as a closed end to the pulse wave. Vasoconstriction here further accentuates the size of the reflected positive wave while dilatation has the reverse effect. Owing to damping, this main reflected wave is normally only some 30 to 40% of the size of the primary. It in turn is "re-reflected" to some extent, etc., but damping again rapidly suppresses these successively reflected waves. Such marked internal damping makes it very unlikely that true standing waves occur in the arterial tree (see McDonald, 1960).

If no reflection occurred the pulse wave would gradually decline as it passed peripherally because of such damping. However, reflection may cause *peaking* of the pulse wave—particularly obvious in the femoral artery where the size and rate of rise of the wave is greater than in the more central vessels. This peaking is mainly due to positive reflection from the "resistance" section and can be further accentuated by constriction of the small peripheral vessels (Fig. 6-6).

The pulse travels at 3 m/sec in the thoracic aorta, speeding to 5 or more m/sec in the muscular arteries, which are stiffer. The length of the pulse wave (5 to 7 m in man) considerably exceeds that of the longest part of the arterial system. The pulse wave velocity is increased when the arterial distensibility is less (because of hypertension, wall sclerosis, or muscle contraction in the arterial wall).

Effects of Pulsatile Pressure on Arterial Flow

Pulsatile flow results from pulsatile pressure, since flow always follows the pressure gradient, and *not* the absolute pressure. Thus, it is not surprising to find that the peak flow may *precede* the peak pressure when both are measured at the same site. When pressure is simultaneously recorded upstream and at the site itself the integration of the two pressure curves gives the *pressure gradient* which drives the flow. It then becomes evident that the pulsatile flow exactly follows this oscillating pressure gradient.

Backflow in the arteries likewise occurs whenever the downstream propagation of the pulse wave momentarily causes the pressure at a site downstream to exceed that in an upstream section. Phasic backflow occurs usually at sites where a considerable peaking of the pulse wave takes place as a result of a strong positive wave reflection. The femoral arteries—wide straight tubes which, during rest, have a relatively small flow and a high peripheral resistance—are characterized by phasic backflow. Other sites include parts of the arterial system where the large arteries are fairly wide but the peripheral flow resistance is high.

Figure 6-7 illustrates the principal relationship between pulsatile pressure and arterial flow in circumstances of vasoconstriction and vasodilatation, respectively. The figure shows how phasic backflow can occur and why it tends to vanish when vasodilatation ensues which is accompanied by an increased flow rate but not by a comparable increase in width of the large artery. The positive wave reflection then decreases while the pressure drop along the large arteries increases. Each of these factors minimizes

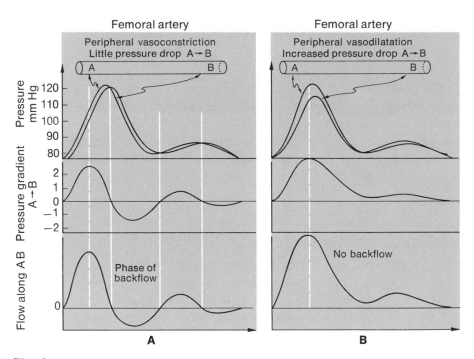

Fig. 6-7. The propagation of the pulse wave along an artery, with deduction of the pressure gradient and the phasic flow. Peripheral dilatation (B) increases the pressure drop along the vessel *AB*, which eliminates the brief phase of retrograde pressure gradient and hence the backflow phase. (Modified from McDonald, 1960. By permission.)

the likelihood of the pressure at a downstream site being greater than that recorded upstream (whatever the phase of the cyclic pressure curve). This explains why backflow is usually not seen in the splanchnic vascular bed. Here the peripheral resistance is low while that of the main arteries is comparatively high. The large flow through these arteries implies a pressure drop sufficient to minimize the likelihood of a pressure downstream ever exceeding that upstream.

Venous Pulsation

The systemic arterial pulse wave—but *not* the pulmonary one—is entirely damped out by the time the capillaries and venules are reached, except at marked vasodilatation. However, the cardiac pulsations are transmitted *backwards* to the central veins, though such pulsations are rapidly damped and delayed, being feeble beyond the thorax. The pressure changes transmitted into the central veins reflect the atrial contraction ("A wave") and the atrial pressure rise when the A-V valves close at the onset of ventricular systole ("C wave"). These pressure changes are immediately followed by a marked pressure drop when, during systole, the ventricles by their recoil are pushed downwards and exert "suction" on the atria, causing their rapid filling from the veins. Then pressure rises again to a transient peak ("V wave"), corresponding to the further entrance of blood into the by now well-filled atria, until the A-V valves are again opened and allow flow into the ventricles (see Chapter 12).

References

Bader, H. (1963). "The anatomy and physiology of the vascular wall," *Handbook of Physiology*, 2, Circulation **II**, 865–90.

Folkow, B., P. Gaskell, and B. Waaler (1970). "Blood flow through limb muscles during heavy rhythmic exercise," *Acta Physiol. Scand.* **80**, 61–72.

Folkow, B., U. Haglund, M. Jodal, and O. Lundgren (1971). "Blood flow in the calf muscles of man during heavy rhythmic exercise," *Acta Physiol. Scand.* In press.

Gaskell, P. (1969). Personal communication.

Gauer, O. H., and H. L. Thron (1965). "Postural changes in the circulation," *Handbook of Physiology*, 2, Circulation **III**, 2409–40.

Harding, V. (1962). "Propagation of pulse waves in visco-elastic tubings," *Handbook of Physiology*, 2, Circulation **I**, 107–35.

Holmberg, A. (1956). "Circulatory changes during muscular work in man," *Scand. J. Clin. & Lab. Invest.*, **8** Suppl., 24.

McDonald, D. A. (1960). *Blood flow in arteries*. London: Arnold.

Remington, J. W. (1963). "The physiology of the aorta and major arteries," *Handbook of Physiology*, 2, Circulation, **II**, 799–838.

Spencer, M. P., and A. B. Denison, Jr. (1963). "Pulsatile blood flow in the vascular system," *Handbook of Physiology*, 2, Circulation **II**, 839–64.

Wiederhielm, C. A. (1968). "Dynamics of transcapillary fluid exchange," Symposium on biological interfaces, flows, and exchanges, New York Heart Assoc.

7

Measurements of Pressures, Flows, and Volumes in the Cardiovascular System

Measurements in the cardiovascular system may be classified as *direct*, entailing catheterisation or cannulation of the vessels, or *indirect*, obtained without such interference.

Pressure Measurements

General Considerations

The *vascular circuits* are characterised by *the central arterial pressure, P_a, the central venous pressure, P_v* (in each case the mean pressure as well as the pulsatile pressure is of importance), and *the mean capillary pressure, P_c*. $P_a - P_v$ is the pressure head, and P_c, when related to P_a and P_v, gives the pre/postcapillary resistance ratio and reflects the current filtration-absorption equilibrium. Measurements at points along the pre- and post-capillary routes provide additional information about the profile of the pressure drop, in turn reflecting the regional resistances within the pre- and post-capillary compartments.

Pressure changes in the cardiac chambers are of the greatest importance in elucidating cardiac dynamics in health and disease.

Indirect Methods

Of the indirect methods, the estimation of *systemic arterial pressure* is by far the most important and routine. The procedure of choice is the auscultatory Riva Rocci method, utilizing the appearance and disappearance of the Korotkow sounds. The principle is simple, but accurate use of this method requires both skill and judgement (for details see Pickering, 1968). When correctly used, the agreement with directly recorded pressure is very good (Fig. 7-1A). In principle, a cuff around the forearm is rapidly inflated, beyond the systolic pressure level, then slowly deflated. The first sounds over the cubital artery signal the *systolic pressure* (P_s). With further cuff deflation the sounds suddenly become muffled and usually disappear within a few mm Hg. Direct pressure recordings indicate that the sudden

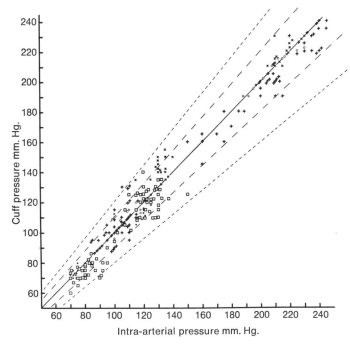

Fig. 7-1A. Correlation between intra-arterially measured blood pressure and pressure measured by the indirect Riva-Rocci method. The dotted lines indicate ± 10% and 20%, respectively. (From Pickering, 1968. By permission.)

decrease of the Korotkow sounds best corresponds to the *diastolic pressure* (P_d), but often both pressure values—where the sound suddenly decreases and where it vanishes—are given (e.g. 120/80–75).

However, in using this method, some turbulence and wall vibrations may occasionally occur in the brachial artery even when it is wide open. The Korotkow sounds in such situations are markedly reduced when the diastolic pressure level is reached, but they do not vanish entirely even at very low cuff pressures which are far below that of the true diastolic pressure.

Mean arterial pressure (P_a) in most cases can be regarded as approximately equal to the *sum* of the diastolic pressure and one-third of the pulse pressure (systolic – diastolic):

$$P_a = P_d + \frac{P_s - P_d}{3}$$

In recent years devices for semiautomatic, intermittent recordings of arterial pressure have been developed. They have the great advantage that the events of the subject's daily life can be followed, and that, therefore, their impact on the blood pressure level can be analysed (see Pickering, 1968; also Fig. 7-1B).

Indirect methods cannot be used for the accurate evaluation of intra-cardiac or central venous pressure. However, a marked rise of central venous pressure may be detected by examining the appearance of the superficial veins in the hand or the neck. When the hand is dependent its veins become well filled; on raising the arm to and above heart level it can be noted at what height the arm veins collapse and empty their contents into the vena cava. If the central venous pressure is pathologically high (a situation mimicked by the Valsalva manoeuvre), the hand must be raised considerably above heart level for venous collapse to occur. This method provides valuable first hand information for the clinician.

Mean capillary pressure (P_c) can also be estimated by indirect methods, though these require such elaborate precautions that reliable information can be obtained only in specific experimental conditions, and then in anaesthetized animals. Tissue weight, or volume (plethysmographic method, see section on Blood Flow Measurement, below), is recorded and a steady state "isogravimetric" or "isovolumetric" condition is established at known arterial inflow and venous outflow pressures, P_a and P_v. The extent by which P_a and P_v have to be changed to produce identical disturbances of the filtration-absorption equilibrium is then determined.

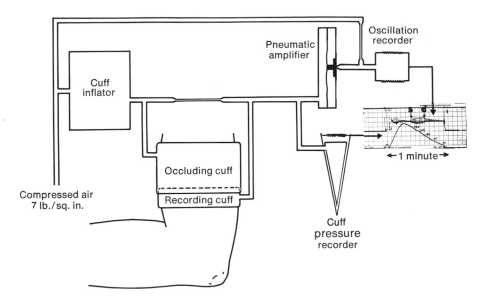

Fig. 7-1B. One of the principles used for semi-automatic measurements of arterial blood pressure in man. (From Pickering, 1968. By permission.)

Provided that autoregulatory precapillary adjustments (Chapter 16) can be avoided (which is difficult, except at maximal dilatation) it can be deduced, for instance, that the pre/postcapillary resistance ratio must be 5/1 if the filtration-absorption equilibrium is equally disturbed by a 50 mm Hg rise of P_a as it is by a 10 mm Hg rise of P_v. Then P_c can be estimated on the basis of the formula (see Chapter 6):

$$P_c = \frac{P_a\left(\dfrac{rv}{ra}\right) + P_v}{\left[1 + \left(\dfrac{rv}{ra}\right)\right]}$$

This indirect method has the great advantage that it provides a "statistical mean value" of the pressure in the whole capillary bed (see Chapter 8). The direct puncture of an individual capillary by a micropipette, though furnishing an exact measurement of the pressure in that capillary, may yield an unrepresentative result for the bed as a whole, or even for that capillary (which has, after all, been slightly injured).

Direct Methods

Since Poiseuille (1831) the U-tube *mercury manometer* connected to a can-nulated artery has been invaluable in the measurement of mean pressure. The mean pressure *drop* across the circuit can be recorded by cannulating both the artery and the vein, using two such manometers. A saline-filled manometer is employed in the low pressure vein to display the pressure variations more sensitively. Venous pressures are thus often referred to in cm H_2O instead of mm Hg.

The inertia of this manometer system causes considerable damping of rapid pressure changes. Only the mean pressure is accurately recorded. In most studies of flow this is actually an advantage, for the purpose is to relate the flow to the driving pressure (the driving pressure being equal to the difference between the mean pressures in the two ends of the circuit). Exact pressure readings necessitate in this (or any other manometer) determination of the correct "zero point". Otherwise hydrostatic pressure factors will impose an error. Further, depending on how the tip of the connecting cannula is placed in relation to the bloodstream in which the pressure is to be measured, it may record the lateral pressure alone or the lateral pressure plus or minus the impact of the kinetic energy (see Chapter 6).

Nowadays there are available new types of manometers, based on the principle that a membrane of small mass and minor displacement can, by electrical transformation (e.g. strain gauge principle) of the displacement produced by the blood pressure, deliver a proportional signal to a suitable recorder. Because of the small mass and displacement of the moveable part, combined with designs suiting different pressure levels and ranges, such modern manometers can accurately record both very rapid and very small pressure changes. Linden (1958, 1963) provides a useful critique of the physical principles in such measurements. The correct recording of rapid pressure changes calls for a manometer system displaying a natural frequency of at least ten times that to be recorded. The oscillations recorded by such manometers can, however, also be damped electronically so that mean pressures can be obtained as well. They have been of the greatest importance—for example, for the correct interpretation of pres-sure events within the heart and adjacent vascular connections. However, Poiseuille's classical mercury manometer still lurks in the background, as most modern manometer systems are calibrated against Poiseuille's.

Blood Flow Measurements

General Considerations

Flows to be measured vary widely, ranging from the cardiac output and the total flow through a single organ to measurements of flow in individual tissue compartments within organs, such as in the grey matter of the brain and the secretory crypts of the intestinal wall, or of flow in individual microvessels.

Both mean and phasic blood flows may be required, as in the left ventricular myocardium, where systolic contraction mechanically affects the vascular bed. In skin it is sometimes necessary to differentiate between nutritional flow, traversing the capillaries, and the true shunt blood flow, passing through specific A-V anastomoses. Such varied requirements presuppose the use of many different methods (see Bruner, 1960; Kramer *et al.*, 1963).

Measurement of Cardiac Output

Although electromagnetic flow probes (see below) can be chronically implanted around the pulmonary artery or aorta, allowing beat-to-beat (stroke volume) measurements, and direct recorders of other types (see below) can be inserted in anaesthetized animals in the pulmonary artery or in the caval veins, so far only indirect methods can be employed in man. Two main techniques are employed, though several other approaches have been explored (see Hamilton, 1962). The two main techniques are Stewart-Hamilton's indicator dilution method and the Fick principle. Both have the disadvantage that they only provide intermittent values; the ideal, of course, would be continuous beat-by-beat recording.

Stewart-Hamilton's Indicator Dilution Method

If a known amount of indicator is quickly injected into a tube system in which fluid is flowing, a segment of the tube downstream will "see" the indicator as a rising concentration which, after reaching its peak, falls off exponentially. The passage time for the indicator is recorded from its first appearance to its final disappearance, and its average concentration during one circulation is deduced from the concentration time curve. (See Hamilton, 1962; Zierler, 1962).

The flow is deduced from the injected amount, I, its time of passage, t, and its average concentration during this time, c. The principle is largely the same as when the size of a pool is deduced by adding to it a known amount of indicator and measuring its concentration after thorough mixing. The trouble is, however, that in the closed cardiovascular system most indicators thus injected reappear (due to recirculation) before the concentration produced by the first slug has fallen to zero. Even so, as the indicator disappearance would otherwise be exponential, it is possible to extrapolate the falling limb of the primary concentration curve fairly accurately by plotting this on semilog paper, since it then forms a straight line (Fig. 7-2A). The time for one circulation is given by the intercept of this line with the abscissa.

A known amount of the indicator is injected intravenously, becomes fully mixed with the blood in the heart, and is then continuously sampled via an arterial catheter, where its concentration curve can be directly

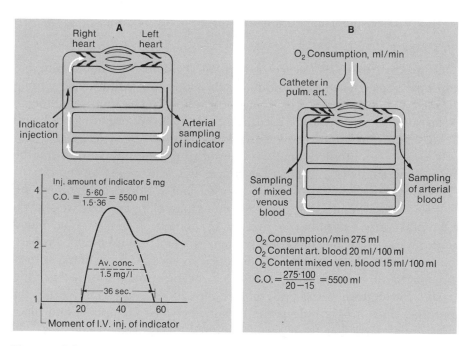

Fig. 7-2. Measurement of cardiac output (diagrammatic). A. Principle of the dye dilution method. B. Fick principle.

recorded, even in the semilog fashion, and, if so, this gives the time t between the appearance and disappearance of the indicator in its first passage, once the falling limb has been extrapolated to the abscissa. Suppose the indicator amount I injected equals 5 mg and that its average concentration c during the primary passage is 1.5 mg/litre of blood and the passage time t is 36 sec. Then

$$\text{Cardiac output} = \frac{I}{ct}$$

$$\text{Cardiac output} \; \frac{5 \times 60}{1.5 \times 36} = 5.5 \; \text{l/min}$$

Indicators most commonly used are Evan's blue (T 1834) or cardiogreen, but also slugs of suitable isotopes, hypotonic or hypertonic salt solutions, or even saline of a different temperature from that of blood can be used. The indicator should not, however, be lost from the blood from the point of injection to the point of sampling, which is partly the case with a "thermoslug", but this can be approximately corrected for and the "thermodilution" variant has the advantage that almost no recirculation occurs so that very frequent measurements can be performed.

The Fick Principle

Outlined by Adolf Fick as early as 1870, this principle was not used in man until the 1940's, when a technique was developed for withdrawing samples of mixed venous blood. The principle is also the basis for a number of "clearance" measurements, used in measurements of organ blood flow in man, e.g. in the kidney or liver (see below).

For cardiac output estimations one measures the uptake of a suitable indicator, usually O_2, and its *mean arterial* and *mixed venous* concentrations. The elimination of CO_2 may also be used, but it is less suitable since pH shifts affect the results. Suppose, in resting man of 70 kg body weight, the O_2 uptake is 275 ml/min, the arterial O_2 content is 20 ml/100 ml blood, and the mixed venous blood O_2 content is 15 ml/100 ml blood. Properly mixed venous blood can only be obtained by means of a cannula with its tip placed in either the right ventricle or the pulmonary artery (Fig. 7-2B). Blood from peripheral veins is clearly *not* representative for this purpose, since it only reflects the balance between O_2 uptake and blood flow in the particular tissue section drained by this vein.

Then $\qquad \text{Cardiac output} = \dfrac{275 \times 100}{20 - 15} = 5500 \; \text{ml/min}$

This method is theoretically impeccable, but to be reliable it obviously calls for a heart catheterization and an arterial puncture, and it can only provide intermittent values. The measurements necessarily require cardiac catheterizations, done in a darkened room where the position of the catheter is determined by X-ray screening, and the whole procedure entails circumstances which may frighten the patient and may then yield higher than resting values of cardiac output.

Measurement of Blood Flow in Organs and Regions

Direct Measurements

Blood flow in organs or regions can be measured directly by interposing a suitable recording unit between the ends of the divided cognate artery or vein. Such recorders are reliable only if collateral flow is prevented and if the recorder does not raise the flow resistance much. Trauma to the vessels, and perhaps to adjacent vasomotor nerves, are disadvantages. The exposure of the blood (which must be heparinized) to foreign surfaces causes damage of the blood cells, with release of vasoactive substances such as adenosine compounds, potassium ions, and serotonin (5-HT) from thrombocytes; cell aggregation may result. It is therefore usually preferable to record *venous outflow* instead of *arterial inflow*; the blood reaching the tissue studied is undisturbed while such damage as the venous blood may experience is minimized by dilution in the heart and by its "clearing" in the lungs.

The "constant perfusion" pumps maintain constant flow, yet they often damage the blood so much that vascular "tone" and its control in the perfused tissue are grossly disturbed, and plugging of microvessels may ensue. In the investigation of some problems, however, such disturbances are relatively unimportant compared with the gains in other respects; here, as always, it is a matter of creating a proper balance between the method chosen and the project under appraisal.

In the automatic *Gaddum recorder* (Fig. 7-3A) venous outflow is intermittently collected in a tube, displacing air to a volume recorder and providing ordinates proportional to the flow. The blood is collected and then emptied via a funnel into the central end of the vein. Such a unit, which is "open", can cover a wide range of flows.

Drop recorders (Fig. 7-3B) can be made closed, so that drops of blood, formed at the end of a venous cannula, fall through a silicon oil column

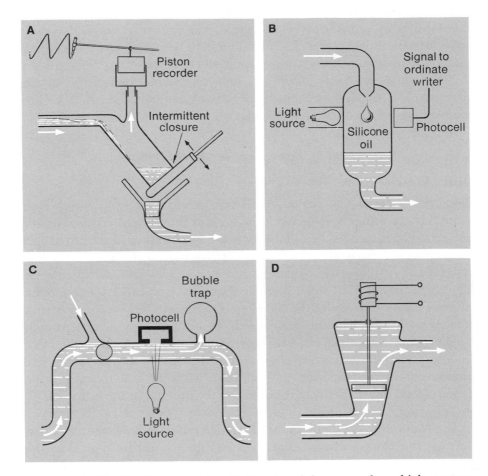

Fig. 7-3. A. The Gaddum recorder. B. The closed drop recorder, which operates an ordinate writer, for example. C. The bubble flow meter. D. The turbo-flow meter.

into a blood pool at an exit cannula; a photoelectric unit signals the fall of each drop to an ordinate writer. Such units, suitable for small flow volumes, can be inserted both on the arterial and the venous sides. The method is most useful, reliable, and accurate; flow is continuously monitored. It requires careful calibration because the size of the drops increase somewhat at increased flows.

A bubble flow meter (Fig. 7-3C), which is often automatized, consists of a tube system of known dimensions and length with a gas bubble trap. The unit is interposed either on the arterial or venous side. Air bubbles are intermittently injected, traverse the tube, and the time for their travel over a given length is signalled photoelectrically, after which the bubble is trapped in a side tube. The tube volume and the transit time are thus known and volume flow is obtained. Though this is an "intermittent" flow recorder, measurements may be automatically obtained so frequently that the device reflects mean flow events almost continuously.

In the *turbo-flow meter* (Fig. 7-3D) blood flowing from below lifts a magnetic cone fitted into a slightly conical cylinder, to a height which largely depends on the rate of flow. The displacement of the magnetic cone is then electronically registered and reflects flow, if properly calibrated. Such devices have the advantage that they can be inserted, for instance, into the root of the aorta in very large animals, to record cardiac output directly.

In the past, recordings of phasic blood flows have been made, using units based on the classical Pitot or Bernoulli principles, and they served well for such purposes. Nowadays, the *electromagnetic flowmeter* (Fig. 7-4A), originally designed by Kolin in 1936, has taken their place (see Kolin, 1960). This unit, though sometimes showing serious calibration problems, has the advantage that it is applied firmly and in close approximation around an *intact* artery. It is based on the principle that the passage of an electrolyte solution within an electromagnetic field generates an electrical potential across the vessel due to electromagnetic induction. With proper electronic magnification and transformation, a signal is obtained which either indicates the pulsatile flow per beat or, if desired, integrates this pulsatile flow to give the mean flow. It can be constructed to fit quite small arteries but is also excellent for cardiac output measurements.

A recorder with similar advantages (and disadvantages) is that based on the classical Doppler principle: sound travels more rapidly *with* the stream than *against* it. It is usually called the *ultrasonic flow meter* (Fig. 7-4B) as it is operated with ultrasonic frequencies. One or two pairs of transmitters and recorders for high frequency operation are mounted on opposite sides of a vessel some longitudinal distance apart; the vessel circumference and the transmitter-recorder distance is known. The faster the flow the greater the difference in wave propagation; this can

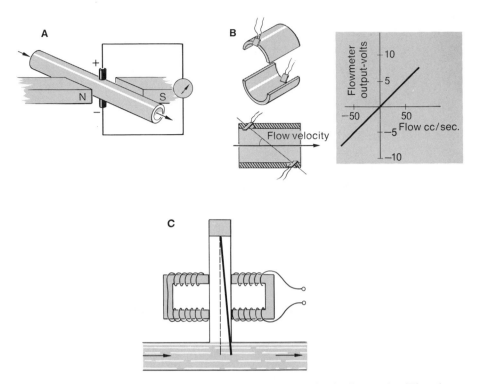

Fig. 7-4. Recorders suitable for measurements of phasic flows. A. The electro-magnetic flow meter. B. The pulsed ultrasonic flow meter. C. The bristle flow meter.

be displayed electronically as a well-calibrated recording of phasic flow (Franklin *et al.*, 1959).

Either of these last two recorders is suitable for use in long-term experiments on intact animals; the perivascular probes are fitted aseptically and the wounds closed to heal without undue fibrous reaction. It is also possible to record such flows by telemetry.

The *bristle flow meter*, based on the pendulum flow meter (in which the flowing blood displaces a pendulum from its resting position according to the velocity of flow; Brecher, 1960), makes use of the RC 5734 valve. The bristle, which projects through the side arm of a T cannula inserted into the vessel, is attached via a fulcrum to the anode of the valve (Fig. 7-4C). Movements of the bristle are thus transmitted to the anode, and displacements of the anode alter the voltage output of the valve. These displacement outputs can be amplified and displayed. This instrument has proved particularly useful in recording phasic changes of flow in central veins.

Indirect Measurements

Plethysmographic methods can be used to measure flow in limbs in man or flow in limbs, organs, adipose tissue preparations, skin flaps, etc., in anaesthetized animals. The *plethysmograph* (Fig. 7-5) is an instrument of

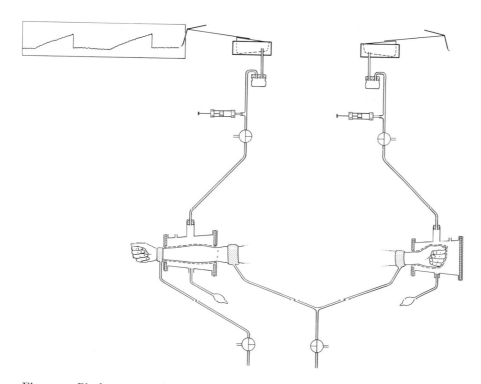

Fig. 7-5. Plethysmographic recordings of forearm and hand blood flows in man. Prior to the recording of forearm flow, blood supply to the corresponding hand is excluded by the wrist cuff. Intermittent venous obstruction is then produced by the proximal cuff and the increase in forearm (hand) volume per unit time is recorded. Knowing the time, and the volume, the rate of blood flow/min/100 ml of tissue can then be calculated. (Modified from Barcroft and Swan, 1953. By permission.)

great value and it has a wide range of usefulness, for it allows the recording not only of flow, but also of regional changes of blood volume and of trans-capillary fluid exchange (Mellander, 1960; see below). It is sensitive, exact, easily calibrated, and involves no trauma when used in man. It is also simple and cheap.

The organ or region is enclosed in a leak-proof fluid-filled or air-filled rigid container which is connected to a volume recorder of the required sensitivity. An inflatable cuff is placed just proximal to the plethysmograph and is intermittently pumped up to a pressure below the diastolic pressure at which venous outflow, but not arterial inflow, is obstructed. Arterial inflow, which reaches the veins, causes the enclosed organ to swell in proportion to this inflow and the volume is recorded on a moving paper. The volume increase per unit time and the tissue volume gives, after calibration, blood flow/min × 100 g tissue; as many as 5 to 6 measurements may be made per minute. Whitney (1953) has modified the device by simply mounting a low-pressure *strain gauge* around the limb which records the change in volume electrically.

Clearance Methods

The Fick principle is widely used for so-called *"clearance" measurements*. The A-V difference of a suitable indicator across an organ is measured while its uptake in, or elimination from, the organ is simultaneously determined. Thus, liver blood flow can be estimated by measuring the clearance of bromsulfalein (BSP), which is removed almost solely by the liver. If the clearance of BSP per unit time from the blood is determined and its arterial and hepatic vein concentrations are known, then the total hepatic blood flow can be calculated by applying the Fick principle (see Bradley, 1963). Similarly, the kidneys excrete paraaminohippurate (PAH) almost quantitatively into the urine. As the urine excretion of PAH per unit time is known, as well as the arterial and renal venous (sensibly zero) PAH concentrations, the renal blood flow can be calculated (see Selkurt, 1963).

Sapirstein (1958) introduced the method of i.v. or i.a. injection of radioactive ^{86}Rb or ^{42}K, after which the animal was immediately killed and the organ contents of the tracer determined. Provided that the capillary transfer of the tracer is rapid and uniform, its tissue distribution would reflect the blood supply to the various organs at the time of injection. However, distortions arise, as the transfer of these indicators is not rapid enough to reflect flow exactly in all situations. On the other hand, when the investigator remembers such pitfalls and uses this approach for the proper purposes, it can be a most useful tool for exploring the approximate distribution of blood supply to the tissues.

Kety (1949) introduced the principle of the *"tissue clearance" of rapidly diffusing, inert isotopes*. Initially ^{21}Na was used, but this has been replaced by the inert, lipid-soluble gases ^{133}Xe and ^{85}Kr (Lassen and Munck, 1955). These elements pass so rapidly from tissue to blood that their elimination is in most situations only limited by blood flow. They are almost totally eliminated in the lungs in the first passage, hence recirculation problems do not arise. Such an isotope is eliminated in the form of a mono-exponential function (giving a straight line when plotted on a semilog paper) in case a tissue is *uniformly* and *constantly* perfused (Fig. 7-6A). This is, however, an idealized situation, as blood flow is usually to some extent uneven.

If there are several tissue compartments with clearly different blood flows and the indicator has been administered intra-arterially, the elimination curve becomes more complex. Even then, however, it may be analysed into its individual components on the semilog plot according to the principle of successively subtracting exponentials (Fig. 7-6B).

This clearance method can also be used after topical administration of the indicator by means of direct injections. If the amount of the tracer injected is minute enough it allows measurements of the blood flow in a very small area. The localisation of the different components of a multi-compartment clearance curve can by such means be ascertained in organs which contain several tissue sections (the intestine, for example; see Lundgren, 1967).

In a constantly and uniformly perfused tissue, where the arterial concentration of the tracer is virtually zero, its exponential elimination from the tissue is described by the formula:

$$C_t = C_0 \cdot e^{-kt} \qquad (1)$$

where C_t and C_0 are the tissue concentrations at times t and zero. k is the "clearance constant", which is closely related to the blood flow and can be determined from the following formula, derived from (1):

$$k = \frac{\ln 2}{t\,1/2} \qquad (2)$$

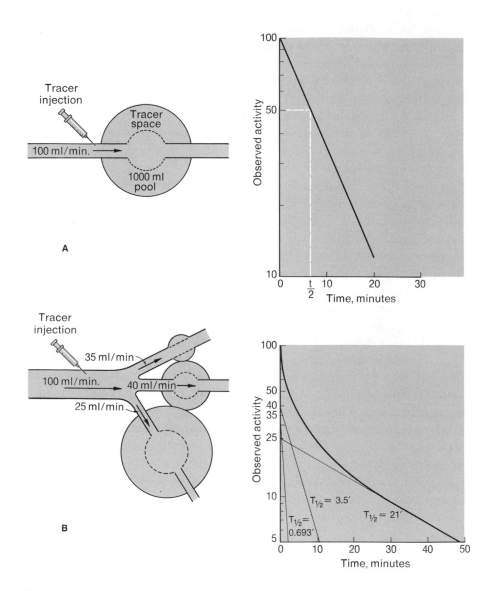

Fig. 7-6. A. Monoexponential wash-out curve in a "uniform" and constantly perfused system (e.g. myocardium or most skeletal muscles).

B. Multiexponential (three components) wash-out curve in a system composed of three tissue compartments, each with a different rate of blood flow. (Modified from Dobson and Warner, 1960. By permission.)

where $t\,1/2$ is the half time of decay in minutes and is calculated from the straight line obtained upon plotting equation (1) on semilog paper. If the tracer leaves the tissue only by the bloodstream and if the concentration gradients in the tissue can be neglected (which usually seems to be the case with ^{85}Kr and ^{133}Xe), then the blood flow, Q, is obtained in ml/min/ 100 g tissue from the formula:

$$Q = k \cdot s \cdot 100 \qquad (3)$$

where s denotes the tissue-blood partition coefficient of the tracer gas, divided by the specific weight of the tissue.

The great advantage of this method—which is readily applicable in man—is that virtually any tissue blood flow can be studied provided that it can be reached by an injection needle for depositing the indicator. The disadvantage is that fairly long periods of recordings in a steady state are needed for the calculation of a single flow figure. Further, artefacts—due, for example, to the widely differing partition coefficients for the gases in water and fat, or to gas diffusion to air from superficial tissues—unless they are taken into account, may seriously complicate the results.

Heat Clearance Methods

Local blood flow changes—in the tip of the finger, for example—can be deduced from measurements of the heat flow and the temperature gradient, though many hazards are involved in the practical situation.

The *"heat clearance" principle* has been utilized in other ways, among them in the form of the Hensel needle (see Golenhofen and Hildebrandt, 1962). Such a variant involves a constant heat source and a temperature-recording thermocouple, both of which are built into the tip of a relatively thin injection needle. The constant heat source warms the surrounding tissues and the adjacent thermocouple, but the more rapid the bloodstream which carries away the heat, the less warm the tissue becomes. Thus the temperature signal can be transformed into a recording device for measuring regional blood flow. Theoretically, this approach is very attractive, but complicating factors are such as to require the utmost expertise on the part of the experimenter.

A unit of this type may be placed in the tip of a cardiac catheter and the thermocouple may be replaced by a more sensitive thermistor. Such a device may then be inserted into a central vessel, but the vascular diameter must be known to give reliable flow figures. This may be achieved if the catheter is fitted with a device which positions the tip in the midline and simultaneously gives a measure of the vascular diameter (Fig. 7-7).

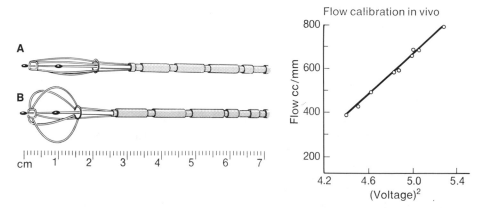

Fig. 7-7. "Isothermal" catheter flowmeter. A heating coil encloses a thermistor at the catheter tip, with the sensing element placed more proximally and held in the centre of the vessel; the vascular dimensions can be evaluated from the position of the five spring wires. The heat production is automatically so adjusted as to keep the thermistor temperature constant; then the heat production varies linearly with flow. (Modified from Mellander and Rushmer, 1960. By permission.)

Measurements of Blood Volume

Total Blood Volume

The total blood volume can be measured in different ways, based on the indicator dilution technique. If a known amount of indicator which does not readily leave the bloodstream (such as Evans blue) is given, it soon becomes evenly distributed in the plasma compartment. Its dilution in the plasma sample, once it is thoroughly mixed but not yet lost in significant amounts from the cardiovascular system, gives the plasma volume directly. A haematocrit estimation then gives the total blood volume. Other indicators of similar principle, such as "Risa" (= radioactive iodinated serum albumin) are used.

One can also use tracers which selectively enter, and thus measure, the cellular compartment of the blood—such as carbon monoxide, which combines with haemoglobin, or radioactive chromium (^{51}Cr), which also binds with haemoglobin (For details see Lawson, 1962; Zierler, 1962).

Estimation of Regional Blood Content

In animal experiments, the plethysmograph, when used only as a *volume* recorder, in combination with recordings of P_a, P_v, and total blood flow, can provide good insight into various aspects of the haemodynamic events (Fig. 7-8). Such a combination of techniques can reveal even minor changes both in regional blood content, as induced, for instance, by vasomotor nerves or exercise, as well as changes in the capillary filtration-absorption equilibrium, secondary to shifts in the pre/postcapillary resistance ratio.

The *total* blood content of the region studied can also be measured by excluding it temporarily from the rest of the circulation while labelling it with ^{51}Cr, for example. Then the excluded region is opened again and the dilution of ^{51}Cr is recorded.

Further, the combined use of external monitoring of ^{51}Cr and plethysmographic measurement of volume changes can differentiate between a tissue volume change that is due to fluid shifts between blood and tissues and one that is due to a changed blood content, such as in exercise (Fig. 7-9). This is of the greatest use in analyses of effects of vasoconstrictor fibres on the mobilization of blood from the capacitance side and the mobilization of tissue fluid as a consequence of reduced capillary pressure, especially when these adjustments are so gradual in onset that a clear distinction between blood volume changes and shifts in the transcapillary fluid exchange is not possible by the volume recording alone.

In man such methods cannot be used, at least not if one wants to measure the blood content of, for example, the pulmonary circuit, which is of considerable interest in many pathophysiological situations. This can, however, be accomplished in the following way (see Zierler, 1962). The blood content of a tube system is its cross-sectional area A times its length L, but neither A nor L can be measured directly *in vivo*. A can be deduced if the flow Q and the mean linear velocity V are known:

$$V = Q/A \tag{1}$$

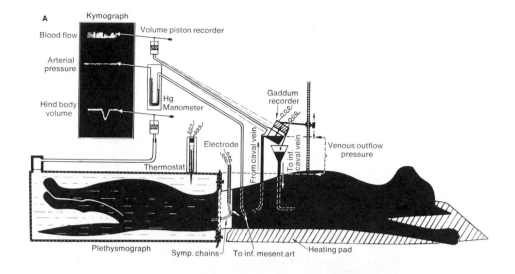

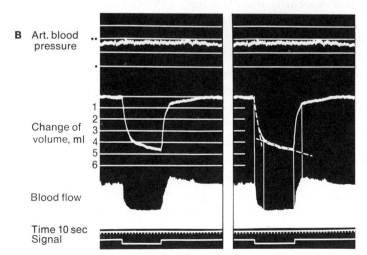

Fig. 7-8A. Simultaneous measurements of blood pressure, flow, and blood volume for analysing resistance and capacitance responses and changes in transcapillary events (filtration/absorption). (From Mellander, 1960. By permission.)

Fig. 7-8B. A recording using the technique shown in A; sympathetic stimulation causes reduced flow, reduced volume, and an absorption of tissue fluid (the slow component of the fall in volume). (From Mellander, 1960. By permission.)

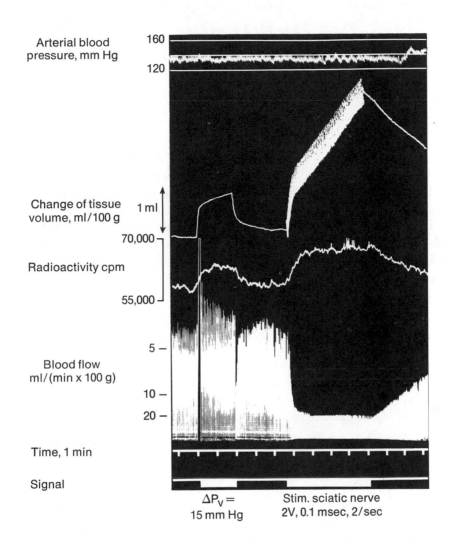

Fig. 7-9. Effect of exercise on blood pressure, tissue volume, erythrocyte content (^{51}Cr activity) in cat's calf, and on blood flow. Before the exercise venous pressure is briefly raised 15 mm Hg, producing filtration and increased blood content. Exercise produces increased blood content (evident from both the recording of tissue volume and erythrocyte content) and a considerable capillary filtration, revealed by the second, slower phase of volume increase, when regional blood volume (erythrocyte content) stays constant. (From Kjellmer, 1965. By permission.)

L can be deduced if the mean transit time MTT is measured, for

$$MTT = L/V \qquad\qquad (2)$$

from (1) and (2)

$$MTT = \frac{L \times A}{Q}$$

$L \times A$ is the regional blood content BV:

$$BV = MTT \times Q \qquad\qquad (3)$$

MTT can be determined by the "*sudden injection method*". A suitable indicator is rapidly injected on the arterial side and its appearance in the venous outflow is recorded as an indicator dilution curve. MTT is equal to the time delay between the moment of injection and the instant at which the *average* concentration of the indicator passes the outflow recording site (Fig. 7-10A). Several methods can be used for measuring Q. For instance, it can be deduced from the indicator dilution curve (Fig. 7-10A). As an example:

> Pulmonary circuit: $MTT = 5$ sec
> Flow $= 6000$ ml/min $= 100$ ml/sec

> Pulmonary blood volume $= 5 \times 100 = 500$ ml

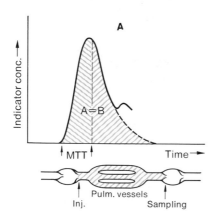

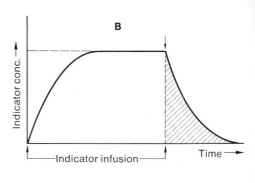

Shaded area x flow = Volume

Fig. 7-10. A. "Sudden injection" method for determination of regional blood volume. B. "Constant infusion" method for determination of regional blood volume. (Modified from Zierler, 1962; for details see this paper. By permission.)

Another way of measuring the regional blood volume is by means of the *"constant infusion method"*. When a constant known blood concentration of an infused indicator is reached in the outflow from the vascular circuit studied the infusion is stopped. The progressive fall in outflow concentration of indicator is recorded simultaneously with the outflow Q itself (Fig. 7-10B). The size of the shaded area is computed, and this, multiplied by the outflow Q, gives the regional blood volume between the sites of infusion and withdrawal.

References

Barcroft, H., and H. J. C. Swan (1953). *Sympathetic control of human blood vessels.* London: E. Arnold & Co.

Bradley, S. E. (1963). "The hepatic circulation," *Handbook of Physiology*, 2, Circulation **II,** 1387–1438.

Brecher, G. A. (1960). "Bristle flowmeter," in *Methods in medical research, Yr. Bk.* **8,** 307–8. Chicago.

Bruner, H. D. (1960). "Peripheral blood flow measurement," in *Methods in medical research, Yr. Bk.* **8,** 222–351. Chicago.

Dobson, E. L., and G. F. Warner (1960). "Clearance rates following intra-arterial injections in the study of peripheral vascular beds," in *Methods in medical research, Yr. Bk.* **8,** 242–48. Chicago.

Franklin, D. L., D. W. Baker, R. M. Ellis, and R. F. Rushmer (1959). "A pulsed ultrasonic flowmeter," *Ire Transactions on Medical Electronics*, ME-**6,** 204–6.

Golenhofen, K., and G. Hildebrandt (1962). "Das Verfahren der Wärmeleit-messung und seine Bedeutung für die Physiologie des menschlichen Muskelkreislaufes," *Archiv für Kreislaufforschung*, **38,** 23–70.

Hamilton, W. F. (1962). "Measurement of the cardiac output," *Handbook of Physiology*, 2, Circulation **I,** 551–84.

Kety, S. S. (1949). "Measurement of regional circulation by the local clearance of radioactive sodium," *Am. Heart J.* **38,** 321–28.

Kjellmer, I. (1965). "Studies on exercise hyperaemia," *Acta Physiol. Scand.* **64,** Suppl., 244, 1–27.

Kolin, A. (1960). "Blood flow determination by electromagnetic method," in *Medical physics*, ed. by O. Glasser. *Yr. Bk.* **3,** 141–55. Chicago.

Kramer, K., W. Lochner, and E. Wetterer (1963). "Methods of measuring blood flow," *Handbook of Physiology*, 2, Circulation **II,** 1277–324.

Lassen, N. A., and O. Munck (1955). "Cerebral blood flow in man determined by the use of radioactive krypton," *Acta Physiol. Scand.* **33,** 30–49.

Lawson, H. C. (1962). "The volume of blood—a critical examination of methods for its measurement," *Handbook of Physiology*, 2, Circulation **I,** 23–49.

Linden, R. J. (1958). *Blood pressure within the atria of canine and human heart*, Ph.D. Thesis, University of Leeds, England.

Linden, R. J. (1963). "The control of output of the heart," Chap. 10 in *Recent advances in physiology* (ed. R. Creese), 8th ed. London: Churchill.

Lundgren, O. (1967). "Studies on blood flow distribution and countercurrent exchange in the small intestine," *Acta Physiol. Scand.*, Suppl., 303.

Mellander, S. (1960). "Comparative studies on the adrenergic neuro-hormonal control of resistance and capacitance blood vessels in the cat," *Acta Physiol. Scand.* **50,** Suppl., 176.

Mellander, S., and R. F. Rushmer (1960). "Venous blood flow recorded with an isothermal flowmeter," *Acta Physiol. Scand.* **48,** 13–19.

Pickering, G. (1968). *High blood pressure*, 2nd ed. London: Churchill.

Sapirstein, L. A. (1958). "Regional blood flow by fractional distribution of indicators," *Am. J. Physiol.* **193,** 161–68.

Selkurt, E. E. (1963). "The renal circulation," *Handbook of Physiology*, 2, Circulation **II,** 1457–516.

Whitney, R. J. (1953). "Measurement of volume changes in human limbs," *J. Physiol.*, **121,** 1–27.

Zierler, K. L. (1962). "Circulation times and the theory of indicator-dilution methods for determining blood flow and volume," *Handbook of Physiology*, 2, Circulation **I,** 585–615.

8

Capillary Function

General Introduction

The term "microcirculation" designates the blood flow through terminal arterioles, metarterioles, precapillary sphincters, capillaries, and post-capillary venules. Terminal arterioles are vessels lined (as elsewhere) by endothelium that is surrounded by a single layer of smooth muscle and by a minimum of supporting connective tissue. The metarteriole is an off-shoot from the arteriole, of similar structure, serving to provide blood via the precapillary sphincters to the capillaries (Illig, 1961; Zweifach, 1961; Wiedeman, 1963; Fig. 8-1A). The precapillary sphincters, each of which is characterised by a local muscular investment, close rhythmically and asynchronously in resting tissue. The precapillary sphincter is the last site of smooth muscle cells in the wall of any of the branches of a terminal arteriole. The EM pictures shown in Fig. 8-1B and C illustrate the situation admirably. The functional activity of the precapillary sphincters determines the number of patent capillaries, and, hence, the perfused surface area of the capillary bed.

For practical purposes we may say that the capillary tubes consist of a wall composed of a single layer of endothelial cells. Such a thin wall is appropriate for an abundant transmural exchange and, indeed, solutes and solvent pass readily back and forth.

Solutes may be conveniently divided into those which are soluble in lipid and those which are soluble in water. This arbitrary distinction is,

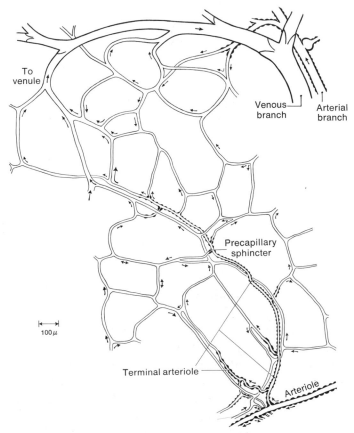

Fig. 8-1A. Example of the arrangement of the microcirculation; in this case in the bat's wing. (From Nicoll and Webb, 1946. By permission). See also Figs. 5-1A and 5-1B.

Fig. 8-1B. Electron micrograph ($\times$ 1750) of a terminal arteriole with an inner diameter of 30 μ, at the point at which a smaller 12 μ terminal arteriole is given off. Direction of blood flow shown by arrows. Smooth muscle cells of a precapillary sphincter (**) indicate the beginning of an arterial capillary (7μ) with an adjacent lymphatic capillary (L). (From Rhodin, 1967. By permission.)

Fig. 8-1C. Enlargement ($\times$ 25,500) of precapillary sphincter area seen in Fig. 8-1B. The lumen and the direction of blood flow are shown by the arrow. The endothelial cell (E) containing mitochondria (M) is separated from the smooth muscle cells (S) by a basement membrane (BM). Short-processes (*) of the endothelial cell pierce the basement membrane to make membranous contacts (myoendothelial junctions) with the smooth muscle cells (S). The two smooth muscle cells seen in this figure correspond to those marked** in Fig. 8-1B. (From Rhodin, 1967. By permission.)

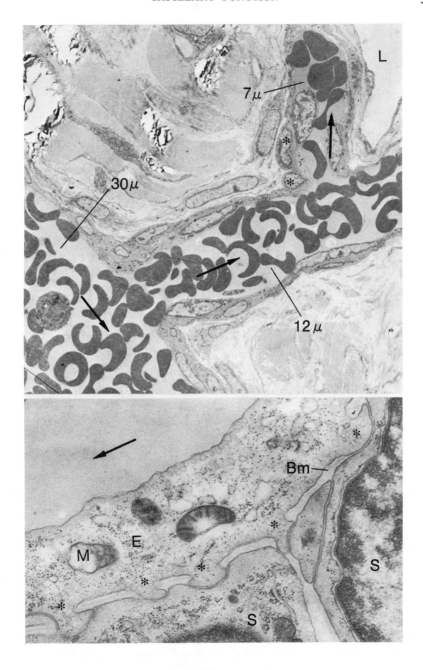

in this case, of enormous functional importance, for whereas lipid-soluble substances (like O_2 and CO_2) can traverse almost the entire capillary wall surface, those soluble only in water (like glucose) are restricted in their passage to "pores" in the wall. Water itself, on the other hand, appears to pass not only through these capillary pores, but also through the endothelial cell membranes per se, by means of routes that are not available for solutes (Yudilevich and Alvarez, 1967).

Obviously, the size of the *capillary surface area* perfused will quantitatively influence the loss and gain of both solvent and solutes, whether such solutes are lipid-soluble or water-soluble. This surface area is itself controlled by the tone of the precapillary spincters. Again, for any given capillary surface area the passage of *water*-soluble substances is determined by the number and size of the pores in that surface area, i.e. by its *permeability*. The density and size of capillary pores differ in the various regional circuits. The permeability of a given capillary surface area is therefore customarily expressed in terms of the measured passage of "tracer" substances which are water-soluble. Local tissue substances, such as histamine and bradykinin, which alter the size and possibly the number of the capillary pores, correspondingly modify capillary permeability.

Various aspects of capillary function are critically surveyed in some recent reviews (Pappenheimer, 1953; Landis and Pappenheimer, 1963, Majno, 1965) and a recent symposium (Crone *et al.*, 1970).

Structural Specialization

Three main types of capillaries are described on the basis of electron microscope studies (see Majno, 1965; Fig. 8-2).

Continuous (Non-Fenestrated) Capillaries

These are found in all types of muscle, the lungs, the central nervous system, and in fat and connective tissue. The single layer of endothelial cells (about 30 microns long, 10 microns wide, and 0.1 to 0.3 microns thick, save at the site of the nucleus where it may be 2 to 3 microns thick) is apparently continuous. The intercellular region is occupied by a homogeneous material of moderate density, some 100Å wide, possibly of mucopolysaccharide nature. Further, it appears that the luminal surface of the

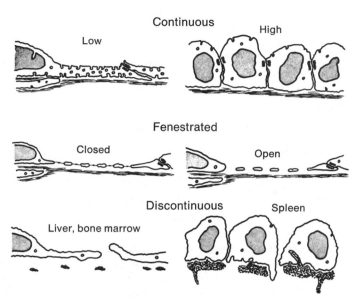

Fig. 8-2. Schematic illustration of the different types of capillaries. (From Majno, 1965. By permission.)

endothelium is normally covered by a very thin coating of the same material, continuous with the intercellular substance. Functional studies, however, have clearly established that the continuous capillaries behave as porous membranes, as will be discussed below: even the effective diameter and density of these pores have been estimated by means of functional studies (see Landis and Pappenheimer, 1963; Crone *et al.*, 1970). Morphological evidence for such pores in the intercellular substance has only recently come to hand. The principal arrangement of the wall in a muscle capillary is shown in Fig. 8-3.

These recent ultrastructural studies of the continuous capillaries of muscle clearly reveal the existence of *intercellular* pore-like channels (Fig. 8-4) which in their narrowest sections have a width of some 40 to 45Å and can be visualized along their entire course with the aid of the tracer peroxidase, administered via the blood (Karnovsky, 1967, 1970). They may occupy up to some 20% of the narrow seams between the endothelial cells. In the cerebral capillaries, on the other hand, there appear to be no intercellular pores since tracers of even fairly low molecular weight do not pass across the junctions between the endothelial cells (Brightman, 1970; see also Chapter 24).

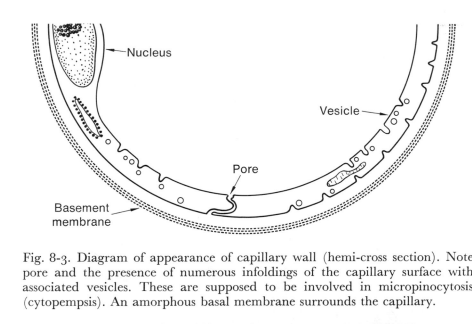

Fig. 8-3. Diagram of appearance of capillary wall (hemi-cross section). Note pore and the presence of numerous infoldings of the capillary surface with associated vesicles. These are supposed to be involved in micropinocytosis (cytopempsis). An amorphous basal membrane surrounds the capillary.

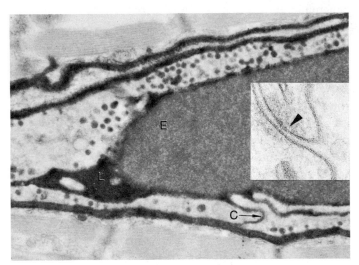

Fig. 8-4. Capillary in heart of mouse sacrificed 10 min after peroxidase injection. Peroxidase is present in the capillary lumen (L) around erythrocyte (E) and also stains the intercellular cleft (C) throughout its length from lumen to basal lamina, which is also stained. Micropinocytotic vesicles stained with peroxidase are seen throughout the endothelial cytoplasm. × 32,000. Insert shows endothelial intercellular junction with a slit of about 40 Å between unit membranes (at arrow). × 150,000. (Courtesy of Dr. M. J. Karnovsky, Harvard Medical School.)

On the outer surface of the endothelial cells there is a basement membrane 200 to 600Å thick, consisting of delicate fibrillary elements embedded in an amorphous, mucopolysaccharide matrix. This basement membrane does not significantly hinder transport. It provides a "rigid jacket" for the wall, being especially thick in capillaries exposed to high transmural pressure, such as those of the glomeruli.

The basement lamina may split to surround an occasional third component of the wall—the pericyte, or Rouget cell (up to 200 μ long, 0.5 μ thick). The pericyte is probably one form of histiocyte and there is no firm evidence either of its contracting or of its contributing to wall permeability.

Fenestrated Capillaries

These occur in the renal glomeruli, in glands, in the ciliary body, in the choroid plexus, and in the intestinal mucosa. They are prominent features of "countercurrent capillary systems" such as those of the vasa recta of the renal medulla and the intestinal villi.

Their endothelial cells show numerous *intracellular* fenestrations (less than 0.1 μ diameter) which may either be open or closed by a very delicate diaphragm. The "functional" dimensions of these openings are, however, probably not very much larger than those of the intercellular pores of continuous capillaries (see below), since "leakage" of proteins is only moderate. Fenestrated capillaries permit exchange of solvent and solutes which is both rapid and large, as exemplified by the exchange in the renal glomeruli. In glomerular capillaries the intracellular fenestrations are 200 to 250Å wide and occupy some 30% of the endothelial wall area. Functional data (Landis and Pappenheimer, 1963) suggest, however, that glomerular capillaries have an effective pore radius of only 45 to 50Å and a combined pore area of 5% of that of the total surface (see Chapter 27). The basement membrane of glomerular capillaries is 3000Å thick—appreciably more than elsewhere. Perhaps this thickness is related to the glomerular intraluminal pressure, which, at 70 mm Hg, is higher than that in any other capillaries.

Discontinuous ("Intercellularly Fenestrated") Capillaries ("Sinusoids")

These possess an endothelial layer with obvious intercellular gaps. Bone marrow, liver, spleen are characterised by this type of capillary, which seems adapted for the transmural exchange, not only of macromolecules, but even of blood cells. Thus, a blood transfusion can be administered via a cannula inserted into the bone marrow. Basement membranes and pericytes are sparse or absent.

Transcapillary Exchange

Three different types of transport are responsible for transmural exchange: filtration-absorption, diffusion, and micropinocytosis (or cytopempsis).

Filtration-Absorption

The Starling Hypothesis

The forces concerned in exchange (Fig. 8-5) are the hydrostatic pressure difference across the wall of the capillary, which favours filtration $(P_c - P_{if})$, and the colloid-osmotic pressure difference $(\pi_{pl} - \pi_{if})$ which favours absorption (Starling, 1896). If filtration and absorption are balanced in any organ, conditions are "isovolumetric" or "isogravimetric", and a "Starling equilibrium" exists. The state of this balance determines the partition of fluid between the vascular bed and the interstitial space and

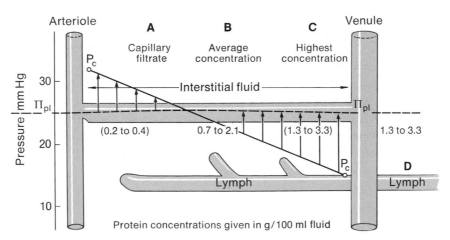

Fig. 8-5. Schematic illustration of the filtration-reabsorption events in an "average" muscle capillary. (From Landis and Pappenheimer, 1963. By permission.)

is therefore of utmost importance for maintaining a constant blood volume and hence cardiovascular homeostasis. It was not until Landis (1930) measured P_c directly that much headway was made in investigating Starling's hypothesis, and the development of modern microtechniques has greatly facilitated detailed studies (e.g. Wiederhielm, 1967).

In man there is a systemic blood flow of 8000 to 9000 litres per day. Only about 20 litres of this fluid is filtered from the capillaries in 24 hours (except for the 170 litres filtered across the glomeruli). Considering the huge capillary surface area (Chapter 5), this small figure illustrates how comparatively constant the capillary pressure level must be kept in the normal individual. Of these 20 litres filtered, 16 to 18 litres are reabsorbed in the distal ends of the capillaries and the remainder returns to the blood via the lymphatic system (Fig. 8-6; see also Chapter 9). The lymphatics, however, return the great bulk of protein, 100 to 200 g, which escapes from the bloodstream per day.

Capillary Pressure Level

Landis showed that the pressure at the arteriolar end of the capillary loop in the human finger held at heart level was about 30 mm Hg and at the venous end of the loop it was 10 to 15 mm Hg. Hence, mean capillary pressure (P_c) has until recently been taken as 20 to 25 mm Hg. However, the mean "effective" hydrostatic pressure in the "exchange" vessels of many tissues may be considerably lower, perhaps as low as 15 mm Hg in the resting situation. The recent viewpoint considers the immediately postcapillary segment of the venules to be part of the "capillary exchange tubes" as pores seem to be abundant here (Chapter 5). Such venular segments do, however, manifest an inevitably lower hydrostatic pressure than that in the capillaries proper, and hence the *mean* hydrostatic pressure of the capillary exchange tubes is correspondingly diminished. The capillary pressure is particularly low in the pulmonary circuit (about 10 mm Hg) and in the liver (6 to 7 mm Hg). The glomerular capillaries, subserving ultrafiltration, form the other extreme (70 mm Hg). Clearly, if the colloid osmotic pressure difference is similar to the mean capillary pressure, the arteriolar end of the capillary loop would lose fluid, whereas the venous end of the capillary would be the site of reabsorption (Fig. 8-5).

P_c is not constant, even in any one tissue, for it depends on the state of tone of the resistance vessels, rising when the tone is lowered, as is seen in muscle capillaries during exercise, or falling when precapillary tone is

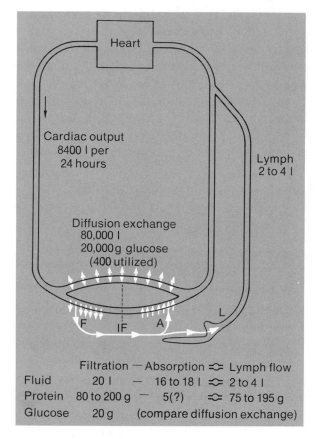

Fig. 8-6. Schematic illustration of the approximate magnitude of cardiac output, diffusion exchange, filtration-absorption exchange, and lymph flow in man during 24 hrs. (From Landis and Pappenheimer, 1963. By permission.)

increased, as is seen in neurogenic arteriolar constriction in skeletal muscles following haemorrhage.

Generally speaking then, for any one tissue, P_c is determined by the ratio between the precapillary resistance (ra) and the postcapillary resistance (rv).

$$P_c = \frac{P_a\left(\dfrac{rv}{ra}\right) + P_v}{1 + \left(\dfrac{rv}{ra}\right)}$$

where P_a and P_v are the central arterial and venous pressures, respectively (Chapter 6).

Interstitial Fluid Pressure Level

P_{if} does not vary much in most tissues, and until recently was thought to be slightly above atmospheric pressure throughout. However, recent studies suggest that P_{if} is normally slightly *subatmospheric* in many tissues (Guyton, 1965). It would be difficult to explain the existence of a subatmospheric tissue fluid pressure, at the known colloid-osmotic pressure differences, were mean capillary pressure as high as it was earlier assumed to be. The kidney, however, enclosed as it is by a fibrous capsule, has a tissue fluid pressure as high as 10 mm Hg. The bone marrow, possessing discontinuous capillaries and enclosed in a rigid box, has a tissue fluid pressure virtually identical with that in the sinusoids.

Standing obviously increases P_c in the feet, for instance, but it does not cause a primary increase of P_{if} except where dense fascia surrounding the tissue and its vessels transmits the increased pressure in the distended veins to the interstitial spaces. In such circumstances the situation approximates that of truly encapsulated organs, such as the brain and, to a lesser extent, the abdominal viscera. Such organs "float" in rigid or semi-rigid fluid compartments and alterations of their position relative to heart level cause almost equal changes in both P_c and P_{if} so that the over-all transmural pressure is little affected.

Plasma Colloid Osmotic Pressure

Plasma contains 300 milliOsmoles/litre of crystalloids. As each 1000 mOsm/l exerts an osmotic pressure of 22.4 atmospheres the total osmotic pressure of plasma is about 6.7 atmospheres. The crystalloids can and do pass back and forth across the capillary wall with great ease, so that they do not contribute to the *effective* osmotic pressure across the wall in a steady state. This effective osmotic pressure results from the plasma proteins, which constitute 7 g/100 ml of plasma and exert an osmotic pressure of about 25 mm Hg (π_{pl}). Of this osmotic pressure 65 to 80% is due to albumin which not only exceeds the globulins in concentration (A/G generally about 1.8), but which possesses a molecular weight of only 70,000 compared with those of the globulins, most of which range from 100,000 to 450,000. It is the number of molecules of solute which is osmotically important. Thus, 1 g albumin in 100 ml exerts an osmotic effect equivalent to 6 mm Hg, whereas the same concentration of globulin gives an osmotic pressure of only 1.5 mm Hg.

The colloid osmotic pressure is not as simply proportional to the concentration of the dissolved protein macromolecules as would be expected from van't Hoff's law. Donnan equilibrium requirements and protein-protein interactions complicate the situation (see Landis and Pappenheimer, 1963). At a total plasma protein concentration of 7 g/100 ml, the colloid osmotic pressure is 25 mm Hg, which is as high as if all the protein content had been made up by an ideal solute of molecular weight 37,000 instead of the actual ones which average a molecular weight of say 80,000 to 100,000. If this deviation from van't Hoff's predictions had not occurred we would require a 12% plasma protein content to yield an osmotic pressure of 25 mm Hg—with a correspondingly higher viscosity and flow resistance.

Interstitial Colloid Osmotic Pressure

Interstitial fluid contains some protein, but never as much as plasma does. Protein in the interstitial fluid exerts a colloid osmotic pressure (π_{if}) in proportion to its concentration and this differs in the various regions. Thus, skeletal muscle has an interstitial fluid protein concentration 10 to 30% of that in the plasma; the intestine shows 40 to 60% and the liver 80% of the protein content of plasma.

The Filtration Process

The hydrodynamic flow, or pore-restricted filtration, essentially obeys Poiseuille's law, providing that the radius of solvent and solute particles is less than 1/20th of that of the pores. Assuming the pores to be cylindrical, effective pore radius has been calculated to be 35 to 45Å; but it is perhaps more likely that they are like *slits*, in which case their width would be about 45 to 55Å (see Landis and Pappenheimer, 1963; Crone *et al.*, 1970). In fenestrated capillaries the pore radii are presumably somewhat higher, though not much, as proteins do not pass freely. The increased permeability of such capillaries may be due mainly to the presence of a greater number of pores per unit area.

The plasma proteins in most capillaries are too big to pass the capillary filters in large amounts, and the protein content of the filtrate is as low as 0.3% in "continuous" capillaries. Hence, proteins exert an effective intravascular osmotic pressure, which tends to counteract the filtration process.

However, there is no doubt that a small amount of protein does traverse the capillary wall during filtration, and to this small amount is added that provided by a very slow transcapillary *diffusion* of protein into the interstitial space. Furthermore, the *relative* concentrations of the various proteins in interstitial fluid are not very different from those in plasma. This may seem surprising—it would seem more probable that molecular sieving in the narrow pores would restrict the transfer of globulins more than that of the smaller albumin molecules. Experimental evidence (Grotte, 1956) suggests, however, that most of the protein transfer which occurs in continuous capillaries takes place through a few "large pores" or "capillary leaks" of considerable dimensions (see below), which are predominantly situated in the venular segments immediately adjacent to the capillaries.

These various mechanisms of protein transport into the interstitium, coupled with the fluid absorption in the distal part of the capillary, results in an interstitial colloid osmotic pressure which cannot be ignored. π_{if} offsets the full effect of the intravascular colloid osmotic pressure. In tissues characterized by continuous capillaries, the π_{if} is low, as mentioned above, whereas the interstitium of tissues with fenestrated capillaries may manifest 50% of the plasma-protein concentration. In tissues with discontinuous capillaries π_{if} approximates that of the plasma.

Bradykinin, kallidin and histamine, locally released, increase capillary permeability reversibly, perhaps widening the venular "leaks"—and probably also the "regular" pores—hence flavouring the loss of protein from the blood (such effects are additional to their vasodilator properties). Kallidin is responsible for the hyperaemia of activated salivary glands, which furnishes the bulk volume needed for salivary secretion. Histamine and bradykinin may contribute to inflammatory oedema and to the increased protein content of the interstitial fluid in such circumstances (see Chapter 16).

Although the protein concentration in the interstitial fluid is not as high as in the plasma the total interstitial fluid volume is 3 to 4 times greater than that of the plasma. Therefore the total interstitial protein bulk, which is slowly circulating back to the blood via the lymphatics, is not dissimilar to that of the plasma. As these proteins serve as substrates for specific enzyme reactions and as hormone carriers, and also take part in immunological reactions, this slow transcapillary exchange of protein is a most important characteristic of capillary function and, indeed, not an "unfortunate leakage".

The Absorption Process

As the protein concentration in the capillaries exceeds that outside, interstitial fluid is absorbed at the latter end of the capillary, where $P_c - P_{if}$ is now below $\pi_{pl} - \pi_{if}$. Such absorption occurs by essentially pore-restricted hydrodynamic inflow, which again obeys Poiseuille's law. Proteins cannot be reabsorbed by the capillaries, except possibly by cytopempsis (see below). Far and away the main route of return of protein to the blood is via the lymphatics.

Interaction Between Filtration and Absorption

Capillary ultrafiltration entails a slight concentration of the plasma proteins in systemic capillaries. In the renal glomeruli, where 20% of the plasma is filtered, this concentration of the proteins is considerable. Plasma colloid osmotic pressure rises more than one might predict from the increase of protein concentration, owing to the deviation of conditions from those calculated from van't Hoff's law. This is usually of trivial significance in any tissue other than that of the kidney, where the rise in plasma colloid osmotic pressure is marked. There the colloid osmotic pressure, instead of rising by 20%, actually rises by 40%, to some 35 mm Hg, and this favours subsequent reabsorption of fluid from the nephric tubules.

A primary change of any of the four pressure parameters of the Starling equilibrium secondary shifts the others and this automatically counters the change. Thus, if P_c increases, P_{if} tends to rise and π_{if} falls because of the dilution of the interstitial protein concentration. Meanwhile π_{pl} rises because of the fluid lost and also because of the deviation from van't Hoff's law. Therefore $\pi_{pl} - \pi_{if}$ will be greater than predicted for conditions in a simple solution.

Measurements of the Filtration-Absorption State

Filtration and absorption quantitatively depend (1) on the size of the pressure forces, (2) on the permeability of the individual capillary, and (3) on the size of the capillary surface area perfused, which varies according to the state of precapillary sphincter activity. If the precapillary sphincter closes, the corresponding capillary content becomes stagnant and local exchange rapidly ceases until flow is re-established.

The regional *capillary filtration coefficient* (CFC) gives a measure of capillary permeability *and* perfused area available for diffusion under the experimental circumstances. CFC—the "hydrodynamic conductivity" of the capillary walls—is measured in ml/mm Hg/min/100 g tissue by record-ing the increase of volume or weight of an organ or limb that is caused by a known increase of P_c.

CFC varies from tissue to tissue. The density of the capillaries and the size and number of the capillary pores per unit wall area, together with the conditions of precapillary sphincter activity, all affect CFC.

If P_c is raised from a value which had previously secured isovolumetric conditions, by say 3 mm Hg, then in a tissue whose CFC is 0.01 there would be a net filtration of 0.03 ml/min per 100 g of tissue. If, on the other hand, CFC is doubled to 0.02 by the relaxation of some of the precapillary sphincters, but at the same time P_c is decreased 3 mm from an earlier isovolumetric state, there would be an absorption of 0.06 ml/min/100 g tissue.

An increase of CFC due to greater capillary permeability cannot be differentiated from one which is due to the opening of more capillaries by CFC measurements alone. However, an increased leakage of proteins will occur in the first case but not in the second, and this may help to distin-guish between them.

Oedema

Oedema is an excess of fluid in the interstitial spaces. Its causes are obvious from what has been discussed above. They may be: hydrostatic, hypoproteinaemic, inflammatory, or lymphatic obstruction.

Hydrostatic oedema may be local or general. In the main the raised P_c is brought about by a rise in venous pressure, as occurs in congestive heart failure, or locally distal to a venous thrombosis. The tendency is for such oedema to have a gravitational distribution (the ankles in ambulant subjects, the buttocks and back in recumbent individuals). It is more prone to occur in lax tissues (vulva, scrotum, dorsal side of the feet, etc.). This type of oedema is characterized by a low protein content.

Hypoproteinaemia oedema usually occurs whenever plasma protein con-centration falls below a critical level of some 5 g/100 ml. Starvation and nephrosis furnish examples of this type of oedema. Such oedema fluid again has a low protein content.

Inflammatory oedema results from an increased capillary permeability caused by inflammatory agents. More protein passes through the capillary wall and this reduces the forces of absorption. The oedema fluid is protein-rich. However, an important factor in establishing inflammatory oedema is simply the osmotic transfer of water. Tissue damage usually implies an increased production of solutes by breakdown of larger aggregates, which raises local osmotic pressure and causes a rapid hydrodynamic water transfer from the blood (Arturson and Mellander, 1964).

Lymphoedema forms another type of protein-rich fluid accumulation, which is in this case caused by an obstruction of the lymphatic vessels (cancer, operations for cancer, filariasis). As proteins drain only by the lymphatics such oedema fluid is characteristically protein-rich.

In oedematous tissues the accumulation of interstitial fluid implies, among other things, an increased distance for diffusion between blood and tissue cells. Supposing oedema doubles the volume of a cutaneous section, where the interstitial space normally accounts for 15% of the total tissue volume. If all the extra fluid is contained within the interstitial space, this must have increased its volume eightfold. The increase of the mean diffusion distance is then at least twofold, which is disadvantageous for cell nutrition.

Diffusion

Free Diffusion

Diffusion is all-important in tissue nutrition. Thermodynamic random movement of all molecules and ions tends to disperse them evenly in any available space. Whenever a concentration difference is created these random movements cause a net transport towards the lower concentration, which persists until equilibrium is restored.

Adolf Fick (1855) formulated the law which governs the free diffusion of uncharged soluble particles.

$$dn/dt = DA(dc/dx)$$

At any given temperature the amount of substance transported, n, per unit time t, is equal to the product of the free diffusion constant, D, the transverse section area available, A, and the concentration gradient (that is, the concentration difference per unit distance), dc/dx.

Each substance has a characteristic diffusion constant, the numerical value of which also depends on the medium, for the diffusion proclivity of the substance is inversely proportional to the molecular radius of the solute and to the viscosity of the medium (providing that the diffusing solute particles are large in comparison with the solvent molecules).

Diffusion Across Capillary Membranes

In considering the diffusion across a capillary wall it is evident that the wall itself provides a hindrance compared with the circumstances prevailing in free diffusion in a monophase solvent compartment. There are two alternatives: passage through the entire wall, and pore-bound passage.

In the first alternative, solute diffusion is nevertheless relatively "free", the solute traversing the endothelial cells themselves, which is the case with lipid-soluble substances, such as CO_2 and O_2. Also water molecules pass, even though more slowly, through the endothelial cells, as indeed through cell membranes generally.

In the second alternative, the case of water-soluble substances, which cannot themselves pass the endothelial cell membranes and can therefore only traverse the pores, diffusion through these pores is still relatively free if the pore radius is large compared with that of the solute particles. Suppose this is the case and that the total pore area is 0.1% of that of the total capillary wall surface (e.g. in muscle capillaries). Then A in the Fick formula approximates 0.1% of the total membrane surface and the "free" diffusion constant for the substance can be used without there being a significant error. However, the total surface area available for such diffusion is, of course, far smaller than that available for lipid-soluble substances. For such reasons lipid-soluble oxygen passes perhaps several hundred times more easily through the capillary walls than do pore-bound molecules of equal size.

Restricted, Pore-bound Diffusion

If pore radius and particle radius become more sensibly equal, free diffusion through pores gives place to *restricted diffusion*. Then the Fick formula is best modified by replacing the "free diffusion constant" with a "restricted diffusion coefficient". Two factors seem to be important in these circumstances: (a) a steric hindrance is created at the entrance, for it seems that passage of the solute through the pore will occur only if a randomly moving solute particle does not collide with the pore edge; and (b) once the solute particle has entered the pore, friction between the particle and the pore channel wall restricts passage through the channel.

In Pappenheimer's original work on capillary transfer mechanisms (see Pappenheimer, 1953, Landis and Pappenheimer, 1963) the functional estimates of the pore radius in continuous capillaries give a figure of some

35 to 45Å, assuming that the pores are cylindrical. However, for several reasons it seems more likely that the pores are like *slits*, in which case the "effective" slit width has been calculated to be some 45 to 55Å. The diffusion of molecules of different sizes was studied and measurements of their restricted diffusion yielded data which, together with other experimental results, were used to estimate both the effective pore radius (slit width) and the combined pore area. Also the pore density was calculated from these results (see Landis and Pappenheimer, 1963). On the whole, these figures based on physiological data agree very well with the recent structural findings by Karnovsky (1967), mentioned earlier. "Pore-bound" diffusion becomes gradually more restricted as molecular size increases. Thus, while glucose (radius 3.5Å) is only slightly restricted and inulin (radius 12Å) moderately so, the "restricted diffusion coefficient" for macromolecules such as haemoglobin and albumin (30 to 35Å) is only 5% or less of the free diffusion constant.

Differences in the free diffusion constant of various molecules and the influence of restricted diffusion help to account for the rapid accumulation of interstitial fluid which occurs in tissue activity or injury. The interstitial and intracellular accumulation of a large number of pore-bound solute particles, which cannot diffuse as rapidly as water, causes an osmotic force which leads to a rapid hydrodynamic pore-bound egress of water from the blood. Similarly, hypertonic solutions, injected intra-arterially, "suck" water from swollen tissues; this property led to their use in alleviating cerebral oedema.

These processes are indeed exceedingly complex because of the unique permeability characteristics of the capillary wall, which in important respects are quite different from those of artificial membranes. As the dimensions of the capillary pores are, relatively speaking, fairly large, the fraction of water transferred by hydrodynamic, pore-bound flow is far larger than that transferred by pore-bound net diffusion, their ratio increasing with the second power of the pore radius (see Landis and Pappenheimer, 1963). However, water has another route available; it also seems to diffuse readily across the endothelial cells proper (Yudilevich and Alvarez, 1967), presumably via numerous but narrow membrane "channels". These "channels" might allow for a substantial transfer of water by means of net diffusion when osmotic gradients are present. However, in this situation they would hardly allow any substantial hydrodynamic flow, simply because they apparently are so narrow (no solutes pass) that the relationship to the second power of the radius here greatly favours the diffusion transfer.

Thus, the surface area available for solvent transfer in capillaries seems to be decidedly larger than that for solute transfer, except for lipid-soluble substances. For this reason the "osmotic reflection coefficient", σ, used to modify van't Hoff's law in deductions of osmotic pressure differences across "leaky" membranes (see Landis and Pappenheimer, 1963), is probably close to unity for water-soluble substances when passing capillary walls:

$$\sigma = 1 - \frac{D'_s}{D'_w}$$

where D'_s and D'_w are the restricted diffusion coefficients for the test solute and for water, respectively. For lipid-soluble substances, on the other hand, σ may even be negative, as such substances are often less restricted than water in their passage through capillary walls. When Pappenheimer's studies were performed neither the passage of water through the endothelial cells nor the influence of σ was known, but happily their impact on deductions of pore size, etc., tends to cancel out. There seems to be little doubt that the general concepts based on his admirable work stand firm; it was a breakthrough concerning our understanding of capillary events.

Capillary "Leaks"

In addition to the greatly restricted diffusion of macromolecules through the ordinary pores of the capillary wall, it has been postulated that "large pores" or capillary "leaks" (200 to 250Å radius) provide an additional and easier passage for such molecules. Molecules of 100Å or more can escape from the normal capillaries and there is evidence that they do so via the large pores. Such large pores or "leaks" constitute only 1/30,000 of the total pore population in continuous capillaries, but fenestrated capillaries, and, particularly, discontinuous capillaries, appear to possess them in greater abundance (Grotte, 1956). In the continuous capillaries they are mostly found in the immediately postcapillary venules.

The bulk of the protein that enters the interstitial fluid does so through these large pores. To call them "leaks" is inappropriate, as the term suggests a defect of the capillary wall and disguises their true physiological role, which is the transfer of the functionally important macromolecules (such as immunological proteins) from blood to tissues. The diffusion processes, and cytopempsis, are schematized in Fig. 8-7.

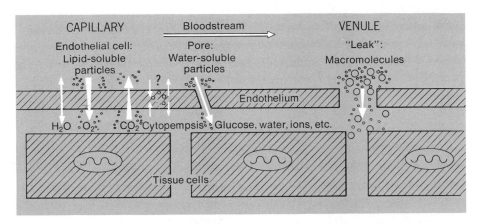

Fig. 8-7. Schematic drawing illustrating the diffusion of lipid-soluble particles (O_2, CO_2) through the entire capillary wall, of water-soluble particles (glucose, ions, etc.) through the pores and "leaks" only, while water itself will to some extent diffuse also across the membranes of the endothelial cells. Macromolecules are mainly confined for their diffusion passage through "leaks" and other wide-bore pores. Whether cytopempsis involves true transcapillary passage, and, if so, what is transported, is not known.

Transinterstitial Diffusion

So far we have discussed only transcapillary diffusion occurring over a distance of less than 1 micron. However, the interstitial space, of complex design and often of greater width, is additionally interposed between the blood and the tissue cells. The interstitial space has a sol-gel ultrastructure and may add a substantial hindrance to diffusion, at least when distances are also considered. Thus, considerable differences may exist between the concentration of some solutes in the venous effluent and in the interstitial fluid even when capillary flow distribution is adequate and uniform. Increased filtration-absorption can considerably improve diffusion exchange and this may reflect a decrease of a "transinterstitial resistance" to diffusion, possibly by a convection influence of the enhanced streaming of fluid in microcanaliculi of the interstitium, aiding solute distribution (Lundgren and Mellander, 1967). This supposed stirring of the contents on the "tissue side" of the capillary walls may have a counterpart on the "blood side", by means of the bolus passage of the erythrocytes, which seems to cause stirring of the plasma columns passing along the capillary. It seems to be increasingly obvious that stirring of the contents close to a membrane greatly aids in the transfer across the membrane (see Crone *et al.*, 1970). It is possible, therefore, that even normal filtration-absorption events in capillaries, greatly enhanced in most states of functional hyperaemia, may constitute a stirring effect of importance for nutritional exchange.

Consequences of Uneven Capillary Perfusion

The commonest cause of substantial concentration differences between solutes in interstitial fluid and solutes in venous blood is simply uneven distribution of capillary flow. In resting tissues the inherently rhythmic alterations of precapillary sphincter tone tend to create such a situation which may be greatly aggravated by excessive neurogenic vasoconstriction which features haemorrhagic hypotension. Such a situation is further exacerbated by rheological disturbances due to aggregation of blood cells with capillary plugging. Some of the tissue cells may thus receive scant perfusion while others may be over-perfused (so-called "functional shunting"). Over-all vasodilatation usually abolishes "functional shunting" but does not eliminate the *true shunting* of blood through A-V anastomoses. "Functional shunting" has often been taken as evidence indicating the presence of true A-V anastomoses, but such specific vascular structures are found in few tissues other than the skin (where they are of great importance in thermoregulation).

Quantitative Aspects

In continuous capillaries, pores occupy only 0.1% of the total capillary surface area—if pore length is considered to be 1 micron. Actually, as the "effective" pore length is probably well below 1 micron as an average, the area occupied by the pores may be even smaller than 0.1%. In any case, skeletal muscle with a total capillary surface area of 7000 cm^2/100 g at maximal vasodilatation would then have a total pore area of 7 cm^2 at most. At first sight it would appear that this small area, divided into numerous narrow passages, would greatly limit diffusion exchange.

However, the capacity for pore-bound diffusion is indeed enormous, as is exemplified in glucose transfer. Heavy aerobic exercise (1500 kilopond metre/minute at an efficiency of 20%) would require 4 g glucose per minute (0.2 mg/sec/100 g of muscle) were it to be covered by blood-borne glucose alone (which it is *not*).

In the Fick formula $A = 7$ cm^2 and the "restricted diffusion coefficient" for glucose is 0.9×10^{-5}/cm^2/sec (Landis and Pappenheimer, 1963). Assuming a pore length of 0.5 micron, a blood-tissue concentration difference for glucose of $\overline{X}$ mg/ml, required for a glucose transfer of 0.2 mg/100 g muscle/sec, can be calculated:

$$0.2 = 0.9 \times 10^{-5} \times 7 \times \frac{\overline{X}}{0.5 \times 10^{-4}}$$

$$\overline{X} = 0.16 \text{ mg/ml}$$

Thus, with an arterial glucose concentration of 100 mg/100 ml, even if the interstitial glucose concentration were as high as 84 mg/100 ml there would still be an adequate transcapillary gradient for the net diffusion transfer of enough glucose to satisfy the entire metabolic demands of skeletal muscles in maximal aerobic activity. Fortunately, however, the muscle cells take up blood glucose quite slowly because their membranes —*not* the capillaries—constitute a considerable hindrance to what otherwise would be a dangerous depletion of the blood glucose concentration, particularly for the brain. Active muscle in fact uses only minor amounts of blood glucose, relying instead on its stores of glycogen and on blood-borne fatty acids.

This theoretical example nevertheless illustrates the capacity of pore-bound diffusion even of molecules of respectable size. Maximal muscle blood flow is about 50 ml/min/100 g with a glucose concentration of 100 mg/100 ml, and hence brings 50 mg of glucose to each 100 g of muscle/min. If the interstitial glucose concentration were to reach zero in muscle, a maximal transcapillary glucose gradient of 1 mg/ml would be established, allowing at this maximal vasodilatation a diffusion transfer exceeding 60 mg/min, i.e. more than can be delivered by the bloodstream. At rest, muscle blood flow is only some 3 ml/min/100 g and the perfused capillary surface area is perhaps 1/3 of maximum. Hence, 20 mg/min glucose *could* diffuse across, but the delivery by the blood is only 3 mg/min. Thus at rest the capacity for transcapillary glucose diffusion is some seven times that of the blood glucose delivery. Molecules smaller than glucose molecules escape even more easily, for their diffusion capacity is larger for a given concentration gradient.

Some tissues—still with "continuous" capillary beds—have an even greater capillary density and therefore a greater diffusion capacity. The total capillary surface area of the myocardium probably exceeds 40,000 cm²/100 g and its maximal flow capacity is 300 to 400 ml/100 g/min (see Chapter 23). If the pore/total surface area ratio is still only 0.1%, the total pore area would be at least 40 cm²/100 g.

Tissues with *fenestrated* capillaries exhibit a potentially greater diffusion transfer, having more and usually somewhat larger pores per unit surface area, and hence allow for a greater transfer of macromolecules also. Further, such tissues are usually characterized by a denser capillary network than those which possess continuous capillaries, and this density further benefits diffusion. Organs that secrete or absorb a large bulk of water and solutes (gastrointestinal glands) or that allow a rapid transference of macromolecules (endocrine organs) are characterised by fenestrated capillaries. *Discontinuous* capillaries are a conspicuous feature of the bone marrow, the liver, and the spleen—organs in which even cells may cross freely between the blood and the interstitium.

Functional Estimates of the Diffusion Surface

Transcapillary diffusion transfer can be calculated if the available surface area, the diffusion coefficient, and the concentration gradient are known. Similarly, the surface area available for diffusion of a given tracer substance could be calculated if the concentration gradient and the transfer rate were known, but unfortunately the concentration gradient cannot usually be determined exactly. Lately a compromise has been reached.

The diffusion transfer of ^{86}Rb (radioactive rubidium)—a pore-restricted ion handled by the tissues in the same way as potassium—has been used for this purpose (Renkin, 1959). Its transport across cell membranes is not a significant rate-limiting factor and the intracellular space acts as an effective "sink", providing that the arterial concentration of ^{86}Rb is low and the extracapillary concentration can be regarded as zero. It should be stressed, however, that the latter assumption is probably an oversimplification in most situations, because of the significant hindrance to diffusion offered by the interstitial space per se.

The clearance of any substance from blood (see Chapter 7) is given by the formula

$$\text{Clearance} = Q \times E \qquad (1)$$

where Q is the blood flow and E is the extraction from the blood by the tissues.

$$E = \frac{A - V}{A} \quad \text{or} \quad V = A - EA \tag{2}$$

Hence
$$\text{Clearance} = Q\frac{A - V}{A}$$

As ^{86}Rb is pore-restricted, its transcapillary diffusion depends on the total pore area exposed to flow, and this area depends on both a capillary permeability factor P (which varies with the size and density of the capillary pores) and on the perfused capillary surface area S (which is determined by the *number* of capillaries open to flow if their lengths and radii are considered equal). P and S cannot be separated by this technique alone, but together they constitute the "PS product", often called the "Capillary Transport Coefficient".

As the diffusion escape of ^{86}Rb from the arterial blood during its capillary passage is described by Fick's law, the "surface area" available for its transfer is PS and the concentration gradient is set by $[C]_b - [C]_{if}$ —the difference between the concentrations of ^{86}Rb in blood and interstitial fluid. $[C]_{if}$ is considered to be virtually zero, which is, as mentioned, not always the case. $[C]_b$ on the other hand, gradually falls during passage of the blood through the tissues as ^{86}Rb diffuses through the pores. The slower this capillary passage the more completely does diffusion transfer reduce $[C]_b$ until the extraction E approaches unity.

From such considerations the following formula can be derived:

$$V = Ae^{-PS/Q} \tag{4} \text{ (Renkin, 1959)}$$

where e is the base of the natural logarithm. As $V = A - EA$ (equation 2),

$$E = 1 - e^{-PS/Q}. \tag{5}$$

If Q (ml/min/100 g tissue) and E are known,

$$PS(\text{ml/min/100 g tissue}) = -Q \ln (1 - E) \tag{6}$$

The blood flow through the denervated vessels of resting muscle is 6 to 10 ml/min/100 g and, with about one-third of the total capillary surface area perfused, PS is 3 to 5. In denervated intestinal vessels, with a flow of 30 to 50 ml/min/100 g, PS is 30 to 50, about ten times greater than that of muscle. As the intestinal mucosa contains fenestrated capillaries, its greater value of *PS* probably reflects not only the greater density of the capillary network but the greater size and density of the pores as well. It is interesting to note that capillary filtration coefficient (CFC) of intestinal vessels is also about ten times that of muscle vessels—presumably for the same reason (Dresel *et al.*, 1966).

"Indicator diffusion methods" are also used; in these, capillary permeability is derived from the time-concentration curves obtained following single injections of molecules to be tested (Chinard *et al.*, 1955). Comparisons of the permeability coefficients for molecules of different sizes, and hence, diffusion constants, may then reveal, for example, the extent of restricted diffusion which they respectively manifest in the capillary

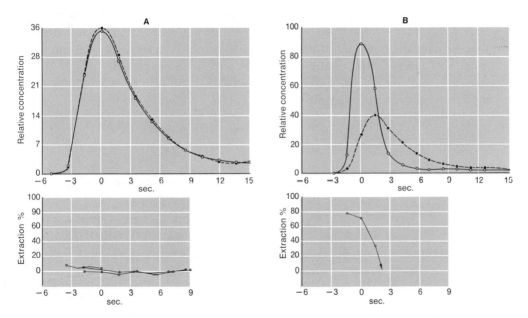

Fig. 8-8. Tissue concentration curves for Evan's blue and inulin in brain (A) and in kidney (B). Evan's blue, which does not leave the vascular bed readily, is only diluted by the blood plasma passing the vascular bed. Hence its dilution curve serves as a "reference" for such substances which pass across the capillaries into the interstitial space (and the tissue cells). Inulin (12 Å) behaves like Evan's blue in the brain thanks to the blood-brain barrier, but passes freely through the glomerular capillaries of the kidney. Note the consequent difference between the two dilution curves in the kidney. (From Crone, 1963. By permission.)

beds studied (Crone, 1963; Fig. 8-8). In recent years considerable progress has been achieved by this type of approach (see Crone *et al.*, 1970).

Cytopempsis or Micropinocytosis

Cytopempsis, in contrast to the passive processes of diffusion and filtration, involves an element of active transport. It is, however, very slow and can hardly be considered to contribute much to the *total* transcapillary exchange. Electron microscope studies reveal "vacuoles" which seem to be in the process of traversing the endothelial cells of the capillary wall (Fig. 8-4). Not only is the direction of the "transport" uncertain—it is not even known whether the "vacuoles" always represent a transport at all—they may only reflect a phagocytosis-like function. Despite these reservations it is possible that cytopempsis may provide an active transport route for macromolecules (such as gamma globulins) which otherwise have limited powers of access to the tissues, mainly by way of the capillary "leaks". It may also provide a route for the transfer of molecules by active expulsion against a concentration gradient—even proteins from the interstitial space might thus be transferred to the blood, though no evidence of any such mechanism exists at present.

References

Arturson, G., and S. Mellander (1964). "Acute changes in capillary filtration and diffusion in experimental burn injury," *Acta Physiol. Scand.* **62,** 457–63.

Brightman, M. W. (1970). "Morphology of the blood-brain barrier including studies with some electron dense larger molecules," in *Alfred Benzon Symposium II on Capillary Permeability*. Copenhagen: Munksgaard Internat. Publ.

Chinard, F. P., G. J. Vosburgh, and T. Enns (1955). "Transcapillary exchange of water and of other substances in certain organs of the dog," *Am. J. Physiol.* **183,** 221–34.

Crone, C. (1963). "The permeability of capillaries in various organs as determined by use of the 'Indicator Diffusion' method," *Acta Physiol. Scand.* **58,** 292–305.

Crone, C., P. Kruhöffer, N. A. Lassen, and H. H. Ussing, eds. (1970). *Alfred Benzon Symposium II on Capillary Permeability*. Copenhagen: Munksgaard Internat. Publ.

Dresel, P., B. Folkow, and I. Wallentin (1966). "Rubidium[86] clearance during neurogenic redistribution of intestinal blood flow," *Acta Physiol. Scand.* **67,** 173–84.

Fick, A. (1855). "Über Diffusion," *Ann. Physik.* **94,** 59–86.

Grotte, G. (1956). "Passage of dextran molecules across the blood-lymph barrier," *Acta Chir. Scand.* **211,** Suppl., 1–84.

Guyton, A. C. (1965). "Interstitial fluid pressure: II Pressure-volume curves of interstitial space," *Circ. Res.* **16,** 452–60.

Illig, L. (1961). *Die terminale Strombahn*. Berlin: Springer.

Karnovsky, M. J. (1967). "The ultrastructural basis of capillary permeability studied with peroxidase as a tracer," *J. Cell. Biol.* **35,** 213–36.

Karnovsky, M. J. (1970). "Morphology of capillaries with special regard to muscle capillaries," in *Alfred Benzon Symposium II on Capillary Permeability*. Copenhagen: Munksgaard Internat. Publ.

Landis, E. M. (1930). "The capillary blood pressure in mammalian mesentery as determined by the microinjection method," *Am. J. Physiol.* **93,** 353–62.

Landis, E. M., and J. R. Pappenheimer (1963). "Exchange of substances through the capillary walls," *Handbook of Physiology*, 2, Circulation **II,** 961–1034.

Lundgren, O., and S. Mellander (1967). "Augmentation of tissue-blood transfer of solutes by transcapillary filtration and absorption," *Acta Physiol. Scand.* **70,** 26–41.

Majno, G. (1965). "Ultrastructure of the vascular membrane," *Handbook of Physiology*, 2, Circulation **III,** 2293–375.

Nicoll, P. A., and R. L. Webb (1946). "Blood circulation in the subcutaneous tissue of the living bat's wing," *Ann. N. Y. Acad. Sci.* **46,** 697–711.

Pappenheimer, J. R. (1953). "Passage of molecules through capillary walls," *Physiol. Rev.* **33,** 387–423.

Renkin, E. M. (1959). "Transport of potassium[42] from blood to tissue in isolated mammalian skeletal muscles, "*Am. J. Physiol.*, **197,** 1205–10.

Rhodin, J. (1967). "The ultrastructure of mammalian arterioles and pre-capillary sphincters," *J. Ultrastructure Res.* **18,** 181–223.

Starling, E. H. (1896). "On the absorption of fluids from the connective tissue spaces," *J. Physiol.* 312–26. (London.)

Wiedemann, M. P. (1963). "Patterns of the arteriovenous pathways," *Handbook of Physiology*, 2, Circulation, **II,** 891–933.

Wiederhielm, C. A. (1967). "Analysis of small vessel function," in *Proc. conf. on physical bases of circulatory transport: regulation and exchange*, ed. by E. B. Reeve and A. C. Guyton, pp. 313–26. Philadelphia: W. B. Saunders.

Yudilevich, D., and O. A. Alvarez (1967). "Water, sodium and thiourea transcapillary diffusion in the dog heart," *Am. J. Physiol.* **213,** 308–14.

Zweifach, B. W. (1961). *Functional behaviour of the microcirculation*. Springfield, Ill.: Charles C Thomas.

9

The Lymphatic System

General Organization

Aselli (1627) first noted the lacteals in the mesentery of a well-fed dog, and later in that of a criminal, executed presumably after a hearty breakfast. Bartholin (1651) and Rudbeck (1653) independently used the term *lymphatic* and discovered the nature of the lymph system.

The lymphatic system is well developed only in homeotherms, and phylogenetically the lymph vessels are modified veins. Histologically the lymphatic capillaries are "closed-ended" endothelial tubes, but they are highly permeable to macromolecules and even to particles (see below). The lymphatic capillaries are otherwise fairly similar to the vascular capillaries, and they are distributed among the tissue cells in the same way as are the vascular capillaries.

The lymphatic capillaries coalesce into larger vessels and myogenically active smooth muscles begin to appear in the walls of these vessels. Gradually the elastic and muscle components increase and the smooth muscles display an adrenergic innervation. Another characteristic feature of the lymphatics is their endothelial valves, monocuspid or biscuspid, which permit flow only towards their drainage into the central veins (see Mayerson, 1963; Rusznyak *et al.*, 1967).

Lymph glands are interposed in the course of the larger lymphatics. On reaching the glands the lymph vessels subdivide into smaller channels which, entering the gland, open into the sinuses of the lymph node. Fine vessels drain these sinuses and, becoming confluent, re-form larger trunks. The lymph nodes, which have a rich blood supply (Lundgren and Wallentin, 1964), contain phagocytic cells which attack and destroy foreign material conveyed to them by the lymph. They also manufacture lympho-cytes and plasma cells and produce antibodies. The lymph nodes form powerful defence stations against invading bacteria.

The two great terminal channels—the right and left thoracic ducts—empty into the right and left subclavian veins, respectively, at their junction with the jugular veins. With a daily lymph flow of 2 to 4 litres and with lymphatic dimensions that are not markedly smaller than those of the vascular system, it follows that the flow of lymph is extremely slow.

Functional Significance

Protein Transport

Some 75 to 200 g of protein return via the lymph channels to the blood-stream in 24 hours, and this protein is contained in 2 to 4 litres of lymph. Both the fluid and the protein of lymph are derived from the vascular bed as a result of filtration and diffusion across the capillaries (Chapter 8). The tissue fluid protein is an important constituent of the normal cell environment, and is thus in slow but continuous circulation from the blood and back to the blood via the lymphatics.

When labelled protein is injected intravenously, the radioactivity of lymph increases and its specific activity (the ratio of labelled and natural protein concentrations) equals that of the plasma within 12 hours. Further samples show a slow and equal decline in activity in the lymph and plasma. Some 20 litres of fluid, with a protein content varying from less than 0.3% (muscle) to about 5 to 6% (liver), escape from the vascular compartment in 24 hours, but, whereas 16 to 18 litres of this fluid is reabsorbed to the blood capillaries, it is doubtful whether any significant fraction of the protein is taken back into the bloodstream directly (Chapter 8).

In most tissue regions, therefore, the lymph is more protein-rich than is the tissue fluid immediately surrounding the capillaries. Moreover, the protein concentration found in lymph varies according to the region or organ. At rest, lymph from the leg contains about 15 to 20% of the protein in plasma. The protein concentration is considerably decreased in exercise due to increased ultrafiltration and osmotic fluid transfer (see Chapter 22). These dilute the proteins, for they mainly permeate the vascular capillaries by slow diffusion.

Lymph from the GI tract usually contains 40 to 50% of the plasma protein concentration, while liver lymph shows the highest percentage, some 85% of that of the plasma. As the liver sinusoids pose little hindrance to macromolecular transfer, and as the liver is the main progenitor of the plasma proteins, this high figure is not surprising. Lymph contains all the proteins present in plasma (Chapter 8); thus it contains fibrinogen and prothrombin and will clot on standing.

The great majority of the protein which has escaped from the vascular capillary walls must be returned by the lymph system to the bloodstream. Blockade of, or serious leakage from, the *main* lymphatic stems is incompatible with life, as the colloid osmotic pressure difference between blood and tissue fluid becomes vanishingly small. Blockage of *regional* lymphatic vessels, draining a limb for instance, causes a brawny oedema with fibroblastic organization due to the failure of the system to remove protein—and, to a less extent, fluid.

Lipid Transport

The intestinal lymphatic carries some 60% of the lipid, mainly long-chain fatty acids, absorbed from the intestine following digestion. Alpha and beta lipoproteins and chylomicrons are found in the lymph.

Enzymes

Certain enzymes are carried from their cells of origin by the lymph to the blood. These include amylase, alkaline phosphatase, and histaminase.

Rate of Lymph Flow

Resting Conditions

The rate of lymph flow, measured in resting patients with fistulae in their left thoracic duct, is 0.5 to 1 ml/min. This would give some 1 to 2 litres/24 hours; the right duct delivers a smaller volume, as it drains a smaller part of the body.

About half of the total lymph flow is derived from the GI tract and liver. The pressures in the lymphatic system vary from 3 to 5 cm H_2O in peripheral trunks to near zero in the thoracic duct. However, considerable phasic changes in pressure naturally occur with movements, which compress the ducts and displace their contents. Sympathetic activity causes a transient increase in lymph flow by decreasing the capacity of the lymphatic vessels.

Venous Obstruction

Venous obstruction markedly increases lymph flow, as Landis (1946) found in man. The capillary pressure rises as a result of venous obstruction, and capillary filtration rate increases correspondingly. A venous pressure of 60 to 70 mm Hg may increase lymph flow tenfold.

Vasodilatation

Vasodilatation, as in muscle exercise, increases both the capillary filtering surface and the filtration pressure. Hyperosmolarity in the activated muscles contributes to the fluid transfer, and lymph flow increases greatly, especially because the rhythmic movements enhance the flow (Chapter 22).

Increased Capillary Permeability

Increased capillary permeability, as caused by locally released histamin, kinins, bacterial toxins and foreign proteins, etc., increase lymph flow. This is due to an increased filtration, to the reduced colloid osmotic pressure difference and, in a tissue lesion, to an osmotic fluid transfer as well.

Glandular Secretion

Glandular secretion is usually accompanied by a marked increase in lymph flow. In salivary glands kallidin is released, increasing the capillary pressure and capillary surface area by means of its vasodilator action, and increasing capillary permeability, as well, by means of its action on the capillary pores. The combined result is a huge transfer of fluid, partly used for secretion production, partly emerging as an increased lymph flow (Chapter 26).

Permeability of the Lymphatic Capillaries

The lymphatic capillaries are characterised by a high permeability for substances which enter them. Thus graphite particles, red cells, lymphocytes, chylomicrons and macromolecules can be shown to enter the capillaries, but such particles fail to *escape* from the lymphatics. The retrograde injection of graphite suspensions into the lymphatics causes no loss of the particles until the pressure is sufficient to rupture the vessels. Mayerson (1963) investigated the situation in two ways: (a) by cannulating a leg lymphatic, infusing substances of different molecular weights, and analyzing samples of thoracic duct and plasma; and (b) by isolating and catheterizing the afferent and efferent vessels of the popliteal node and infusing and collecting test substances.

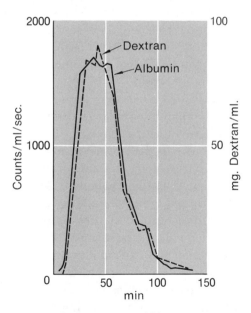

Fig. 9-1. Concentration of dextran and ^{131}I albumin in lymph and plasma. Dextran and ^{131}I albumin infused centrally into leg lymphatic of anaesthetized dog at zero time at 0.5 ml/min. Both infusions stopped after 50 min. and 0.9% saline infusion started at same rate for the next 100 min. (From Mayerson, 1963. By permission.)

In the first group of experiments radioactive iodinated albumin was infused centrally into the leg lymphatic and a typical pattern of appearance of the tagged molecule in the thoracic duct lymph developed (Fig. 9-1). Within ten minutes radioactive material appeared in the thoracic duct lymph. The concentration rose abruptly to reach a plateau which was maintained for the 50 minutes of albumin infusion and for the 10 minutes of a subsequent saline infusion. The radioactivity then sharply declined, and it fell to zero after 150 minutes. Plasma radioactivity rose to a maximum (which was less than 0.1% of that in the thoracic lymph) in 60 to 90 minutes and remained at this level for the rest of the experiment. Dextran behaved similarly. Clearly, there is no loss of these high-molecular-weight substances from the lymphatic system except at the point of egress represented by the thoracic duct. All macromolecules of M.W. 6000 or higher behaved in this fashion.

On the other hand, small molecules like urea, glucose, ions, etc. are freely permeable, so that the lymph is largely in equilibrium with the surrounding tissue fluid in these respects. A dextran molecule of M.W. 2300 also left the lymphatic vessels to gain access to the tissue fluid like the small molecules. The limit of permeability "inside and out" thus lies somewhere between the molecular weights of 2300 and 6000. The isolated lymph node experiments gave similar results.

Additional studies have suggested that large particles and molecules gain easy access to the lymphatic capillaries through wide gaps between the cells, and perhaps by cytopempsis as well. The relative contribution provided by these two routes to the inflow of such particles is at present unknown. The failure of large molecules and particulate matter to leave the lymphatic appears to be easily explained. Mayerson suggests that although the smallest terminal lymph capillaries are freely permeable to such molecules in either direction, the larger walls are not. Compression of the lymphatic capillaries will, of course, force their contents in all directions but the easiest direction is centripetally into the larger vessels. The valves in such vessels prevent backflow and thus there is no longer any chance of escape of the macromolecules.

To sum up, the lymphatic system plays an important role in the regulation of blood volume. The amount of lymph returning by the thoracic ducts in 24 hours is approximately equal to the plasma volume. Of great significance is the return of protein to the blood via the lymph channels, for there is no other route of consequence for such a return of plasma proteins which have escaped from the blood capillaries. The whole of the protein content of the plasma is returned by the lymph vessels every 24 hours.

References

Asselli, G. (1627). "In lactibus sive lacteis venis, quarto vasorum mesaraicorum genere, novo invento." *Dissertatio*. Milan: Biddellium Mediolani.

Bartholin, T. (1651). *Anatomia, ex Caspari Bartholini parentis Institutionibus, omnium recentiorum, et propries observationibus tertium ad sanguis circulationem reformata*. Leyden: Hack.

Landis, E. M. (1946). "Capillary permeability and the factors affecting the composition of capillary filtrate," *Ann. N. Y. Acad. Sci.* **46,** 713–31.

Lundgren, O., and I. Wallentin (1964). "Local chemical and nervous control of consecutive vascular sections in the mesenteric lymph nodes of the cat," *Angiologica*, **I,** 284–96.

Mayerson, H. S. (1963). "The physiologic importance of lymph," *Handbook of Physiology*, 2, Circulation **II,** 1035–74.

Rudbeck, O. (1653). *Nova exercitatio anatomica, exhibens ductus hepaticus aquosus, et vasa glandulorum serosa*. Uppsala.

Rusznyák, I., M. Földi, and G. Szabó (1967). *Lymphatics and lymph circulation*. Oxford: Pergamon.

10

Veins and Venous Return

General Organization of Systemic Veins

From the capillaries the blood passes via venules to successively larger veins and thence back to the heart. The venules first display connective tissue elements which envelop the endothelial tubes; muscular elements later appear in the walls as the vessels grow bigger. Further junctions of these venules form veins of 0.3 to 1 mm diameter, and it is in vessels of this size, particularly in those of the limbs, that valves first appear as intimal folds. These valves permit the flow of blood only in the direction of the heart. In man they are more prominent in the veins of the leg than in those of the arm and are found both in the deep and superficial venous systems of the leg. They also abound in the communicating vessels between the superficial and deep leg vessels and permit the flow of blood from the superficial to the deep veins. The femoral vein possesses three valves, one at the inguinal end, one just below the mouth of the profunda junction, and one at its lower end. Some veins (venae cavae, hepatic, portal, pulmonary, cerebral, and superficial veins of head and neck) either have no valves or display only small intimal folds which are often functionally incompetent.

While the transverse section area of the venules and small veins is far larger than that of their arterial counterparts (Chapter 5), the big regional veins are more similar in size to the corresponding arteries. However, their walls are much thinner than those of the arteries, containing much less of elastic tissue and muscle (see Fig. 5-5; page 47). For these reasons—and because their transmural pressure is usually often quite low —the veins collapse easily and in doing so their cross-sectional profile alters from one nearly circular to one which is elliptical. This change of geometrical configuration is of considerable importance in both venous capacitance and venous resistance to flow. A number of recent reviews cover most aspects of venous function (Gauer and Thron, 1962; Alexander, 1963; Guyton, 1963; Folkow and Mellander, 1964).

Pressure-volume Characteristics

In supine man, when the right atrial pressure is near zero, the pressure in the systemic venules is about 15 mm Hg. As the venous return is equal to the cardiac output in a steady state, it follows that the resistance offered by the veins to the flow of blood is very low, only some 15% of that on the arterial side of the systemic circulation. Considerable changes of blood flow can and do occur in the intact circulation without there being significant changes in either peripheral or central venous pressure, which indicates that capacitance is the main function of the venous bed and its contribution to *total* resistance is of little relevance. Its flow resistance is of importance mainly because it is the denominator in the pre/postcapillary resistance ratio (see Folkow and Mellander, 1964). The adjustments of this ratio, again, indirectly serve mainly a *capacitance* function, for they help to determine the fluid distribution between blood and interstitial fluid (Chapter 8).

As has been stated, veins may show the profile of a flattened ellipse or that of a circle, depending on the transmural pressure. Clearly, as a venous segment with a circular profile changes to one of increasingly elliptical profile but of the same circumference, flow resistance increases and capacitance decreases because the cross-sectional area of the ellipse is smaller. Most veins appear to exhibit this change when their transmural pressure falls below 6 to 9 cm H_2O, which accounts for the steep part of the pressure-volume curve for veins; their true distensibility is usually quite limited (see Fig. 5-10, page 54).

These marked increases in venous volume for moderate increases in transmural pressure create one of the major problems in cardiovascular regulation in man. The erect position puts the greater part of the venous capacitance section below the heart level and the raised transmural pressure changes the veins from semicollapse to distension. This situation is strikingly different from that in most animals, where the great majority of the venous capacitance compartment is placed at, or even above, heart level (Fig. 10-1). As Amberson (1943) put it: "When man's subhuman ancestors dared to rise and walk upon their hind legs, they essayed a physiological experiment of no mean difficulty". If blood circulated in a system of *rigid* tubes mere changes of posture would offer no problem, for in assuming the upright position the hydrostatic pressure effect on the arterial and venous sides would be identical and no luminal changes could occur.

It follows that the characteristic tendency of the thin-walled veins—to collapse when the transmural pressure falls, and to become circular and to distend when this pressure rises—completely alters the results from those which can be predicted in a rigid tube system. Thus, the veins below the

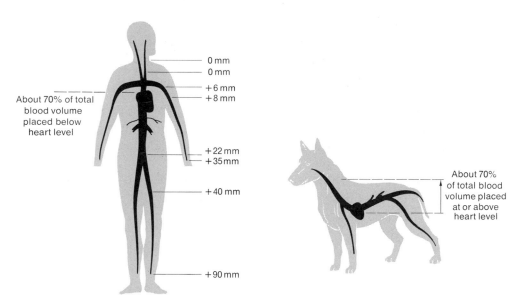

Fig. 10-1. Schematic illustration of the location of the venous blood volume in relation to the heart in man as compared with most animals, including even giraffes. The only animals equivalent to man's situation in the erect position would be the charging bear or gorilla, or the giant kangaroo standing at attention.

level of the heart increase their volume during quiet standing by some 500 ml, or even more when the cutaneous veins are dilated. It is this which may cause dizziness and even fainting in circumstances when standing is prolonged, particularly when thermal stress has already induced reflex cutaneous vasodilatation. The failure of venous return in such situations has therefore nothing whatsoever to do with "the blood having to go uphill"; the problem is the raised *transmural* pressure, the consequent venous distension, and blood pooling.

Flow and Volume in Dependent Veins

When a man stands *quietly*, the "zero" effective pressure level is in his right atrium. If a vein on the dorsum of his foot is connected to a manometer via an intravenous needle the hydrostatic level registered is 85 to 100 mm Hg. The mean arterial blood pressure in the foot is likewise 85 to 100 mm Hg above that registered at heart level. Thus, the pressure head responsible for pushing the blood round is unaltered, for each pressure increases by the same amount. The only difference is that the pressure of blood in the patent capillaries of the foot is also increased by 85 to 100 mm Hg, and this greatly increases the transcapillary filtration pressure and favours transudation of fluid. It would cause considerable swelling of the feet if there were not efficient compensatory mechanisms (see Chapter 16).

Therefore, if the limbs are kept *motionless* the presence of valves in the limb veins does not prevent the full hydrostatic effect of the continuous column of blood between heart and foot from being exerted. However, even slight movements exert external pressure on the veins and their content is then pushed towards the heart because the valves hinder backflow. This reduces the pressure in the muscle veins just after the compression until they are again filled from the capillaries and from the superficial veins via communicating veins, which are also provided with valves permitting only unidirectional flow. The more frequent and powerful the movements are, such as in walking, the more efficient this venous "pumping" (see Fig. 6-3, page 62). As Greenfield (1962) has pointed out, drainage of blood from superficial to deep veins ceases to be an apparent anomaly when it is remembered that the *mean* pressure in the heart ventricles greatly exceeds that in the veins and atria from which they receive their inflow.

Pollack and Wood (1949) measured the venous pressure in a vein of the dorsum of the foot and showed that even one step lowered the pressure by 50%, whereupon it returned to the initial level of 90 mm Hg at a rate which was determined by the blood flow through the leg. Repetitive movements, such as walking, could lower the venous pressure in the foot to approximately 30 to 40 mm Hg, providing that the successive steps occurred before the venous columns in the thighs and calves were refilled (Fig. 10-2).

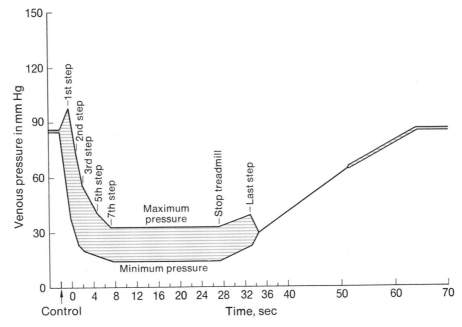

Fig. 10-2. Average changes (10 subjects) in venous pressure at ankle, produced by walking. (From Pollack and Wood, 1949. By permission.)

Thus the lowering of the venous pressure in dependent tissues by movements aids the filling of the heart, lowers the high capillary pressure in these tissues, and can enhance their effective perfusion pressure. On the other hand, the last factor is of relevance only when exercise is intense enough to be accompanied by maximal vasodilatation; otherwise flow is as effectively adjusted to the current needs by changes in flow resistance and changes in perfusion pressure are then not necessary.

However, another problem arises in heavy rhythmic exercise where maximal dilatation already prevails so that flow can only be further increased *if* the effective perfusion pressure is raised. In this situation we may question whether the contraction phases empty the veins enough to accommodate the huge inflow which occurs during the relaxation phases, without there being an immediate resumption of the high venous pressure seen in the motionless, dependent leg. This is in fact a most complex haemodynamic situation, in which the outcome is dependent on the balance between the high rate of inflow during the relaxation phase, the

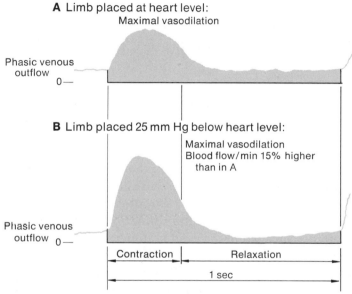

Fig. 10-3. Actual recordings of phasic venous outflow from calf muscles in the cat during heavy rhythmic exercise (0.25 sec at 60 imp./sec and 0.75 sec relaxation) with the vessels maximally dilated. Arterial pressure 100.
A. Limb at heart level. Flow during exercise 85% of that during a brief cessation of the exercise, as the contractions impede the inflow.
B. Limb placed *below* heart level (25 mm Hg), everything else remaining the same including the pressure head when *no* contractions are performed. Flow during exercise now *equal* to that during a brief cessation of the exercise, and about 15% larger than that during exercise in A. Thus, the 25% addition of transmural pressure has evidently been transformed into 60% of effective pressure head (15 out of 25) due to the muscle pump in this state of maximal flow and work. (From Folkow et al., 1969. By permission.)

duration of this phase, and the venous capacitance during this phase, which again depends on the extent and duration of the venous compression during the contraction phase. Recent studies—utilizing the cat's lower limb as a model, with phases of contraction-relaxation similar to those of rapid running or cycling in man and later confirmed in man (Fig. 10-3)— show that even during maximal dilatation, some 60% may be added to the effective perfusion pressure in the rhythmically contracting calf muscles of man (Folkow et al., 1970, 1971). This implies, of course, a marked gain in blood supply to the leg muscles during heavy rhythmic exercise, such as running, skiing, bicycling. In fact, even with the leg at heart level some increase of effective perfusion pressure may be gained. The reason is that venous pressure in this situation of marked precapillary dilatation is perhaps doubled compared with that at rest, due to the changed profile of pressure drop along the circuit (see Fig. 6-1, page 58).

Hydrostatic Effects in Other Venous Compartments

Cerebral Vessels

The cerebral vessels of course show intraluminal pressure changes on tilting, and these are the opposite of those already considered. Both arterial and venous pressures drop by as much as 35 to 45 mm Hg in the upright position, but so does cerebrospinal fluid pressure. As the veins and cerebrospinal fluid are enclosed in the rigid cranium, their pressures therefore change together, so that the transmural pressure remains about the same. The cerebral venous pressure, however, is considerably subatmospheric in this position and the transmural pressure approaches zero in the larger intracranial veins. These, the venous sinuses, are held open by surrounding tissues, but when the veins emerge from the skull they tend to collapse because they are no longer supported.

On the other hand, as long as the volume of the cerebrospinal fluid remains unaltered, the venous plexuses of the cranium and spinal cord and the intervertebral veins serve as an incollapsible communication system for venous return, and the venous flow from the brain is therefore little affected by gravitational forces per se. However, if, during an intracranial operation, a venous sinus is inadvertently punctured, then air may be sucked into the sinus causing a serious air embolism, which may be fatal.

Abdominal Vessels

In the abdomen, venous distension in the erect position is minimized by the increase in intra-abdominal pressure, which occurs on tilting the subject into the head-up position. Measurements of the intra-abdominal pressure at the level of the iliac fossa show that the hydrostatic pressure approximates that which would be produced if the abdomen were filled with fluid. The abdominal organs have a specific gravity similar to that of blood. The pressure in the abdominal veins exceeds the intra-abdominal pressure measured at the same level by only 5 to 10 cm H_2O, whatever the position of the body. Even when the individual voluntarily raises his intra-abdominal pressure, such as when straining at stool, although the pressure in the abdominal veins greatly increases, the blood cannot pass backward into the legs because retrograde flow is prevented by the iliac and femoral valves.

Thoracic Veins

In the thorax the extramural pressure is usually subatmospheric, owing to the tendency of the elastic lungs to collapse. This subatmospheric extravascular pressure of course increases the transmural pressure in the veins entering the thorax, so that they become distended relative to the extrathoracic veins. A "waterfall" phenomenon tends to occur just where the veins enter the thorax, with intermittent collapse of the extrathoracic

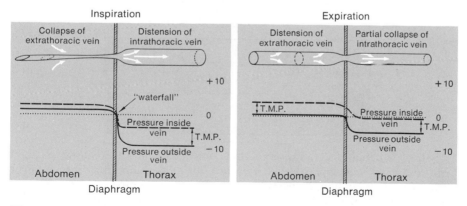

Fig. 10-4. Schematic illustration of transmural pressures (TMP) and venous configuration outside and inside the thorax during inspiration and expiration.

segments during inspiration (Fig. 10-4). The *intravascular* venous pressure inside the thorax is often slightly below atmospheric pressure and this favours the pressure difference between the periphery and the right atrium, thus assisting venous return. Intrathoracic pressure in quiet breathing varies between 5 cm H_2O subatmospheric in expiration and 10 cm H_2O subatmospheric in inspiration. As the intrathoracic pressure falls in inspiration the intra-abdominal pressure rises and the increase in pressure gradient facilitates venous return to the thorax. Conversely, expiration reduces the onward flow of blood from the abdomen to the thorax.

This means that there is an inrush of blood into the right heart during inspiration and a consequent increase of right ventricular stroke volume, because of the Frank–Starling relationship (Chapter 12). However, as the capacitance of the pulmonary circuit increases during inspiration, venous return to the *left* ventricle nevertheless decreases somewhat during the inspiratory phase and so does left ventricular stroke volume. During expiration, when venous return to the right ventricle falls, that to the left

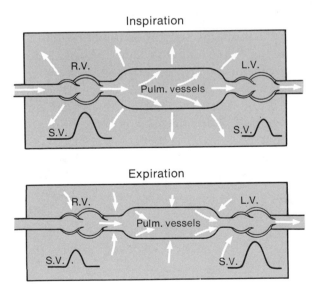

Fig. 10-5. Schematic illustration of how *inspiration* increases filling of right heart and right ventricular stroke volume, but at the same time increases the capacity of the pulmonary vascular bed; hence the filling of the left heart decreases and so does left ventricular stroke volume. At *expiration* the process is reversed: right ventricular stroke volume decreases while that of the left ventricle increases.

ventricle increases phasically, because of the reduced blood content in the recoiling lungs. In this phase, therefore, the right ventricular stroke volume declines while that of the left ventricle increases. Thus, the stroke volumes of the two ventricles are regularly "out of phase" with each other in the course of the respiratory cycle, due to the opposite effects of the respiratory movements on their respective venous returns (Fig. 10-5).

Moreover, venous return to the heart, although mainly dependent on the *forward push* of the force from behind (*vis a tergo*)—provided intially by the heart and transmitted in the form of a positive pressure across the capillaries—can nevertheless be assisted phasically by a *suction force* (*vis a fronte*), exerted by the contraction of the ventricle. Brecher (1956) has produced cogent evidence of ventricular suction, showing that subatmospheric or "negative" pressures may be recorded in the ventricle when the A-V orifice is temporarily clamped. Bloom (1956) excised a rat heart and

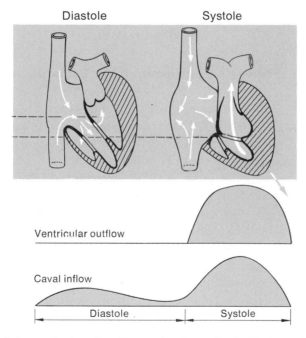

Fig. 10-6. Schematic drawing illustrating how the ballistic action of the blood ejection pushes the ventricles downward during their systole. This distends the atria so that blood rushes into them from the veins, in phase with the ventricular ejection.

immersed it, still beating, in a beaker of saline. With each systole fluid spurted from the aortic stump and with each diastole a flap of the atrial wall was sucked into the mitral orifice. The heart moved around the fluid in a jet-propelled manner. The hydrostatic pressure was the same inside and outside the heart, so the energy for filling the ventricle was provided by the *"elastic recoil"* accompanying ventricular relaxation. These effects of the *vis a fronte* are most manifest when a small heart beats quickly and strongly.

Other factors, perhaps still more important, aid in filling the atria during ventricular systole. As the ventricular systole, by the ballistic action of the blood ejection, pushes the ventricles downwards, they exert traction on the atria so that they elongate (Fig. 10-6). This causes an abrupt fall in atrial pressure (Chapter 6) and blood rushes in from the veins to fill the atria just before ventricular relaxation leads to opening of the A-V valves. These factors, creating a *vis a fronte*, assist in promoting venous return. But the *vis a tergo* is always more important.

Neurogenic Compensatory Mechanisms

The reduction of venous return because of pooling when the subject is in the erect position is partly offset by reflex sympathetic venoconstriction (Chapters 17, 18). However, active venoconstriction is really efficient in decreasing venous blood content only when the veins are well filled and distended, as occurs in the erect position. Even strong contractions of venous smooth muscle, exert only feeble effects on venous content if the transmural pressure is low enough to render the veins semicollapsed. Venoconstriction may then even *increase* the local venous capacity slightly, by stiffening the wall and thereby making the lumen more rounded and larger, even though the *circumference* is decreased. For decades such complications have contributed to the confusion that has existed concerning venous control; with due precautions however, "active" and "passive" changes in venous content may be distinguished and measured separately (Fig. 10-7).

The increase of efferent sympathetic discharge which accompanies an assumption of the erect posture is partly due to a lowering of the mean pressure in the carotid sinuses and partly to effects on the other mechanoreceptors in heart and aortic arch. In an erect man, the carotid mechano-receptors are some 30 cm above the level of the heart, so their intraluminal mean pressure drops from 100 to perhaps 75 mm Hg as compared with a man in the horizontal position. The afferent discharge of the mechano-receptors diminishes, as does their inhibitory effect on vasomotor discharge, and sympathetic constriction of both arterioles and veins results (Chapters 17, 18). The mean arterial blood pressure is thus better sustained and the normal subject so tilted experiences only a momentary dizziness and usually does not faint. Cardiac output measurements show

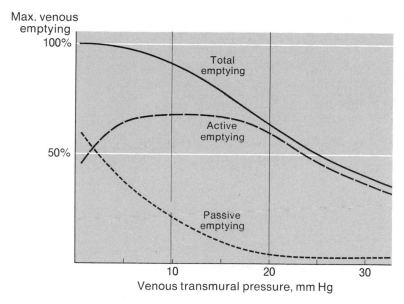

Fig. 10-7. Relationship between active and passive emptying of the venous vascular compartment of the cat's limb as a result of standardized vaso-constrictor fibre stimulation and at various levels of venous transmural pressures. Note that passive factors (venous collapse) dominate if the transmural pressure is initially low, because the upstream constriction produces a further fall in capillary and venous pressures. At pressures at which the veins are kept well rounded (above 10 mm Hg), the venous emptying is almost only due to smooth muscle constriction. Also this active response fails gradually at transmural venous pressures above 20 mm Hg, which are abnormally high for cats. This is probably *not* the case in man, where the leg veins are morphologically adjusted for much higher pressures; the same curve in man would thus presumably be much extended towards the right. (Modified from Öberg, 1967. By permission.)

that, in the vertical position, output is only 75 to 80% of that in the horizontal, so—as the arterial mean pressure at heart level is sensibly the same—there must be an increase in peripheral resistance. Some venous pooling in dependent parts does occur so that venous return to the heart is reduced. Nevertheless, the accompanying reflex venoconstriction, which partly offsets this pooling, is of great importance, as can be shown simply by repeating the tilting experiment in a subject who has been given sympatholytic drugs to abolish this neurogenic vasoconstriction. On tilting such a subject, his arterial blood pressure falls drastically and he faints because his cerebral blood flow is reduced. However, if the subject is first fitted with the trousers of a "g-suit" and these are inflated to a pressure of as little as 20 mm Hg, then, on tilting, he does not faint. The pressurized suit minimises venous pooling in the dependent parts.

In aviation or in space flight the g-suit is of fundamental importance. Centrifugal force towards the feet causes blackout, and if the force is 3 to 4 g all subjects faint after half a minute unless a g-suit is fitted and suitably inflated. In this situation, where there is abnormally increased transmural pressure in "dependent" veins, the relatively weak smooth muscle cover of these veins cannot withstand the distension, even when maximally excited via their vasoconstrictor fibres.

References

Alexander, R. S. (1963). "The peripheral venous system," *Handbook of Physiology*, 2, Circulation **II**, 1075–98.

Amberson, W. R. (1943). "Venous return," *Bull. School of Med. Univ. Maryland*, **27**, 127.

Bloom, W. L. (1956). "Diastolic filling of the beating excised heart," *Am. J. Physiol.* **187**, 143–44.

Brecher, G. O. (1956). *Venous return*. London: Grune and Stratton.

Folkow, B., and S. Mellander (1964). "Veins and venous return," *Am. Heart J.* **68**, 397–408.

Folkow, B., P. Gaskell, and B. Waaler (1970). "Blood flow through limb muscles during heavy rhythmic exercise," *Acta Physiol. Scand.* **80**, 61–72.

Folkow, B., U. Haglund, M. Jodal and O. Lundgren (1971). "Blood flow in the calf muscles of man during heavy rhythmic exercise," *Acta Physiol. Scand.* In press.

Gauer, O., and H. L. Thron (1962). "Properties of veins *in vivo*: integrated effects of their smooth muscle," *Physiol. Rev.* **42,** Suppl., 5, 283–303.

Greenfield, A. D. M. (1962). "Physiology of the veins," in *Cardiovascular functions*, ed. by A. A. Luisada. New York: McGraw-Hill.

Guyton, A. C. (1963). "Venous return," *Handbook of Physiology*, 2, Circulation **II,** 1099–1133.

Oberg, B. (1967). "The relationship between active constriction and passive recoil of the veins at various distending pressures," *Acta Physiol. Scand.* **71,** 233–47.

Pollack, A. A., and E. H. Wood (1949). "Venous pressure in the saphenous vein at the ankle in man during exercise and changes in position," *J. Appl. Physiol.* **I,** 649–62.

II

Structural and Functional Characteristics of the Heart

Structure of the Heart

The Muscle Fibre

Light microscopy reveals that the myocardium consists of columns of striated muscle fibres of cylindrical shape, each some 100 μ long and 15 μ broad. The fibres branch and are surrounded by a rich capillary network. Every muscle fibre consists of a surface limiting membrane (sarcolemma) which surrounds numerous longitudinally disposed myofibrils, themselves striated and containing the contractile proteins; sarcoplasmic constituents; mitochondria sarcoplasm; and a centrally placed nucleus. The muscle fibres that initiate the inherent activity of the heart (*"junctional tissue"* or *"pacemaker"* cells) are somewhat thinner than the ordinary fibres. Those which are specialized for the rapid spread of the excitation to the ventricles (*"Purkinje fibres"*) are somewhat larger and broader than the ordinary ones. All these specialized muscle fibres have relatively few myofibrils but a greater content of sarcoplasm and glycogen. They are generously endowed with capillaries and autonomic nerve fibres.

The myofibrils are approximately 1 μ broad and each consists of a series of repeating structures (longitudinally disposed) 1.5 to 2.5 μ long, the *sarcomeres.* The sarcomere is the fundamental unit of structure and contraction. The sarcomere is delineated by two dark lines (1.5 to 2.5 μ apart), the Z lines (Fig. 11-1). Electron microscope studies show that the sarcomere consists of alternate light and dark bands between the Z lines. This appearance, which confirms and extends the studies of light microscopy, is due to the presence of two types of protein myofilaments, as diagrammed in the lower part of the figure.

The central A band (1.5 μ long) contains filaments (10 mμ diameter) of the protein *myosin*. The I bands which flank the A band contain filaments (5 mμ diameter) of the protein *actin*. The actin filaments usually overlap the myosin filaments within the A band. The centre of the A band contains the H zone, which comprises (a) the central M line, a region in

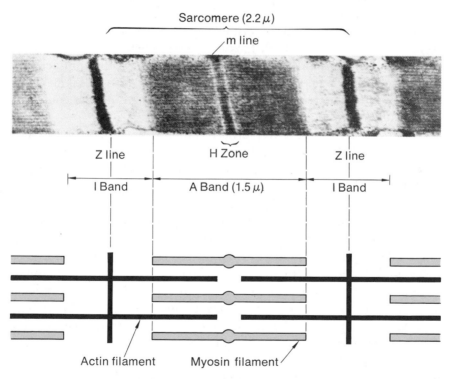

Fig. 11-1. Schematic representation of the filamentous fine structure of the sarcomere (below) in relation to the sarcomere band pattern (above). (From Spiro and Sonnenblick, 1964. By permission.)

which there is a localised thickening of the myosin filaments and, additionally, cross bridges or lateral connections on these filaments; and (b) the L line which represents the termination of the actin filaments of a sarcomeric length of 2.2 μ.

Myosin that is confined to the A band has two important properties: (a) it can split ATP into ADP and inorganic phosphate, i.e. it acts as an adenosinetriphosphatase; and (b) it can combine reversibly with actin to form actomyosin.

Studies on model systems have revealed that muscle contraction is due to the reversible combination of actin and myosin to form actomyosin (with the splitting of ATP to ADP) in the presence of Ca^{++}. H. E. Huxley and J. Hanson (1954) and A. F. Huxley and R. Niedergerke (1954) have independently proposed a sliding filament hypothesis for skeletal muscle contraction. The hypothesis suggests that there is an interaction between the myosin and actin filaments due to the presence of specific force-developing cross bridges formed between them (see A. F. Huxley, 1957; A. F. Huxley and H. E. Huxley, 1964). These cross bridges of the myosin filaments form attachments at specific sites on the thin actin filaments and draw them a short distance. The thick myosin filaments and the thin actin filaments each remain constant in length during contraction (H. E. Huxley, 1964).

The sarcoplasmic reticulum (SR) forms a complex network of anastomosing intracellular tubules that encircles the myofibrils (Fig. 11-2). Part of this network of freely anastomosing membrane-lined tubules is mainly disposed along the myofibrils and has no *direct* continuity with the extracellular space. These tubules are designated the *longitudinal component of SR*. However, there is also a system of sarcoplasmic reticular tubules *transversely* disposed whose components extend into the sarcomeres at the region of the Z line. These tubules represent invaginations of the sarcolemma and *their lumina are in continuity* with the extracellular space. Contiguous (but not continuous) with these transverse tubules at each Z line are the so-called "terminal cisternae" of the longitudinal tubular reticulum. If a section is made along the line of the longitudinal tubules the transverse tubule at each Z line is cut in cross-section and its lumen is seen as a central hole on either side of which terminate the terminal cisternae of the two longitudinal channels. These three structures are known as a *triad* (Fig. 11-2). There is no direct communication between the transverse and longitudinal components in either skeletal or cardiac muscle. H. E. Huxley soaked thin pieces of *skeletal* muscle in solutions containing ferritin for an hour. He then sectioned the muscle and examined it in the electron microscope after fixation. Ferritin was present in the transverse tubular lumina, but *not* in the terminal cisternae.

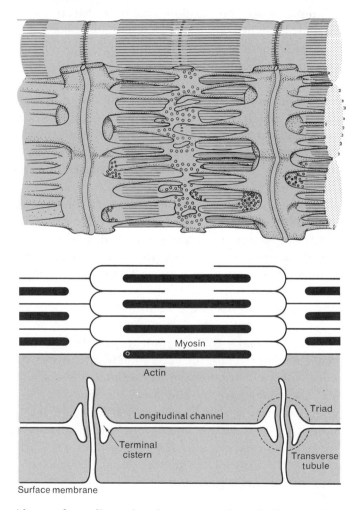

Fig. 11-2. Above: three-dimensional reconstruction of a few myofibrils running from left to right, with endoplasmic reticulum in close contact. Two triads are seen at the upper edge of the picture, each with a central T tubule and two adjacent cisternae. (From Peachey, 1965. By permission.) Below: two-dimensional diagram showing connection between fibre surface and the endoplasmic reticulum. (Modified from Weidmann, 1967. By permission.)

Evidently the transverse tubular system communicates directly with the extracellular space and provides an important pathway for the distribution of substrate material to the myofibril. It is implicated in an even more important role—that of *excitation-contraction coupling*. Depolarization of the sarcolemma causes the development of an electrotonic potential which, conducted along the transverse (T) system, depolarizes the cisternal membranes, causing them to release calcium ions. Calcium diffuses into the myofibrils and activates myosin, which then splits adenosine triphosphate (ATP). The hydrolysis of ATP by myosin yields the energy required for the formation of the actomyosin complex and sequentially for contraction of the muscle. The sarcoplasmic reticulum then takes up Ca^{++} from the solution so that the $[Ca^{++}]$ is lowered below that compatible with interaction between actin and myosin and, hence, the contractile state. Presumably the electrical signal of depolarization temporarily inactivates this uptake ("pumping") mechanism.

Studies made with the light microscope showed that cardiac muscle possesses a branching or syncytial arrangement. This network, however, was additionally characterized by the presence of *intercalated disks* orientated transversely across a bundle of approximately parallel fibres longitudinally disposed. The intercalated disk seen under the electron microscope consists of two apposing cell membranes with an intervening intercellular space. There is no structural continuity of the myocardial fibres across the intercalated disk. The heart muscle is thus not a *structural* syncytium, as was previously thought; but it is important to realize that it *functions* as a syncytium. Thus, the activation of one myocardial fibre by another occurs with ease because the intercalated disks are sites of low impedance, as has been shown by functional studies.

Numerous mitochondria (which occupy some 40% of the myocardial fibre cell volume) subserve the function of converting food substrate energy via oxidative phosphorylation into the synthesis of ATP, the "energy coinage" of the cell. Intracellular inclusions of glycogen and lipid are plentiful in the cardiac cells, providing local stores of substrate.

The Special Junctional and Conduction Tissues

The heart is inherently rhythmic; indeed, the simple cardiac tube formed in the 19th day of foetal life in the human embryo already displays rhythmic contraction (see Chapter 14). If the heart of the amphibian is supplied with Ringer-Locke perfusion fluid it will beat for days outside the body. The mammalian heart is nourished by a coronary circulation, but it too will beat for some hours when removed from the body, if suitably perfused through its coronary circulation. The initiation and propagation of this inherent activity occurs in specialized types of muscle fibres, the *junctional* and *conduction tissues*.

The initiation of the heart beat occurs at the *sino-atrial (S-A) node* in the mammalian heart. The excitation process spreads from here across the wall of the atria to the *atrioventricular (A-V) node*. Thence it is propagated by the *bundle of His* and its ramifications to the subendocardial surface of the ventricles, finally to be conducted throughout the ventricular myocardium (see Scher, 1962), which contracts in response to its arrival (Fig. 11-3).

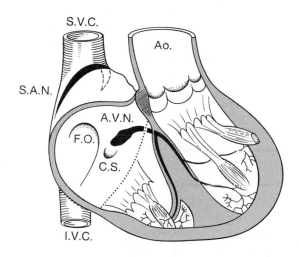

Fig. 11-3. The specialized tissue of the mammalian heart. The pulmonary trunk and part of the right ventricle have been removed. Ao = aorta. AVN = atrio-ventricular node giving origin to the a.v. bundle. Note how the bundle passes beneath the attachment of the tricuspid valve (the septal cusp of which has been removed) and then, after a short course below the membranous part of the interventricular septum, divides straddlewise over the fleshy septum. CS = opening of coronary sinus. FO = fossa ovalis. IVC = inferior vena cava. SAN = sino-atrial node (note its horseshoe shape). SVC = superior vena cava. (Drawn by Professor E. W. Walls. From Keele and Neil, 1965. By permission.)

The sino-atrial node is situated at the junction of the superior vena cava and the free border of the right atrial appendix and extends down along the sulcus terminalis for some 2 cm. It is 2 mm wide and is characterized by elongate plexiformly arranged muscle fibres which are thinner than the usual myocardial cells. It is richly supplied both by nerves and by capillaries. Its vagal innervation is predominantly from the right vagus, for the S-A node is developmentally a right-sided structure. The vagus slows the rate of the impulse generation by the node (see Chapter 12). The post-ganglionic sympathetic fibres also innervate the S-A node. Their influence is the opposite of that of the vagus nerves; the sympathetic fibres quicken the rate of impulse production by the node.

The atrioventricular node is situated at the posterior right border of the inter-atrial septum near the mouth of the coronary sinus. Its histological structure closely resembles that of the S-A node. The A-V node is developed as a left-sided structure from tissue in the vicinity of the entrance of the left great veins which become the coronary sinus. The A-V node receives predominantly left vagal fibres and also enjoys a sympathetic innervation.

The bundle of His passes from the A-V node and runs upward to the posterior margin of the membranous part of the interventricular septum and then courses forward below it, ensheathed and isolated in a canal. At the anterior border of the membranous septum in front of the attachment of the septal cusp of the tricuspid valve to the atrioventricular ring, the bundle divides into left and right branches. The left branch pierces the membrane and then runs along the upper border of the muscular septum to enter the subendocardial space of the left ventricle beneath the union of the anterior and right posterior cusps of the aortic valve. The right division passes down the right side of the septum and forms the so-called *moderator band*. Both branches arborize to form a plexus of subendocardial fibres which in turn distribute terminal fibres throughout the ventricular myocardial wall.

The Cardiac Chambers

The heart contains four chambers—two thinwalled atria separated from each other by an inter-atrial septum and two thicker walled ventricles which have a common wall in the interventricular septum (Fig. 11-4). The bundle of His constitutes the only *muscle* connection between the atria and ventricles, which are joined by a fibrous A-V ring. This ring is penetrated on the right side by the tricuspid valve and on the left by the mitral or bicuspid valve. These atrioventricular valves consist of three triangular flaps on the right side and two on the left side of the heart. The cusps are thick at the valve ring but thin and quite flexible at their free border. They are strong and relatively indistensible. At the free edge of the valve cusps, chordae tendinae are attached, which in turn take their origin from papillary muscles arising from the inner border of the ventricle. When the atrial pressure exceeds that in the ventricle, the valves open, allowing blood to enter the ventricle. When the ventricle contracts, the

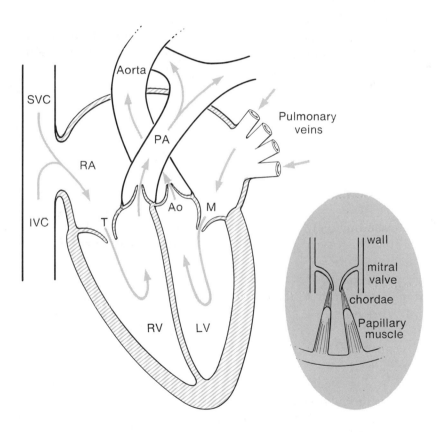

Fig. 11-4. Bloodflow through the heart.

valves close, preventing reflux of blood. The chordae tendinae then act like guy ropes, ensuring that the valves are not inverted.

The semilunar valves, each consisting of three flaps, guard the pulmonary orifice on the right side and the aortic orifice on the left side. These valves open during ventricular ejection and close when the arterial pressure in the relevant vessel exceeds that in its corresponding ventricle. The closure of the atrioventricular valves is accompanied by the first heart sound and the closure of the semilunar valves is accompanied by the second heart sound.

The atria subserve a capacitance function as well as that of contraction. Their thin wall consists of two main muscular systems:—one encircles both atria, and the other, arranged at right angles to this, is independent for each atrium. The excitation process responsible for contraction arises at the S-A node and spreads like the ripples over a pond through the atrial wall to the A-V node at a rate of 1 metre per sec. The contraction of the atrium resembles a peristaltic wave.

The ventricles contain much more muscle, and as might be expected, the left ventricle, which has to do the larger amount of work, is thicker than the right. It is customary to describe four groups of fibres (Fig. 11-5), all arranged spirally:

(a) *Superficial bulbospiral fibres*, arising from the left side of the ventricular-aortic ring and the mitral ring, terminate in the interventricular septum after following a posterior and obliquely downward course.

(b) *Superficial sinospiral fibres*, originating from the back of the tricuspid valve, pass obliquely over the front of the right ventricle to the cardiac apex and thence turn inward to terminate in the anterior papillary muscles of the left ventricle.

(c) *Deep sinospiral fibres* encircle the bases of both ventricles and contribute importantly to the ejection of blood into the arteries.

(d) *Deep bulbospiral fibres* form a thick cuff round the mitral and aortic orifices and are restricted to the left ventricle. They form a "canal" for left ventricular ejection and perhaps contribute to the closure of the mitral valve.

The arrangement of the superficial spiral bundles in particular ensure that on ventricular contraction blood is virtually wrung out of the heart, but it must be clearly understood that the ventricles do not empty themselves completely. After systole there is a residual volume of blood left (end-systolic volume) which varies in amount. When the ventricles con-

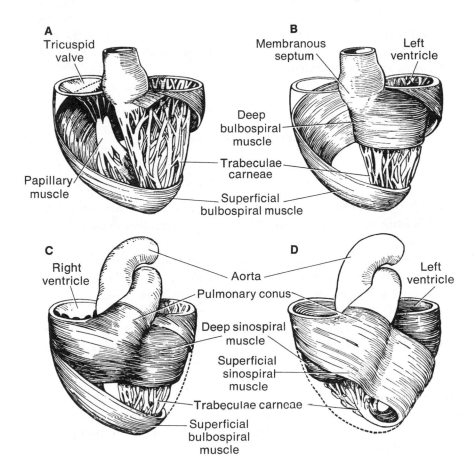

Fig. 11-5. A. The superficial bulbospiral muscle arises principally from the mitral ring and forms the external investment for portions of the left and right ventricles as the bundles spiral towards the apex. Emerging from the vortex on the inside of the chambers, these muscle bundles spiral back toward the valve rings either as trabeculae carneae or as papillary muscles which are joined to the valves through chordae tendinae.

B. The deep bulbospiral muscle encircles the basilar portions of the left ventricle.

C. The deep sinospiral muscle encircles both the right and the left ventricular chambers.

D. The superficial sinospiral muscle is a counterpart of the superficial bulbospiral muscle. The anatomic distinction between the superficial sinospiral and bulbospiral muscles is arbitrary and functionally unimportant. (From Rushmer, 1961. By permission.)

tract, their base (the A-V ring) is pulled downward and the heart rotates to the right so that the apex is pushed forward in closer approximation to the chest wall in the region of the fifth intercostal space, causing the "apex beat", which can be palpated.

Function of the Heart

The Electrocardiogram

Although the electrocardiogram (ECG) is discussed separately (Chapter 13), it is important to correlate it with the mechanical events described below.

The P wave precedes and signals atrial systole and its duration is 0.1 sec approximately. The QRS, which represents the invasion of the ventricle by the excitation process, consists of Q, which is probably associated with the excitation of the upper interventricular septum; R, excitation of the apical septum and apices of the ventricular walls; and S, the excitation of the more basal parts of the ventricle. The QRS complex is complete just *before* the semilunar valves open. The T wave is complete by the time the semilunar valves close (Fig. 11-6A). The P-R interval, lasting 0.13 to 0.16 sec, gives an indication of the conduction velocity from atrium to ventricle, including that in the bundle of His. A P-R interval of >0.2 sec indicates delayed conduction, which usually occurs in the bundle of His or its branches.

Pressure Changes in the Cardiac Chambers and Related Vessels

Using catheters and high fidelity manometers, optical or electrical, the sequence of events in the various chambers that occur during cardiac action can be clarified (Fig. 11-6A).

At the beginning of the cardiac cycle, both atria and ventricles are relaxed and filled with blood by venous return achieved by the *vis a tergo*. Atrium and ventricle on each side are in continuity as the A-V valves are open, and the pressure in each cavity is almost identical. Following the impulse generation of the S-A node, the atrial muscle contracts and P_A rises with P_V following. As P_A is greater than P_V, atrial contraction adds to the diastolic volume of the ventricle, but hardly more than about 15%. The atrial contraction wave (1) lasts about 0.1 sec in a cardiac cycle of 0.8 sec (rate = 75/min). As the wave passes off, the pressure in both atrium and ventricle falls.

The ventricle has meanwhile been invaded by the excitation process which has spread from the S-A node across the atrial muscle to the A-V

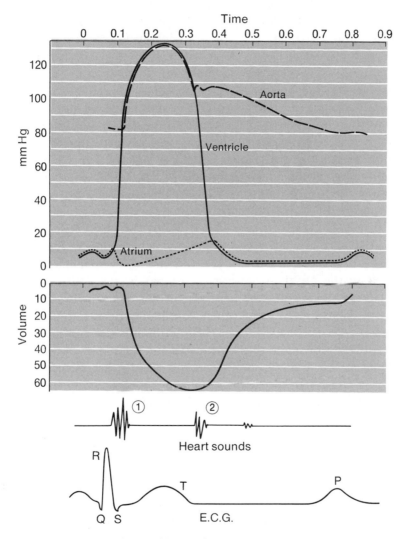

Fig. 11-6A. Events in the cardiac cycle.

node and thence via the bundle of His and the Purkinje tissue. Ventricular contraction begins and P_V immediately exceeds P_A and the A-V valves close (causing the first heart sound). The ventricle is now a closed chamber and the pressure rises promptly during the *"isometric contraction phase"*, which lasts about 0.05 sec. The ventricular pressure then rapidly exceeds that in the artery and the semilunar valve opens.

The *ejection phase* follows, and during this phase the rise of the arterial and ventricular pressures follow each other closely. Initially in this phase ejection is rapid, as evidenced by the ventricular volume tracing, and the arterial pressure rises because blood enters the vessel faster than it can escape via the peripheral arteriolar branches. The summit of the pressure curves is reached when aortic entry and run-off become equal; the pressures subsequently decline as the ventricular contraction begins to subside, while flow from the artery to its peripheral branches continues to be high. The total period of *ventricular systole* is 0.3 sec; when this period ends the ventricular pressure drops sharply. The arterial pressure is better sustained, however, owing to elastic recoil of the vessel wall, and almost immediately the arterial pressure exceeds that in the ventricle, thereby causing closure of the semilunar valve and the sharp second heart sound.

The initial part of ventricular diastole which follows is the *"isometric relaxation phase,"* lasting some 0.08 sec and ending in opening of the A-V valve because the atrial pressure exceeds that in the ventricle. During ventricular systole the atrium has become distended with blood (see Chapter 10). When the A-V valve opens this blood surges into the ventricle for 0.1 to 0.13 sec (*"rapid filling phase"*) although the pressure in both chambers still falls owing to the continued rapid relaxation of the ventricle (see volume curve). Finally, the *"slow filling phase"* (diastasis), which lasts about 0.2 sec, terminates the cardiac cycle. This slow filling is due to the continued venous return, filling both atrium and ventricle and readjusting the end diastolic volume of the ventricle. In a cardiac cycle of 0.8 sec, *ventricular diastole* lasts 0.5 sec: 0.08 sec (isometric relaxation) + 0.12 sec (rapid filling) + 0.2 sec (diastasis) + 0.1 sec (during *atrial* systole).

Obviously, when the heart beats at 180/min (*as during heavy exercise*) with a total cardiac cycle of only 0.33 sec, these periods of systole and diastole given for a heart rate of 75/min are shortened, systole to about 0.2 sec. and diastole to about 0.13 sec. Thus, diastole suffers particularly, and herein lies the danger of pathological tachycardia:—The heart is inadequately filled and its output rapidly declines if the filling phase is reduced below some 0.12 sec.

The atrial pressure curve shows three well-marked waves, A, C, and V, as briefly mentioned in Chapter 6.

1. The first is due to atrial systole and has already been described.

2. With the onset of ventricular systole there is a rise of pressure due to bulging of the A-V valve into the atrium. This is soon succeeded by a sharp fall of atrial pressure beginning at the time of onset of ventricular ejection. The abrupt fall of pressure is attributed to the passive lengthening of the atrium caused by the downward movement of the A-V ring as the ventricular contraction proceeds. The atrial pressure is now exceeded by the venous pressure and rapid atrial filling takes place.

3. The rising phase of the atrial wave is due to venous return. The atrial pressure eventually exceeds that in the ventricle and the opening of the A-V valves, which follows as a simple physical consequence, terminates the phase of ventricular isometric relaxation. As the atrial blood passes into the relaxing ventricle, atrial pressure falls, to rise again during the phase of diastasis.

Changes in Ventricular Volume

A glass container is fitted with a rubber diaphragm perforated by a central hole to permit the fitting of the ventricles: the rubber diaphragm fits snugly round the A-V ring to provide an airtight seal. The glass container is connected by tubing to a piston recorder and the changes in ventricular volume during the cardiac cycle are recorded graphically. With the onset of atrial systole, ventricular volume increases. At the beginning of ventricular systole and closing of the A-V valve there follows the period of isometric contraction, during which ventricular volume does not change, of course. The *onset* of ejection is accompanied by quite a minor change of ventricular volume—this initial expulsion mainly has the effect of expanding the ascending aortic wall. Subsequently, however, ventricular volume falls more sharply, and then the rate of ejection subsides (Fig. 11-6A). The end of ejection occurs simultaneously with the incisura, but the volume remains unaltered, indicating the isometric relaxation phase, which is terminated by rapid filling of the ventricle. Subsequently, slow filling restores the ventricular volume. From the pressure and volume curves the mechanical work of the heart (see page 188) can be computed (Fig. 11-6B).

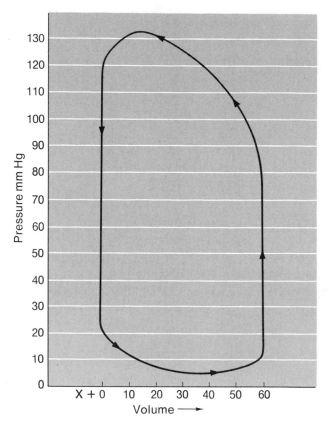

Fig. 11-6B. Work diagram of the heart, constructed from the pressure and volume curves shown in Fig. 11-6A.

Heart Sounds

The heart sounds may be heard by placing the ear on the chest wall or by using a stethoscope. They may be "displayed" by using a recording microphone on the chest wall connected with suitable recording equipment (phonocardiogram; see Lewis, 1962).

The first heart sound is due partly to vibrations of the A-V valves and the adjacent cardiac wall on closure of the valves, and due partly to turbulence.

The second heart sound is due mainly to coaptation of the valves. If the pressure in the aorta or pulmonary artery is unusually high the corresponding sound is excessively loud, as the rebound of the valves is more pronounced than normal.

These are the classical heart sounds. The first sound has a frequency of 30 to 80/sec and a duration of 0.05 sec and is commonly described as "lubb". That due to closure of the tricuspid valve is most audible at the right sternal border in the fourth intercostal space; that of the mitral is best heard at the apex of the heart. The second sound has a higher pitch, with a frequency of 150 to 200/sec and a shorter duration, 0.025 sec. It is commonly described as "dup". The pulmonary second sound is best heard in the parasternal line in the second left intercostal space, and that of the aortic valve in the second intercostal space near the right side of the sternum. The third and fourth "sounds" are less important, being usually inaudible—although they can be detected on the phonocardiogram. The third sound is due to vibrations of the cardiac walls produced by the rapid filling phase of the ventricles. The fourth sound, of low frequency and amplitude, occurs during atrial systole (see Lewis, 1962).

The two first heart sounds signal the duration of ventricular systole (Fig. 11-6A). The characteristics of the sounds are of course clinically important. A split first sound is not uncommon and merely indicates that, as is the case physiologically, the mitral valve shuts after the tricuspid does. A split *second* sound, on the other hand, is suggestive of delayed conduction in the right or left branch of the bundle of His.

Murmurs are heard whenever turbulence becomes excessive. Any increase in the velocity of blood flow favours turbulence (Chapter 3) and consequently such sounds are heard in strenuous exercise, in anaemia, in thyrotoxicosis, etc. If the valve aperture is narrowed (stenosis) the velocity of flow and hence the turbulence of flow increase. Mitral stenosis causes a diastolic (or presystolic) murmur which converts the first mitral sound into *rr*ubb. Aortic stenosis causes a systolic aortic murmur, *rr*up. Incompetence of the valves produced by disease allows regurgitation of blood and mitral incompetence thus causes a systolic mitral murmur which is described as "lusti" in sound. Aortic valvular incompetence causes a softening and prolongation of the second sound during early diastole. In disease both stenosis and incompetence may coexist.

Biophysics of Isolated Cardiac Muscle

General Principles

Hill (1938, 1949) first conceived of skeletal muscle in terms of a model consisting of a contractile element (CE) arranged in series with a passive elastic component (SE). Another passive elastic element—the parallel elastic component (PE)—is arranged in parallel (Fig. 11-7).

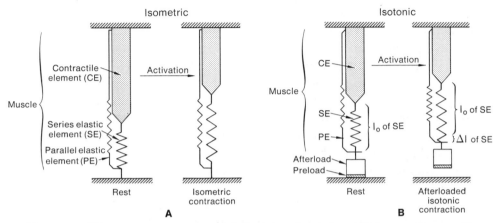

Fig. 11-7. Three-component model for muscle (after Hill). 1. Contractile component (CE). 2. Elastic component in series with contractile component (SE). 3. Elastic component (PE) in parallel with 1 and 2. A: isometric contraction; B: isotonic contraction. (From Sonnenblick, 1962b. By permission.)

Resting tension is sustained primarily by PE, for CE at rest is believed to be quite extensible and the length-resting tension relationship describes the properties of PE. When the muscle is stimulated, CE shortens, develops force, and stretches SE. The force registered at the ends of the muscle depends on three factors: the shortening properties of CE, the elastic properties of SE, and the time allowed for the interaction between the lengthening of SE and the shortening of CE. This last factor is referred to as *the duration of the active state*. The active state—which characterizes the properties of the activated CE—may be defined as a mechanical measure of the chemical processes in the CE which generate force and shortening. This performance of the active CE element can be expressed in terms of four dimensions; force, velocity, instantaneous muscle length, and time (see also Leonard and Hajdiu, 1962).

Papillary muscle from the canine right ventricle provides a longitudinally oriented parallel arrangement of cardiac muscle fibres which is reasonably thin and which serves as a paradigm of cardiac muscle performance, avoiding the complexities of the intricate geometrical disposition of myocardial fibres. The muscle is arranged so as to record force and displacement simultaneously.

Stimulation of the muscle is achieved by numerous electrodes placed at intervals along the length of the muscle, thereby ensuring simultaneous contraction of all the muscle fibres. Displacement of the isotonic lever and the force delivered to the tension transducer are simultaneously recorded (Sonnenblick, 1962a, b).

The initial length of the muscle is established by a small *preload* and fixed by the micrometer stop above the lever (Fig. 11-8). Thereafter, additional loads added to the preload can have no effect on the resting muscle length, but are encountered by the muscle only with the onset of contraction. Such additional loads are called *afterload*. The total load during muscle shortening equals the preload plus the afterload.

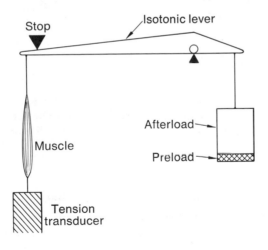

Fig. 11-8. After-loaded isotonic contraction. Papillary muscle is connected to isotonic lever. Initial length of the muscle is established by a small preload. A stop is then set which keeps initial length of the muscle constant prior to contraction. Loads added to preload are only encountered by the muscle with the onset of contraction. (From Sonnenblick, 1962b. By permission.)

Isometric Contraction and Length-tension Relations

When the isotonic level is fixed, thereby preventing external shortening of the muscle, recording is isometric. Fig. 11-9 shows the effect of increasing the initial length of the muscle on the isometric twitch tension developed during stimulation. As the length increases, so does the force of contraction, as revealed by the greater peak tension developed. In this respect, cardiac muscle behaves like skeletal muscle and, indeed, this simple preparation shows results which are in keeping with Starling's Law of the Heart (see Chapter 12).

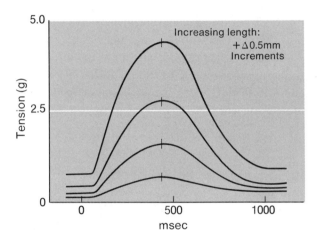

Fig. 11-9. Four superimposed isometric muscle twitches obtained from a cat papillary muscle. From below upwards the four twitches were obtained at initial lengths of 8.5, 9.0, 9.5, and 10.0 mm. (From Sonnenblick, 1962a. By permission.)

Unlike most skeletal muscle, however, cardiac muscle shows an increased force of contraction from the same initial length when catecholamines are added to the solution in the bath surrounding the papillary preparation (Fig. 11-10).

When the initial length of the resting muscle is increased, the rate of development of tension and the peak tension developed are greater, but the time taken from the onset of contraction to the maximal tension development is not changed so long as the frequency of stimulation is kept constant. When the frequency of stimulation is raised there is a substantial shortening of the time taken to reach peak tension in any one contraction (Abbot and Mommaerts, 1959; Sonnenblick, 1962a, b).

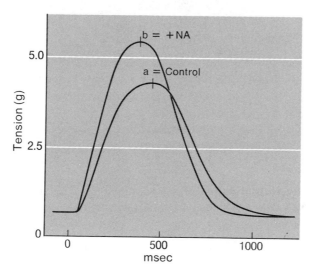

Fig. 11-10. Two isometric twitches obtained at same initial length. "a" is control twitch; "b" twitch obtained when noradrenaline was added to the bath solution in a concentration of 0.5 µg/ml. (From Sonnenblick, 1962a. By permission.)

Isotonic Contraction and Force-velocity Relations

In isotonic recording, once the force that is generated by shortening of CE matches the load, the load moves and SE is first stretched by a constant force equal to the load, after which the length of SE remains constant as a function of this load. Hence, the course of shortening of the muscle during this isotonic phase of the contraction expresses the movements of CE, independent of SE.

Fig. 11-11 shows the force-velocity relation of the active CE. As the load increases, the initial velocity of shortening and the extent of this shortening become progressively smaller until finally only isometric force is developed. When external shortening is zero, the maximal isometric force developed is referred to as P_0. Conversely, when the load is zero, maximal velocity (V_{max}) is approached.

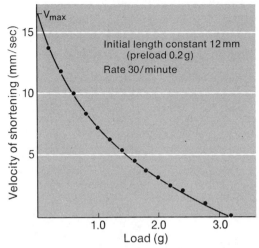

Fig. 11-11. Force-velocity relation of cat papillary muscle. Abscissa: afterload (grams). Ordinate: initial velocity of isotonic shortening. (From Sonnenblick, 1962b. By permission.)

The force-velocity curve derived from studies of papillary muscle is only approximate because the contractions are non-tetanic and the curve is both length-dependent and time-dependent. It is length-dependent, in that shortening of CE occurs at the expense of SE during the isometric phase of contraction even though the over-all length of the muscle is constant; it is time-dependent in both the onset of the active state during the initial phase of contraction and in the decay of the active state during relaxation of the muscle. If, for instance, the active state lasted for such a brief time that relaxation began before the development of maximum ("tetanic") force, P_0 determined from the twitch contraction would be less than the true tetanic P_0.

Experiments in which the initial length of the muscle is altered show that the force-velocity relationship is changed by varying the muscle length. Fig. 11-12 reveals that, although an increase in muscle length increases P_0 and increases the velocity of shortening at any muscle load less than P_0, it does not increase V_{max}. Such a result suggests that, although increasing muscle length causes an increase in the number of force-generating sites in CE, it does not alter the maximal rate at which chemical energy is converted to mechanical energy at any individual contractile site.

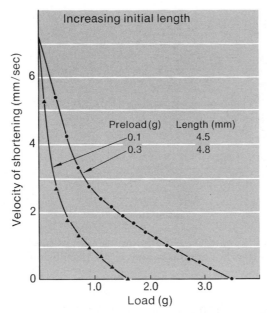

Fig. 11-12. Cat papillary muscle. Increasing initial muscle length by increasing preload increases developed force (ρ_0 on the load axis) without change in the maximum velocity of shortening (V_{max}). (From Sonnenblick, 1962b. By permission.)

When the frequency of contraction is increased, however, P_0 remains unchanged, but V_{max} is increased. Such results suggest that an increased frequency of contraction is causing a greater rate of turnover from chemical to mechanical energy, without necessarily affecting the number of force-generating contractile sites.

When catecholamines are added to the bath, the muscle responds to stimulation by contraction (under afterloaded conditions) with an increased velocity of shortening. Both P_0 and V_{max} are greater (Fig. 11-13). Again, this increase in V_{max} indicates that catecholamines accelerate the rate determining processes of the contractile mechanism of cardiac muscle. The concentration of calcium ions also increases V_{max} and P_0. Like the catecholamines, raised [Ca^{++}] causes an increase in the extent of shortening, and hence the work, at any one afterload. Thus, cardiac muscle, unlike skeletal muscle, can alter its work and power at any one load and muscle length by the nature of its changing force-velocity curves

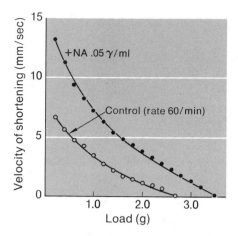

Fig. 11-13. Cat papillary muscle. Noradrenaline (NA) causes an increase both of ρ_0 and of V_{max}. (From Sonnenblick, 1962b. By permission.)

in different chemical environments and also with different frequencies of contraction.

Work per contraction is thus a complex function of initial muscle length, load, and the force-velocity curve on which the cardiac muscle is operating (Sonnenblick, 1962a, b). In the intact heart these parameters can be correlated with the ventricular filling pressure (left ventricular end dia-stolic pressure—LVEDP), the ejection resistance (aortic pressure), and the inotropic state of the myocardium.

References

Abbott, B. C., and W. H. F. M. Mommaerts (1959). "A study of inotropic mechanisms in the papillary muscle preparation," *J. Gen. Physiol.* **42,** 533–51.

Hill, A. V. (1938). "Heat of shortening and dynamic constants of muscle," *Proc. Roy. Soc. London (B),* **126,** 136–95.

Hill, A. V. (1949). "Abrupt transition from rest to activity in muscle," *Proc. Roy. Soc. London (B),* **136,** 399–420.

Huxley, A. F. (1957). "Muscle structure and theories of contraction," *Prog. Biophys.* **7,** 255–318.

Huxley, A. F., and H. E. Huxley (1964). "A discussion on the physical and chemical basis of muscular contraction," *Proc. Roy. Soc. (B),* **155,** 455–77.

Huxley, A. F., and R. Niedergerke (1954). "Structural changes in muscle during contraction," *Nature,* **173,** 971–77.

Huxley, H. E. (1964). "Evidence for continuity between the central elements of the triads and extracellular space in frog sartorius muscle," *Nature,* **202,** 1067.

Huxley, H. E., and J. Hanson (1954). "Structural changes in muscle during contraction", *Nature,* **173,** 978–87.

Keele, C. A., and E. Neil (1965). *Samson Wright's Applied Physiology,* 11th ed. London: Oxford University Press.

Leonard, E., and S. Hajdu (1962). "Action of electrolytes and drugs on the contractile mechanism of the cardiac muscle cell," *Handbook of Physiology,* 2, Circulation **I,** 151–97.

Lewis, D. H. (1962). "Phonocardiography," *Handbook of Physiology,* 2, Circulation **I,** 695–734.

Peachey, L. D. (1965). "The sarcoplasmic reticulum and transverse tubules of the frog's sartorius," *J. Cell. Biol.* **25,** 209–31.

Rushmer, R. F. (1961). *Cardiovascular Dynamics,* 2nd ed. Philadelphia: Saunders.

Scher, A. M. (1962). "Excitation of the heart," *Handbook of Physiology,* 2, Circulation **I,** 287–322.

Sonnenblick, E. H. (1962a). "Force-velocity relations in mammalian heart muscle," *Am. J. Physiol.,* **202,** 931–39.

Sonnenblick, E. H. (1962b). "Implications of muscle mechanics in the heart," *Fed. Proc.* **21,** 975–90.

Spiro, D., and E. H. Sonnenblick (1964). "Structure and function of the heart muscle cell," in *Cyclopedia of Medicine, Surgery and Specialities,* **III,** 9–53.

Weidmann, S. (1967). "Cardiac electrophysiology in the light of recent morphological findings," *The Harvey Lectures,* Series 61, pp.1–16. New York: Academic Press.

12

The Heart as a Pump; Myocardial Metabolism

Performance of the Intact Isolated Heart

The Influence of End-diastolic Fibre Length on Stroke Volume

Fick, in 1882, and Blix, in 1895, disclosed the fundamental relationship between initial length of skeletal muscle and force of its contraction, which Frank, in 1895, proved to be valid for the myocardium as well (see Sarnoff and Mitchell, 1962).

The heart-lung preparation (Fig. 12-1), perfected by Starling and his colleagues (see Starling, 1918), allowed a quantitative appraisal of the effects of increasing the diastolic volume of the ventricle on the stroke output of the heart. Starling showed that if the diastolic filling of the heart is increased (by raising the height of the venous reservoir) the heart increases its stroke output. He also demonstrated that an artificial rise of arterial resistance caused an increase in the diastolic volume of the ventricles, which initially empty less completely, and the volume that remains is added to the volume provided by venous filling from the reservoir. Within a few beats the increased diastolic volume secures an increased force of contraction and the stroke volume is restored to its "control" value. The heart thus does more work at a greater diastolic volume, which presumably can be related to the greater initial length of the ventricular fibres.

Starling thus stated that "The law of the heart is therefore the same as that of skeletal muscle, namely that the mechanical energy set free on passage from the resting to the contracted state depends on the area of 'chemically active surfaces', i.e. on the length of the muscle fibre".

As Linden (1963) has pointed out, the arguments which have raged about the applicability of Starling's law in the description of the performance of the heart in the intact animal have arisen because of the difficulty of measuring the two parameters—the initial muscle length and the energy

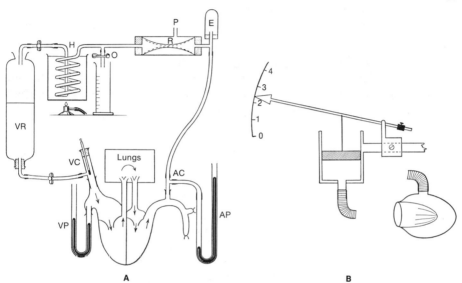

A   B

Fig. 12-1A. Knowlton-Starling heart-lung apparatus (after Hemingway). AC, arterial cannula; E, air-chamber, to give elasticity; H, heating apparatus; O, outlet for determination of output (when determining output this clip is opened for a given time and outlet to venous reservoir closed); P, to pressure-bottle; R, peripheral resistance (dotted line shows position during increased resistance); VC, venous cannula; VR, venous reservoir; VP, manometer to record venous pressure (regulated by screw clip on tube from reservoir); AP, manometer to record arterial pressure. (From McDowall, 1951. By permission.) Fig. 12-1B. Cardiometer—composed of piston recorder and heart chamber. The chamber is made of glass. One opening leads to the recorder and the heart is inserted into the other. In some forms the latter has a thin rubber diaphragm which has a hole in the centre and which fits accurately round the base of the heart, but in other forms the heart fits into a thin rubber sheath (as shown) which does not impede its action. For longer records the rubber is perforated at the apex and the chamber has an inferior opening by which pericardial fluid may be drained away.

of contraction. Linden and Mitchell (1960) devised an instrument which indicated the change in distance between two points in the ventricular myocardium, using a lever-potentiometer principle. This gave reliable quantitative information of the segment length at the end of diastole and showed that sympathetic stimulation in the paced heart caused a decrease in this length both in diastole and systole, and, *simultaneously*, a reduction of the left ventricular end diastolic pressure. They made no claims for its instrumental frequency response during ventricular systole or early diastole when rapid changes were occurring.

Starling himself had used the *right* atrial pressure as an index of the end-diastolic volume of the ventricle and measured the stroke output of the *left* ventricle. Sarnoff (1955) originally suggested the measurement of the mean *left* atrial pressure as the better indication of the left ventricular end-diastolic volume or "initial length." However, it has been shown that even this is inadmissible, for the changes in mean atrial pressure and in

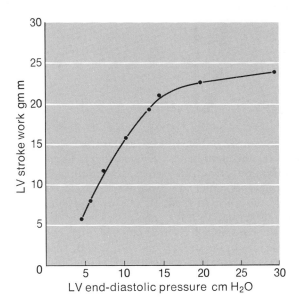

Fig. 12-2. Relationship between left ventricular stroke work (gm m) and end-diastolic pressure in the left ventricle (cm H_2O). Different end-diastolic pressures obtained by infusion and haemorrhage. (From Sarnoff *et al.*, 1960. By permission.)

end-diastolic ventricular pressure are not only of different magnitudes, but these two pressures may sometimes change in opposite directions.

Present opinion is that the *left ventricular end-diastolic pressure*, accurately measured by recording at high sensitivity, is the best index of a change in length. Sarnoff (1955) introduced the graphic plot of left ventricular work (stroke volume × mean aortic pressure) against the left ventricular end diastolic pressure (LVEDP) and used the term *"ventricular function curve"* (VFC) to designate this.

Figure 12-2 shows the intrinsic response of the left ventricle to changing the LVEDP from 5 cm H_2O to 20 cm H_2O. It can be seen that the ventricle contracts more powerfully as LVEDP is increased, although at pressures

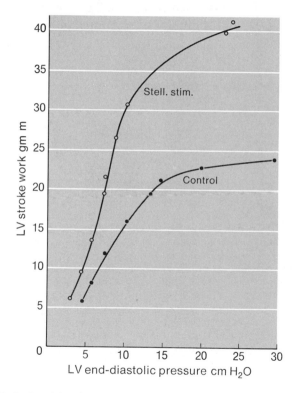

Fig. 12-3. Relationship between left ventricular stroke work and LVEDP before (closed circles) and during (open circles) stimulation of the left stellate ganglion. Both vagi cut. Heart rate constant at 171/min throughout. (From Sarnoff *et al.*, 1960. By permission.)

above 20 cm H_2O the further increase of stroke volume and work is only
slight. Hence the ventricular output per beat is related to the accepted
index of initial length of the myocardial fibres, as was seen in the case of
the isolated papillary muscle. This may also be called the *"heterometric
autoregulation"* of the heart, to distinguish it from the *"homeometric autoregulation"* (see below).

The Influence of Sympathetic Stimulation on Ventricular Function

Further studies have shown that the sympathetic nerves which supply the
heart via the stellate ganglia profoundly influence the stroke work at any
one LVEDP. Thus, Fig. 12-3 shows the ventricular function curves obtained in an anaesthetized dog (in which the heart rate was maintained
constant) with and without stimulation of the stellate ganglion.

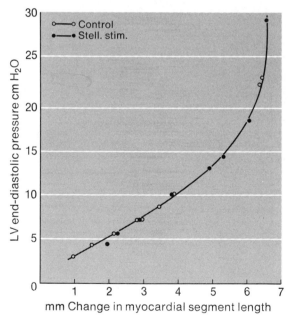

Fig. 12-4. Relationship between end-diastolic pressure in the left ventricle and
the changes in length of a segment of the left ventricular myocardium before
(closed circles) and during (open circles) stimulation of the left stellate ganglion.
(Same experiment as in Fig. 12-3.) (From Sarnoff *et al.*, 1960. By permission.)

Sympathetic stimulation obviously increases the work done by the ventricle at any given LVEDP. The effect of sympathetic stimulation cannot be ascribed to any increase of distensibility of the ventricular fibres during diastolic filling. If such were the case then the diastolic length of the fibres would be greater at any given LVEDP. However, Mitchell, Linden, and Sarnoff (1960) proved that sympathetic stimulation did not alter the relationship between myocardial segment length and LVEDP (Fig. 12-4).

It follows therefore that sympathetic nerve stimulation (and the release of catecholamines from the adrenal medulla) causes a positive inotropic effect on the performance of the ventricles in the intact heart, just as was shown in isolated papillary muscle (Chapter 11). *This influence of the sympathetic innervation enables the ventricles to contract more strongly even though their initial length has not increased.*

"Starling" and Sympathetic Effects in Unison

Linden (1968) has elegantly shown how the two mechanisms—the effect of increasing diastolic length and the positive inotropic influence of the sympathetic postganglionic release of catecholamines—may operate together in the intact animal (Figs. 12-5, 12-6, 12-7). A heart-lung preparation was used; both the vagi and the ansae subclaviae, whence course the cardiac sympathetic nerves, were sectioned. When the inflow to the right atrium was raised (see Fig. 12-5), the venous pressure, and hence the diastolic volume, increased, whereupon the stroke volume increased from 15 ml to 20 ml. This stroke volume was maintained until the right atrial pressure was reduced to its control value, whereupon the stroke volume was restored to approximately the same end-diastolic volume as before.

Figure 12-6 shows the effect of stimulating the sympathetic supply to the same heart; the heart rate was maintained constant at 104 ml/min; the stroke volume was 14 ml. A few seconds after stimulation began, end-diastolic volume and end-systolic volume fell and the right atrial pressure was reduced. The stroke volume at first increased slightly, even though the inflow from the venous reservoir remained the same, because a little more blood was ejected as the heart size adjusted to its smaller end-diastolic volume. As essentially the same stroke volume was achieved at a smaller end-diastolic volume, the figure shows clear evidence of a positive inotropic effect.

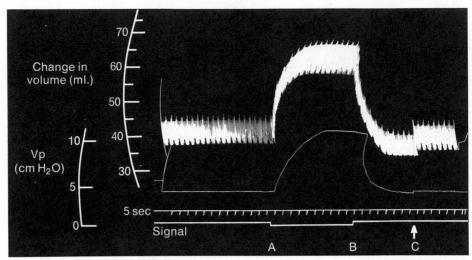

Fig. 12-5. Example of the Starling mechanism. From above downwards: cardiometer trace, indicating change in volume of both ventricles; venous pressure (from right atrium); time marker, 5 seconds; signal marker. Both vagi and both ansae subclaviae were sectioned. During the signal, the inflow to the right atrium was suddenly increased. (From Linden, 1968. By permission.)

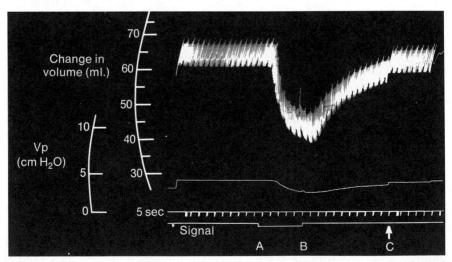

Fig. 12-6. Stimulation of the sympathetic nerves to the heart. Records as in previous figure. During the signal the left ansa subclavia was stimulated supramaximally at 4 pulses/sec. (From Linden, 1968. By permission.)

Finally, Fig. 12-7 illustrates how these two mechanisms may work in unison. After a control period, sympathetic stimulation was performed (at signal mark A) and the stimulation continued until signal mark C. This sympathetic stimulation caused a fall in both end-diastolic and end-systolic volumes, and evoked a fall in the venous pressure. It did not, however, reduce the stroke volume. At signal mark B the venous reservoir was raised to the same height as that used to obtain the record shown in Fig. 12-5. The increase in venous return, however, only raised the venous

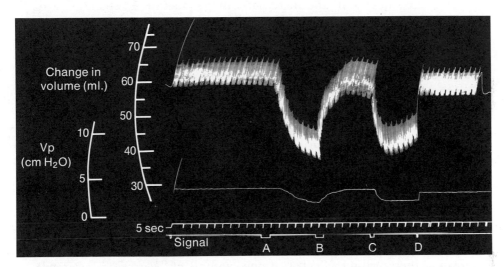

Fig. 12-7. Combined effect of stimulation of sympathetic nerves and Starling mechanism. Records as in the two previous figures. At signal A the left ansa subclavia was stimulated *and this stimulation continued until signal C.* At signal B the inflow to the right atrium was increased and this increase was maintained until signal C. At signal C both stimulus and extra inflow stopped. At signal D recording stopped for 2 mins. (From Linden, 1968. By permission.)

pressure to a level similar to that seen in the control period and increased the end-diastolic volume above that of the control level; the end-systolic volume remained below that of the control period. Thus, the simultaneous operation of the two mechanisms caused an increased stroke volume from a slightly increased end-diastolic volume and a smaller end-systolic volume (hence a bigger beat output) although the venous pressure was much the same as that during the control period. At signal mark C sympathetic stimulation ceased and the venous reservoir was returned to its control height. The "Starling effect" was abolished promptly, but the inotropic influence exerted by catecholamine release abated more slowly. At signal mark D the record was stopped for two minutes, following which the volumes and pressures returned to their control values. As Linden suggests, the volumes and pressure recorded between the second (B) and third (C) signal marks could represent those which occur during the increased output of exercise in the intact animal when the two mechanisms—sympathetic stimulation and increased filling—operate together.

Other Positive Inotropic Effects on Ventricular Performance

Positive inotropic effects may be produced by influences other than those listed as due to the catecholamines in the section on isolated muscle and in that on the heart-lung preparation. That of calcium on isolated papillary muscle has been described. It is doubtful whether this is of much importance in affecting the performance of the *intact* heart, although it can be demonstrated "pharmacologically". Two influences that may play a physiological role, however, are those exerted by increasing the frequency of the heart beat and by increasing the aortic pressure, respectively. An increased heart rate causes an increased contractility of the ventricle which develops progressively over a number of beats. This "staircase phenomenon", or "Treppe", was first described by Bowditch and is also known as the Bowditch effect. It is one example of "*homeometric autoregulation*", as defined by Sarnoff *et al.* (1960).

As a result of this positive inotropic effect the heart maintains an LVEDP and fibre length more nearly similar to those which characterize the period prior to the increase in its activity. Various causes of the phenomenon have been advanced. Hajdu and Leonard (1959) noted that potassium leaves the myocardial cell with each contraction and re-enters the cell during diastole. Hence, the higher the rate and the shorter the period of diastole, the less the time available for re-entry of the potassium lost, thereby lowering the intracellular $[K^+]$ in the new equilibrium state. This situation is known to increase myocardial contractility. Sarnoff and Mitchell (1962) have suggested that the phenomenon of homeometric autoregulation may depend on the amount of tension developed by the myocardium per unit of time—the tension time index (see p. 191). Another example of a staircase phenomenon or of homeometric autoregulation is the "Anrep" effect. Here, an increase in aortic pressure in the heart-lung preparation causes at first an increase in the diastolic volume. The increase in contractility thus induced diminishes the proportion of the total cardiac cycle that systole would otherwise require.

In the intact animal these two staircase mechanisms probably contribute to the increased contractility of the myocardium in exercise, which is brought about by the greater sympathetic activity, for both an increase in rate and an increase in aortic pressure are characteristics of the exercise, but it is difficult to assess their relative importance. Their separate effects on the performance of the ventricle in the anaesthetized dog have been studied by Linden and his colleagues (Linden, 1968). They recorded the rate of change of pressure (dP/dt) during the isometric contraction of the ventricle and found that dP/dt_{max} (peak rate of change in ventricular pressure during isometric contraction) gave an excellent indication of the inotropic response of the ventricle. However, whereas stimulation of the

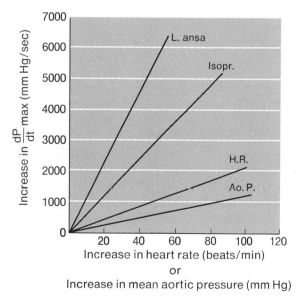

Fig. 12-8. Diagram of comparison of inotropic response to increasing the after load (mean aortic pressure, Ao.P.) on the heart rate (HR) with the inotropic response to increasing stimulation of the left ansa subclavia or infusion of isoprenaline. (From Linden, 1968. By permission.)

left cardiac sympathetic nerves or the infusion of isoprenaline yielded marked positive inotropic effects, those caused by increasing the afterload (mean aortic pressure) or by increasing the frequency of contraction (heart rate) were of much less importance (Fig. 12-8).

The Vagi and Ventricular Performance

In most mammals, few, if any, vagal fibres seem to reach the muscle fibres of the heart ventricles. Provided that the heart rate is kept constant by pacing the heart artificially, it appears that vagal stimulation reduces the cardiac output by depressing the contractility of the atrial muscle alone (Linden, 1963). Thus, according to most studies, the vagi do not significantly alter the distensibility or the contractility of the ventricles (Fig. 12-9). However, according to de Geest et al. (1965) a weak, negative inotropic effect of vagal origin may be obtained in the ventricles of the dog,

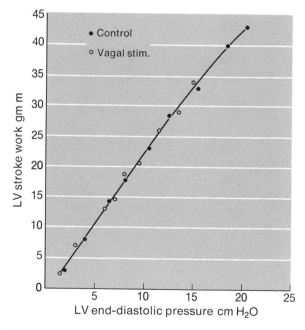

Fig. 12-9. Relationship between left ventricular stroke work and LVEDP before (closed circles) and during (open circles) peripheral vagal stimulation. Both vagi cut in neck. Heart rate kept constant at 187/min by stimulation of left atrium. (From Sarnoff et al., 1960. By permission.)

and in diving species this type of vagal influence seems to be profound (Folkow and Yonce, 1967), but so is here the vagal effect on heart rate.

The vagal nerves do, of course, supply cholinergic fibres to the sino-atrial node and atrioventricular nodes and cause a powerful negative chronotropic effect which is by far the most important vagal influence on the heart. However, in the experiment shown in Fig. 12-9, this effect has been excluded by artificially pacing the heart. The vagi also innervate atrial muscle and depress its contractility, and this negative inotropic effect can, in the paced heart, reduce cardiac output say 5 to 10%, an effect that seems to be predominantly due to the vagal depression of atrial contraction. Whether, and/or to what extent, vagal fibres exert any negative inotropic effect on the heart ventricles in man is not known; it seems likely that their effect is weak or even negligible, as it is in the dog.

Heart Rate and Cardiac Output of the Heart-lung Preparation and of the Anaesthetized Animal

Starling himself showed that if the venous filling and the arterial resistance were held constant in the heart-lung preparation, alterations of heart rate did not change the cardiac output until the rate became very fast, at which point the output fell.

The ventricles can only fill in diastole. For many years it was asserted that the ventricle did not suck blood into it, but was filled only by positive pressure from the atria, which in turn was a manifestation of the *vis a tergo* of the circulation. Certainly, if the heart is suddenly thrown into asystole by artificial vagal stimulation, the right atrial and right ventricular pressures rise sharply. *Vis a tergo* nowadays is still accepted to be the main force responsible for cardiac filling. However, as outlined also in Chapter 10, ventricular action docs contribute to the subsequent filling of the ventricle by exerting "suction" on the atrium. Thus, during atrial systole, superior vena caval blood flow falls to zero, but is greatly increased with each right ventricular ejection, although the tricuspid valve is closed at this time. The reason is that the atrioventricular junction is drawn down during ventricular systole, enlarging the atria and sucking blood into them.

When the atrioventricular valves open the rapid venous filling is mainly due to the *vis a tergo*, but it is also due to ventricular diastolic suction. Thus, Bloom (1955) showed that ventricular relaxation involves some "elastic recoil", at least for the thick-walled left ventricle. He used an excised beating rat heart in a vessel containing Ringer's solution. With each beat, fluid was ejected from the aortic stump and the heart moved as if jet-propelled in the solution. The atrial wall was drawn into the mitral orifice in each diastolic period. As there was no hydrostatic pressure between the cardiac interior and the solution, the energy required for ventricular filling must have been derived from the elastic recoil of ventricular relaxation. The presence of left ventricular suction has been confirmed and further studied by Brecher and Kissen (1958; see also Brecher, 1958). "Negative" pressures of as much as 11 cm H_2O may be observed in the *left* ventricle of the dog when the mitral orifice is temporarily clamped and under hydrostatic conditions similar to those of Bloom's experiment.

Ventricular filling in diastole occurs in two phases: *rapid filling*, which is of major importance (see Fig. 11-6, page 157), and *slow filling*, or diastasis, which is of minor importance and which, moreover, can only be distinctly seen at slow heart rates, less than approximately 110/min in the dog (see Linden, 1963). A slight increase of heart rate from a figure of, say, 80/min would encroach only on the period of diastasis and would impair ventricular filling only slightly. At this stage, as the beat rate *is* increased, an increased cardiac output per minute might result, but a further cardiac acceleration would now encroach upon the *rapid* filling time. It then reduces the end-diastolic volume, and hence the stroke volume, so that the output per minute may not increase. When the heart is paced at high rates cardiac output will *decrease* because of a serious reduction of the rapid filling time.

In summary, an increase in heart rate of itself may, by reducing the end-diastolic volume, decrease the stroke volume, and the resulting cardiac output may only increase moderately and may even decrease.

When, however, the increased heart rate is accompanied by the positive inotropic effect of catecholamines, such as occurs during sympathetic stimulation, the result may be a considerable increase in stroke volume, but this can only be *maintained* if the venous return is boosted—otherwise the heart "uses up" its residual volume. (In the *intact* animal, undergoing muscular exercise, the increased activity of the skeletal muscle pump to a great extent provides this boosting).

As sympathetic stimulation causes an increased rate of contraction and relaxation in each cardiac cycle of the artificially paced heart, although the cycle length of course remains the same in this situation, the diastolic filling time of each cycle is increased.

Figure 12-10 shows that sympathetic stimulation in a paced heart produces an increase in aortic pressure and a decrease in the end-diastolic pressure and a doubling of the diastolic period. When the heart rate is not controlled, sympathetic stimulation causes an increased heart rate, a shorter systole, and a relatively longer proportion of the total length of the cycle available for diastolic filling than if there had been no inotropic effect on the ventricle accompanying the chronotropic influence.

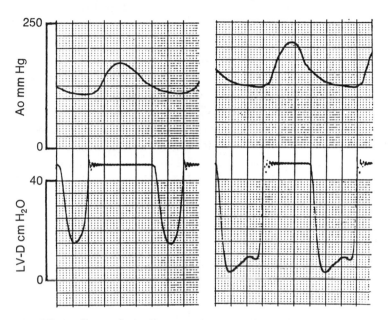

Fig. 12-10. The effect of an increased sympathetic activity on ventricular "filling time." From above down: aortic blood pressure, pressure in the ventricle recorded only during diastole. Left panel, control. Right panel, during stimulation of the left stellate ganglion. The heart rate was held constant throughout at 180 beats per minute by stimulating the left atrium. (From Sarnoff and Mitchell, 1962. By permission.)

The Heart in Exercise

Starling (1918) envisaged the changes in cardiac output in exercise thus: "If a man starts to run, his muscular movements pump more blood into the heart. As a result the heart is overfilled. Its volume, both in systole and diastole, enlarge progressively until by the lengthening of the muscle fibres so much more active surfaces are brought into play within the fibres that the energy of the contraction becomes sufficient to drive on into the aorta during each systole the largely increased volume of blood entering the heart from the veins during diastole".

Starling understood that the greater diastolic size which he postulated in the early stage of exercise was transient, for he stated: "The physiological condition of the heart is thereby improved and the heart gradually returns to its normal volume even though it is doing increased work". These quotations from his Linacre Lecture may be followed by another from a lecture to the Royal Army Medical Corps in 1920: "In studying the reactions of the isolated heart, dilatation of the heart seems to be the only mechanism of the unfailing response of this organ to any increase in the demands made upon it. But the effort of throwing this organ into the circle of control by the central nervous system is that it is kept in rest or activity in an equable condition and the dilatation, which was so marked a condition of its reaction when isolated, is reduced to such small dimensions in the heart, reined in and controlled by the cardiac centres and helped by the correlated changes in other organs that it becomes imperceptible in the intact animal, and is not revealed, for instance, by any radiographic study of the heart during exercise".

The difficulty in interpreting the role of the "Starling" mechanism in exercise in animals and in man himself stems from the uncertainties of measurement of the cardiac volumes. These have been calculated from the length, breadth and area of the X-ray silhouette. Liljestrand et al. (1938) calculated changes in stroke volume in man from two simultaneous photographs taken at rest and during exercise and found the stroke volumes to average 44 ml at rest and 88 ml during exercise, 1260 kpm/min. (The calculated resting stroke volume is unduly low.) They found an increase in the volume of heart from 581 ml ($\pm$ 8 ml) at rest to 673 ml ($\pm$ 21 ml) during the above mentioned work load. Linden (1963) has suggested that this total increase of volume of 91 ml represents one of 25 ml or so in that of the left ventricle. As the *stroke* volume increased from 44 ml (rest, probably too low a figure) to 88 ml in exercise, this indicates that up towards 20 ml of the increase in stroke volume was secured by encroaching upon the left ventricular residual volume (end-systolic volume).

At this stage it is important to realize that the heart does *not* empty itself completely with systole, either in resting conditions of the body or during exercise. Some blood remains in the ventricle. This has been described as the *systolic reserve* (Rushmer, 1961).

In exercise conditions the two factors—increased sympathetic activity (on the heart *and* on the vascular system, both arteries and veins) and the increased *vis a tergo*, which boosts venous return from the active muscles and thereby contributes to an increased diastolic filling of the heart, both contribute to the augmentation of cardiac output which occurs. The simple experiments using the heart-lung preparation indicate how an interplay of these two factors may account for the exercise performance of the heart.

The cardiac output is linearly related to the oxygen consumption. At rest, with a cardiac output (standing) of 5 l/min, the oxygen consumption

Table 12-1. Standing Man

	Resting	*Exercising*
Oxygen uptake	400 ml/min	3–3$\frac{1}{2}$ l/min
Cardiac output	5 l/min	25 l/min
Heart rate	70	180
Stroke volume	70 ml	140 ml
Residual (end-systolic) volume	75 ml	40 ml
End-diastolic volume	145 ml	180 ml
Cycle time	0.85 sec	0.33 sec
Ventricular systole	0.3 sec	0.2 sec
Ventricular diastole	0.55 sec	0.13 sec

is some 400 ml/min. Table 12-1, slightly modified from Linden (1965), shows the changes in some of the features of cardiac activity between rest in standing and severe exercise.

The figures in Table 12-1 are, of course, only *sample* figures. For instance, the heart of a trained athlete—particularly one who indulges in "endurance" sports—may beat at only 40 to 45/min at rest. The resting cardiac output of such individuals is of the same order as that of the untrained individual, and the stroke volume must therefore be 120 to 125 ml. Such subjects have larger and more powerful hearts and feature an end-systolic volume of as much as 120 ml compared with that of 50 ml in the untrained person. They begin, therefore, with a greater systolic reserve than do the untrained.

The maximal heart rate of which either trained or untrained man is capable is about 180/min, or slightly higher. The main difference in performance of the two lies in the ability of the trained subject to supply a bigger stroke volume for any given heart rate, including the highest ones. It is likely that the maximal cardiac output of the professional skier or cyclist can reach 35 l/min—which necessitates a *stroke volume* approaching 200 ml, probably in excess of even the maximal end-diastolic volume of most untrained but healthy subjects when exercising to their fullest powers. The great increase in the systolic reserve of the top athlete makes these astounding performances possible. In more moderate degrees of exercise the trained athlete can draw upon his greater systolic reserve and perform the exercise with a relatively trivial increase of heart rate, whereas the untrained man responds with a steadily increasing heart rate without much increase in stroke volume (for a critical survey of the extensive literature see Bevegård and Shepherd, 1967; Åstrand and Rodahl, 1970).

Despite these reservations about the differing nature of the cardiac response to exercise in trained and untrained subjects (and we do not fully understand the reasons for the difference in the chronotropic response of the two in mild or moderate exercise), the data provided in Table 12-1 suggest that the increased stroke volume of severe exercise is derived both from an encroachment of the systolic reserve (end-systolic volume) and an increased contribution from a greater end-diastolic volume. Both the Starling effect (enhanced venous return thanks to the "muscle pump") and the positive inotropic effect of sympathetic stimulation contribute to the greater stroke volume of severe exercise as compared with that during quiet standing. Any increase in the end-diastolic volume, thereby stretching the myocardial fibres, will increase the force of contraction of the ventricle.

Hamilton (1955) has pointed out that the Starling mechanism presumably forms the basis also of preserving the balance between the pumping of the right and the left ventricles: "this balance must be exact and since the two ventricles are subject to the same hormonal and nervous influences they each act as a control for the other ... only a delicate adjustment of strength of contraction to degree of filling serves as an hypothesis to explain their maintained balanced output in face of the fact that left ventricular pressure load and coronary supply are much more variable than right". This must hold in resting conditions and equally so in exercise.

The sympathetic effect is to increase the speed of myocardial contraction and the output per beat by a positive inotropic influence on the ventricle and also to increase the filling of the ventricle per beat by actions on the diastolic filling time, ventricular suction, and atrial contraction. To these may be added its positive chronotropic influence on the rate of the beat. It is likely that the sympathetic stimulation of the heart in exercise is mainly due to the liberation of catecholamines from the cardiac sympathetic nerve endings and is less due to the effects of catecholamines released into the blood from the adrenal medullae.

The mode of *initiation* of the increase in sympathetic activity in exercise is not entirely clear. It may, at least in part, be due to cortico-hypothalamic discharge (see Chapter 19). Rushmer *et al.* (1960; see also Rushmer, 1961) have shown that stimulation delivered by chronically implanted electrodes, whose tips lay in the region of the H_2 field of Forel and in the periventricular grey matter of the brains of conscious dogs, produced changes of left ventricular performance very similar to those produced by the same dogs when working on the treadmill. The diencephalic sites of stimulation required to evoke these changes were closely adjacent to, perhaps identical with, the "defence area" from which sympathetic vasodilator responses can be evoked; it is known that even light "alerting" stimuli activate this area (see Chapter 19).

It has been suggested that the cardiac acceleration of exercise may be simply due to an abolition of efferent discharge in the cardiac vagi caused by cortico-hypothalamic inhibition of the cardio-inhibitory centre (see Chapter 19). It is most likely that vagal activity is reduced or abolished in this way, but beyond doubt the positive chronotropic effect of the sympathetic discharge greatly contributes to the increased heart rate. This latter influence is further necessary to explain the improvement in ventricular contractility which occurs in exercise and which is a prerequisite for making the tachycardia efficient; systole *must* be shortened if a rate increase is to lead to a substantial gain in output.

Besides the probable involvement of cortico-hypothalamic influences, Ledsome and Linden (1964) have shown that distension of the pulmonary vein-atrial vagal receptors on the left side of the heart causes a powerful tachycardia which is abolished by section of the cardiac sympathetic nerves or by the abolition of sympathetic efferent activity to the heart by the injection of bretylium. This reflex pathway might be the sole explanation of the classical Bainbridge effect—cardiac acceleration ensuing upon an increased venous return (see Chapter 18). The contribution of this reflex to the sympathetic acceleration of exercise is of course undecided, but Linden and his colleagues (personal communication) have proved that the reflex provokes only a sympathetic chronotropic response and does not alter ventricular contractility (dP/dt_{max} is unchanged).

Whenever pH of the blood is decreased in exercise as a result of lactate production, etc., it can be expected that a chemoreceptor drive contributes as well (see Chapter 18). It is thus likely that both central and reflex influences are involved in the establishment of tachycardia during exercise. As discussed briefly in Chapter 18, evidence is accumulating that there might be receptors in tissues such as skeletal muscle, signalling e.g. increased metabolism by sensing local chemical change, which might have a reflex excitatory influence on sympathetic discharge. If so, such peripheral receptors might add also to the neurogenic drive of the heart during exercise. But it is too early to make any definite statements.

Myocardial Oxygen Usage: Cardiac Work and Efficiency

External Work of the Heart

Two tug-of-war teams who strain unavailingly to reach a dead-heat do no mechanical work, although it would only be safe to tell them so when they collapse utterly exhausted at the end of the match. As physiologists we would admit and could indeed confirm by measurement that their oxygen usages had risen startlingly, for muscles in isometric contraction require energy from oxidative and anaerobic processes to sustain the tension they develop.

The physicist defines mechanical or external work as the product of force and the distance moved by the point of application of that force. In the case of a pressure moving a fluid the work done would be pressure times the volume of fluid displaced. The ventricle ejects blood into the aorta, and the amount of work in any small fraction of time is:

$$\Delta W = P_V \times \Delta V$$

Over the period of systolic ejection it is

$$W = \int P_V dV.$$

Fig. 11-6B (page 160) shows the net mechanical work of the ventricular cycle plotted from the pressure volume relations which were determined experimentally. Otto Frank gave a complete expression of the work of the heart, but many of the factors, such as those of the potential energy developed by the elastic physical forces in the ventricular wall, the elastic strains developed in the ventricular wall, and the potential and kinetic energies required for producing movements of parts of the ventricle without degradation into heat, could not be estimated. Most workers have resorted to a simple formula:

$$\text{Mechanical work per beat} = QP + \frac{mv^2}{2}$$

where Q = stroke volume in ml, P = mean arterial pressure (metres of water), m = mass of blood (grams), and v = velocity.

The term $mv^2/2$, which expresses the kinetic energy imparted to the blood, accounts for only some 5% of the external work of the left ventricle beating in resting conditions and can be disregarded for the moment.

External cardiac work then is governed by the product of mean pressure and the stroke volume. Whether the one or the other increases, as long as the product remains the same, then, disregarding the kinetic factor, the external work must be identical. If one were to suppose that the oxygen consumption of the heart were to be devoted only to the performance of *external* work, then the myocardial oxygen usage per minute should be the same whether the mechanical work $\int PdV$ achieved were performed by increasing the volume or the pressure. Measurements of oxygen usage refute this.

Haemodynamic Determinants of Myocardial Oxygen Usage

Even the quiescent left ventricle with no ejection or arterial pressure uses 1.5 to 2 ml O_2/100 g/min. This surprisingly high basal figure will be referred to again later. When the heart beats normally in the intact circulation of the resting dog or man the left ventricular oxygen usage is 8 to 10 ml/100 g/min. Studies of the performance of isolated supported hearts by Sarnoff *et al.* (1958a, b) have revealed the respective effects on myocardial oxygen usage of increasing external work by raising the pressure against which the heart beats or by raising the stroke output.

When the left ventricular work is increased by raising the mean aortic pressure while keeping the stroke volume and heart rate constant ("pressure run"), the increase of cardiac external work is paralleled by the increase of oxygen usage so that the myocardial efficiency (here expressed as external work/O_2 usage) is unaltered (Fig. 12-11).

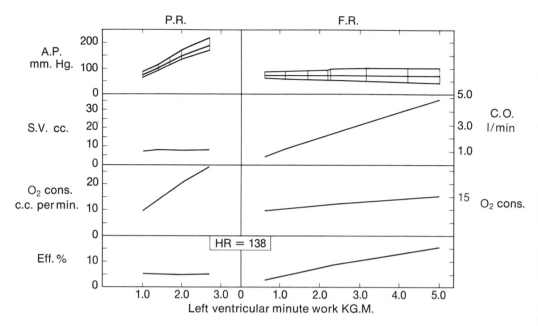

Fig. 12-11. Contrasting effects on myocardial oxygen consumption of increasing work by increasing mean aortic pressure (pressure run, P.R.) and increasing work by increasing cardiac output (flow run, F.R.). Heart rate was held constant at 138/min throughout. A.P., Aortic pressure; S.V., stroke volume; Eff., per cent efficiency. (From Sarnoff *et al.*, 1958. By permission.)

In contrast, when work is increased by raising the stroke volume while keeping aortic pressure and heart rate constant ("flow run") the oxygen usage of the heart increases only slightly and hence the efficiency rises strikingly.

Finally, the mean aortic pressure was held constant at 120 mm Hg and the cardiac output was progressively increased from 1.2 to 4.9 l/min at a constant heart rate of 120/min. This sequence was repeated at heart rates of 160 and 200/min, respectively. At any given mean aortic pressure and cardiac output a higher heart rate was accompanied by a greater oxygen usage and therefore by a lower myocardial efficiency.

These results show that myocardial oxygen usage bears little relationship to the *external* work of the heart *per se*. Sarnoff concluded that they indicated that the myocardial oxygen usage was most closely related to *the total tension developed by the myocardium* insofar as this is reflected by the total area beneath the systolic portion of the systolic pressure pulse. The term *"tension time index"* (TTI) refers to this parameter. TTI is calculated as the product of the mean systolic pressure, the duration of systole, and the heart rate. The cardiac muscle requires an increased rate of energy transformation (O_2 usage) proportional to the tension it develops even when it achieves no external work. Most of the oxygen used by the heart beating normally is needed for *tension development* and only a relatively small fraction of the oxygen consumed is devoted to the performance of external work. Cardiac metabolism is almost entirely aerobic, so the total energy transformation achieved by the beating heart may be calculated from the oxygen usage, remembering that 1 ml oxygen has an energy equivalent of about 2 kpm. The equation for mechanical efficiency is

$$M.E. = \frac{External\ work}{Total\ energy\ transformed}$$

$$\%\ Efficiency = 100 \times \frac{External\ work\ (kg\ m/min)}{2 \times O_2\ (kg\ m/min)}$$

Gregg (1966) has pointed out that the oxygen usage of the quiescent ventricle may be some 25% of the value at normal working level and this should be subtracted from the denominator, otherwise the efficiency calculated from the above equation is too low. However, the main point is that the external work of the heart is a much smaller item in its energy turnover than is the TTI, and the "efficiency" calculated is correspondingly small (say 10%) because the numerator is small compared with the denominator of the equation. If the external work is increased by increasing the stroke volume the efficiency of the heart is greatly increased because, although the numerator is markedly affected, the over-all increase of the denominator is relatively trivial.

Burton (1965) has drawn attention to this importance of keeping the total load of the heart low rather than focussing attention on the small requirements of the external pumping of the heart. As he states, the external work required for mild exercise in the cardiac patient is of much less moment than is an increase in the total load resulting from the raised blood pressure and heart rate associated with angry emotional scenes. (John Hunter was well aware of the danger of the latter factor; see Chapter 23.)

Braunwald *et al.* (1967) have shown that not even the importance of the TTI entirely explains the requirements of the intact heart. Myocardial oxygen usage is increased by positive inotropic influences such as sympathetic nerve stimulation, catecholamine infusion, or exercise, even when the TTI was sometimes reduced. Ventricular oxygen usage can even be increased by noradrenaline when the ventricle is empty and is developing little tension. They have suggested that the level of contractile state as reflected in V_{max} may provide a more complete description of the mechanical determinants of ventricular oxygen usage than does TTI, but, as they say, "further quantitative studies in the intact heart will be required before the relative metabolic costs of wall tension, fibre shortening and the level of the contractile state with its mechanical correlates can be fully assessed".

Myocardial Metabolism

Coronary sinus catheterization studies (see Bing, 1965) have revealed that the heart can use a variety of foodstuffs as metabolic substrate. The catabolism of fat, carbohydrate, and protein produces free energy, of which some 50% is dissipated as heat. The remainder is captured as phosphate bond energy which is employed for the work of the muscle cells and for the synthesis of glycogen, lipids, and proteins.

After a meal, or following the infusion of glucose, metabolism is predominantly that of carbohydrate (glucose, pyruvate, and lactate) with a respiratory quotient of above 0.9. It is notable that the myocardium, in contrast to skeletal muscle, readily utilizes lactate. Fasting, however, reduces the utilization of carbohydrate, and prolonged fasting is attended by a myocardial respiratory quotient of 0.7 with a maximal extraction of fatty acids and ketones. Bing *et al.*, have shown that the human myocardium can derive up to two-thirds of its energy from the oxidation of fatty acids and the source of these fatty acids is the plasma albumin-bound nonesterified fatty acid (NEFA) fraction (see Bing, 1965). Plasma amino acids do not contribute significantly to the energy production of the heart.

The substrates of oxidative metabolism provide the energy for oxidative phosphorylation. In cardiac muscle, as elsewhere, adenosine triphosphate forms the energy currency of the cell.

Myocardial contraction leads to the reaction

$$ATP \xrightarrow[\substack{\text{actomyosin} \\ \text{ATPase}}]{} ADP + P_i$$

$$ADP + PC \rightleftharpoons ATP + C$$

Phosphocreatine rapidly regenerates the ATP (Lohmann reaction); the catalysing enzyme is creatine phosphotransferase:

$$K = \frac{[ATP][C]}{[ADP][PC]}$$

This transphosphorylation is reversible, and its equilibrium constant K is 20.

From the concentrations present in the myocardium it can be calculated that, of the ATP split, approximately 99% is restored at the expense of PC. Hence, as the ATP content of myocardium is tiny compared with that of creatine phosphate, the ATP concentration falls appreciably only when the PC concentration is reduced to a small fraction of its normal value. Enough of the enzyme creatine phosphotransferase (CPT) is present to ensure that the transphosphorylation proceeds rapidly during the contraction itself.

However, it has recently been found that the enzyme CPT can be selectively inhibited by fluorodinitrobenzene (FDNB) and it has been demonstrated that skeletal muscle treated with FDNB can be made to contract normally for a few twitches. During the course of these contractions ATP is indeed broken down, but CP is not. Similar observations have now been made on cardiac muscle. It is clear that the energy-rich phosphate primarily concerned with the contraction process is ATP.

Ischaemia of the heart and acute myocardial hypoxia cause a striking drop in the PC concentration and a marked rise in inorganic phosphate. The ATP/ADP quotient of the myocardium falls.

The myocardial metabolism of the energy-rich phosphate compounds and their catabolic produces seems to be related to the regulation of coronary blood flow as well (Berne, 1964). Thus, ^{14}C-labelled adenosine added to the perfusion fluid is rapidly incorporated by the isolated perfused heart into myocardial ATP and ADP in the presence or absence of oxygen. Adenosine is a potent coronary vasodilator, and the evidence just cited indicates that it can cross the myocardial membrane with ease. Berne has postulated a scheme whereby a reduction in myocardial pO_2 induced by increased cardiac work or by hypoxaemia or by coronary ischaemia causes a breakdown of ATP to adenosine. Adenosine diffuses out of the cells and causes coronary vasodilatation—which raises the myocardial pO_2 and slows the degradation of ATP (see Chapter 23). Unfortunately, no one has successfully demonstrated the presence of adenosine in coronary sinus blood. This may be due to the rapid deamination which adenosine suffers from the enzymatic action of blood or tissue fluid. It is interesting that whereas skeletal muscle is rich in adenylic acid deaminase, which transforms AMP (6 aminopurine riboside) into inosinic acid (6 oxypurine riboside phosphate), cardiac muscle contains little of this enzyme. If the myocardial cell *did* contain adenylic acid deaminase, then inosinic acid, inosine, or hypoxanthine would be formed in the cell itself and liberated from it. None of these compounds has anything like the coronary vasodilator potency of adenosine. Inosine and hypoxanthine are found in the coronary sinus blood during myocardial hypoxia, but it is believed that they are formed by deaminases in the tissue fluid or blood rather than in the cell.

The myocardial cell contains phosphorylase. This enzyme exists in an inactive form, phosphorylase b (sometimes called dephosphophosphory-lase) and an active form, phosphorylase a. Phosphorylase b can be activated by the addition of cyclic adenylic acid. Cyclic adenylic acid (cyclic 3′5′ AMP) in turn can be formed from ATP by the enzyme adenyl cyclase.

$$\text{ATP} \xrightarrow{\text{adenyl cyclase}} 3'5' \text{ AMP}$$

Adrenaline powerfully activates adenyl cyclase and increases the formation of 3′5′ AMP. Cyclic adenylic acid then accelerates the formation of phosphorylase a from phosphorylase b, by activating the enzyme phosphorylase phosphatase (PR enzyme).

$$2 \text{ Phosphorylase b} \xrightarrow{\text{Phosphorylase phosphatase}} \text{Phosphorylase a}$$

Phosphorylase a breaks down glycogen to give glucose-1 phosphate, and this is converted to glucose $6PO_4$ by phosphoglucomutase. Glucose $6PO_4$ is then dissimilated to yield metabolic energy. It is tempting to suppose that these series of reactions set in motion by the activation of adenylcyclase by adrenaline provide some biochemical background for the positive inotropic action of the catecholamines; however, although sympathetic stimulation increases the myocardial content of phosphorylase a, it is unlikely that the inotropic effect of adrenaline on the myocardium can so simply be explained, for adrenaline exerts similar effects on the phosphorylase of skeletal muscle and usually the catecholamine exerts no inotropic action in this latter tissue.

The Failing Heart

There are two schools of thought about what the underlying cause of myocardial failure may be. One group believes that there may be inadequate energy *production*; the other, that there may be inadequate energy *utilization* (for lit. see Davis, 1965).

Fleckenstein *et al.* (1967) have classified experimental heart failure into two types:

(a) The first type shows a reduction of cardiac contractility due to a deficiency of energy-rich phosphates—such a situation can be created by hypoxia, by ischaemia, by uncoupling agents such as dinitrophenol, and by cyanide.

(b) The second type is characterized by an adequate supply of energy-rich PO_4, but a deficient utilization of these compounds. This type of failure may be caused by interference with Ca^{++} in the excitation-contraction coupling and responds to therapy with Ca^{++}, cardiac glycosides, or sympathetic amines.

Fleckenstein considers that clinical congestive heart failure in man is more related to type (b). He has suggested that the enlarged fibre diameter and the increase in the mass and thickness of the myocardial fibrils might lead to difficulties in the excitation-contraction coupling by reducing the availability of Ca^{++} for the contractile system—perhaps simply because of the increased distance over which the Ca^{++} has to move.

As Bing (1965) states, the fact that there is no change in the extraction of metabolic substrates by the failing heart in man renders it unlikely that a disturbance in energy production is responsible for failure. Moreover, the patient, even with decompensated heart disease, may have a normal coronary blood flow and only a mild increase in his myocardial oxygen usage per unit weight of muscle, despite his increased diastolic heart size. His oxygen usage increases with exercise, so there appears to be no real impediment to the delivery of oxygen to the heart cells, and there is no clear evidence of myocardial anoxia in patients suffering from congestive failure.

Some attempts to implicate changes in the contractile proteins of the myofibril as a causative factor in heart failure have not yielded convincing evidence. As Bing writes, "our ignorance of the metabolic and structural factors that lead to myocardial failure has led to a Babel of theories and hypothesis".

References

Åstrand, P.-O., and K. Rodahl (1970). *Textbook of Work Physiology*. New York: McGraw-Hill.

Berne, R. M. (1964). "Regulation of coronary blood flow," *Physiol. Rev.* **44,** 1–29.

Bevegård, B. S., and J. T. Shepherd (1967). "Regulation of the circulation during exercise in man," *Physiol. Rev.* **47,** 178–213.

Bing, R. J. (1965). "Cardiac metabolism," *Physiol. Rev.* **45,** 171–213.

Bloom, W. L. (1955). "Demonstration of diastolic filling of beating excised heart," *Am. J. Physiol.* **183,** 597.

Braunwald, E., J. Ross, Jr., and E. H. Sonnenblick (1967). "Mechanisms of contraction of the normal and failing heart," *New England J. Med.* **277,** 794–800, 853–63, 910–20, 962–71, 1012–1022.

Brecher, G. A. (1958). "Critical review of recent work on ventricular diastolic suction," *Circ. Res.* **6,** 554–66.

Brecher, G. A., and A. T. Kissen (1958). "Ventricular diastolic suction at normal arterial pressures," *Circ. Res.* **6,** 100–106.

Burton, A. C. (1965). *Physiology and biophysics of the circulation*. Chicago: Year Book Med. Publ.

Davis, J. O. (1965). "The physiology of congestive heart failure," *Handbook of Physiology*, 2, Circulation **III,** 2071–2122.

De Geest, H., M. N. Levy, H. Zierke, and R. F. Lipman (1965). "Depression of ventricular contractility by stimulation of the vagal nerves," *Circ. Res.* **17,** 222–35.

Fleckenstein, A., H. J. Döring, and H. Kammermeier (1967). "Experimental heart failure due to inhibition of utilization of high-energy phosphates," in *Coronary Circulation and Energetics of the Myocardium* (ed. G. Marchetti and B. Taccardi), pp.220–36. Basel: Karger.

Folkow, B., and L. R. Yonce (1967). "The negative inotropic effect of vagal stimulation on the heart ventricles of the duck," *Acta Physiol. Scand.* **71,** 77–84.

Gregg, D. E. (1966). "The output of the heart and the regulation of its action, Chap. 44 in *The physiological basis of medical practice* (ed. C. H. Best and N. H. Taylor), 8th ed., pp.795–812. Edinburgh: Livingstone.

Hajdu, S., and E. Leonard (1959). "The cellular basis of cardiac glycoside action," *Pharmacol. Rev.* **11,** 173–209.

Hamilton, W. F. (1955). "Role of Starling concept in regulation of the normal circulation," *Physiol. Rev.,* **35,** 160–68.

Ledsome, J. R., and R. J. Linden (1964). "A reflex increase in heart rate from distension of the pulmonary vein-atrial junctions," *J. Physiol.* **170,** 456–73.

Liljestrand, G., E. Lysholm, and G. Nylin (1938). "The immediate effect of muscular work on the stroke and heart volume in man," *Scand. Arch. Physiol.* **80,** 265–82.

Linden, R. J. (1963). "The control of the output of the heart," Chap. 10 in *Recent advances in physiology* (ed. by R. Creese), 8th ed., p. 330. London: Churchill.

Linden, R. J. (1965). "The regulation of the output of the mammalian heart," *Scient. Basis Med. Ann. Rev.* 164–85. London: Athlone Press.

Linden, R. J. (1968). "The heart-ventricular function," *Anaesthesia,* **23,** 566–84.

Linden, R. J., and J. H. Mitchell (1960). "Relation between left ventricular diastolic pressure and myocardial segment length and observations on the contribution of atrial systole," *Circ. Res.,* **8,** 1092–99.

McDowall, R. J. S. (1951). *Handbook of physiology,* 41st ed. London: Murray.

Mitchell, J. H., R. J. Linden, and S. J. Sarnoff (1960). "Influence of cardiac sympathetic and vagal nerve stimulation on the relation between left ventricular diastolic pressure and myocardial segment length," *Circ. Res.* **8,** 1100–1107.

Rushmer, R. F. (1961). *Cardiovascular dynamics,* 2nd ed. London: Saunders.

Rushmer, R. F., A. O. Smith, Jr., and E. P. Lasher (1960). "Neural mechanisms of cardiac control during exertion," *Physiol. Rev.* **40,** 27–34.

Sarnoff, S. J. (1955). "Myocardial contractility as described by ventricular function curves: Observations on Starling's law of the heart," *Physiol. Rev.* **35,** 107–22.

Sarnoff, S. J., and J. H. Mitchell (1962). "Control of function of heart," *Handbook of Physiology,* 2, Circulation **I,** 489–532.

Sarnoff, S. J., E. Braunwald, G. H. Welch, Jr., R. B. Case, W. N. Stainsby, and R. Macruz (1958a). "Haemodynamic determinants of oxygen consumption of the heart with special reference to the tension-time index," *Am. J. Physiol.* **192,** 148–56.

Sarnoff, S. J., R. B. Case, G. H. Welch, Jr., E. Braunwald, and W. N. Stainsby (1958b). "Performance characteristics and oxygen debt in a nonfailing, metabolically supported, isolated heart preparation," *Am. J. Physiol.* **192,** 141–47.

Sarnoff, S. J., S. K. Brockman, J. P. Gilmore, R. J. Linden, and J. H. Mitchell (1960). "Regulation of ventricular contraction: Influence of cardiac sympathetic and vagal nerve stimulation on atrial and ventricular dynamics," *Circ. Res.* **8,** 1108–22.

Starling, E. H. (1918). *The Linacre Lecture on the law of the heart.* London: Longmans, Green.

Starling, E. H. (1920). "On the circulatory changes associated with exercise," *J. Roy. Army M. Corps.* **34,** 258–75.

13

Cardiac Electrophysiology and the Arrhythmias

Intracellular Recordings of the Membrane Potential

Basic Features of the Membrane Potential in Nerve and Muscle Cells

General Considerations

No hospital has a clinical ward 13, and many cardiovascular physiologists, after glancing hurriedly through the pages in the accompanying section, might quickly conclude that the same should obtain for the present Chapter 13. S. J. Perelman, in his masterly series of essays published under the title *Crazy like a Fox*, claimed to know so little about electricity that were he to receive a wrapped parcel from an electrician's shop, by so much as carrying it across the room in its wrapping he could be guaranteed a third-degree burn by the time he arrived at the far side. Some people whose expertise extends over the cardiovascular system as a whole nevertheless affect a profound disinterest in cardiac electrophysiology. For such the following text will arouse scant enthusiasm. Nevertheless, we feel that some account of the mechanism of initiation of the heart beat and the performance of one of the most important pacemaker mechanisms yet developed, is obligatory; our advice is "courage mes enfants".

When a membrane separating two solutions is permeable to only one species of ion, say K^+, a potential difference develops across the membrane.

$$E_m = \frac{RT}{F} \log_e \frac{[K^+]_o}{[K^+]_i}$$

$$= 61 \log_{10} \frac{[K^+]_o}{[K^+]_i} \quad \text{mV} \qquad \text{(at } 37°\text{C)}$$

This is an example of the Nernst equation. E_m is the equilibrium potential —that at which the concentration gradient exerts a force balanced by the force exerted by the voltage gradient which tends to move the ion in a direction opposite to that of the concentration gradient. In the case of a cation such as K^+ its equilibrium potential can be written as E_K. As $E_m = E_K$, and E_m is the inside potential relative to that outside, then $E_m = E_K$ must be negative, because the ratio

$\frac{[K^+]_o}{[K^+]_i}$ is less than unity ($[K^+]_o = 5$ mM/l, $[K^+]_i = 150$ mM/l).

If potassium were in equilibrium across the membrane, the membrane potential E would be:

$$E = 61 \times \log \left(\frac{1}{30}\right) \text{mV}$$

$$= -61 \times 1.478$$

$$= -90 \text{ mV}$$

Thus, the actual potential difference recorded (-70 to -80 mV) is not far from that of equilibrium for the potassium ion.

In the case of the sodium ion, however, matters are very different. At equilibrium E_{Na} would be:

$$E_{Na} = 61 \times \log_{10} \frac{[Na^+]_o}{[Na^+]_i}$$

$$= 61 \times \log \frac{150}{15}$$

$$= +61 \text{ mV.}$$

It is now known that the resting membrane of nerve or muscle is not solely permeable to K^+ ions but is also permeable to Cl^- ions and is not wholly impermeable to Na^+ ions. The potential developed across a membrane permeable to all these ions was calculated by Goldman (1943), who assumed a uniform gradient throughout the membrane. His equation gives:

$$E_m = \frac{RT}{F} \log_e \frac{P_K[\text{K}^+]_0 + P_{Na}[\text{Na}^+]_0 + P_{Cl}[\text{Cl}^-]_i}{P_K[\text{K}^+]_i + P_{Na}[\text{Na}^+]_i + P_{Cl}[\text{Cl}^-]_0}$$

Where the P values are those of permeability coefficients—i.e. the number of equivalents of an ion passing through 1 cm^2 of membrane per sec at zero potential difference when the concentration difference of the ion in the solutions is 1 equiv/ml. Obviously, if one ionic permeability coefficient is far greater than the others the Goldman equation reduces to that of Nernst.

Nerve Fibres

In a nerve fibre the resting membrane potential is of the order of -70 to -80 mV, as measured by direct impalement of a single cell by a micro-electrode connected through a galvanometer with an external electrode. It is reasonable to argue then that the value recorded at rest is *approximately* that expected from the Nernst equation and hence that K$^+$ ions are passively distributed. If this is so then the resting membrane potential should be influenced by variations of the extracellular [K$^+$], and such has been shown.

The resting polarized membrane is relatively permeable to K$^+$. When the membrane is *depolarized* by an outward flow of current, provided, say, by an applied cathode, sodium permeability increases fulminantly and a net inward movement of Na$^+$ occurs down the concentration gradient. If the initial depolarization is large enough, Na$^+$ ions enter faster than the K$^+$ ions can leave and this causes the membrane potential to drop still further —from -80 mV to zero, and thence beyond to positive values of $+30$ to $+40$ mV, which approach that of the sodium equilibrium concentration. This extra depolarization increases the sodium permeability even more and accelerates the change of membrane potential in a "positive feedback" manner. However, as the membrane potential approaches E_{Na}, i.e. at the peak of the spike of the "action potential", the rise of sodium permeability is inactivated, whereas potassium permeability now increases. In nerve, this increase of potassium permeability restores the resting potential within 3 to 4 msec, but in heart muscle, this restoration takes as much as 300 msec (for reasons which will be discussed later). According to this ionic hypothesis the nerve membrane can be represented by an equivalent electric circuit (Fig. 13-1).

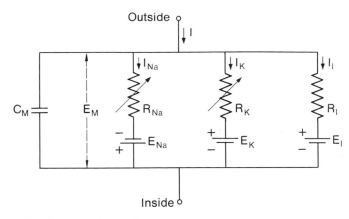

Fig. 13-1. Equivalent circuit for the nerve membrane. R_{Na} and R_K vary with membrane potential and time; the other components are constant. (From Hodgkin and Huxley, 1952. By permission.)

In Fig. 13-1 the membrane conductances are shown as parallel resistors in which $R_{Na} = 1/g_{Na}$, etc., and the diffusion tendency for each ion is shown as a battery of voltage equal to the equilibrium potential for that ion. From Fig. 13-1 it is obvious that the resting membrane would be negative inside, because R_{Na} would be high relative to R_K and R_{Cl} and its battery E_{Na} would exercise little influence on the net potential developed. Once R_{Na} becomes low, as during activation of the membrane, the sodium battery secures a positivity of the "inside" compartment.

Hodgkin, Huxley and Katz (1952) used the voltage clamp technique in order to measure variations in sodium and potassium permeabilities as functions of time and membrane potential. The method involves changing the membrane potential uniformly over a fixed area in a predetermined manner and measuring the resultant current flow through the membrane.

Hodgkin and Huxley (1952) showed that for squid nerve in sea water the permeability of the membrane to Na+ and K+ was best described in terms of the contributions which these ions make to the membrane conductance. The individual ionic conductances are defined by the equations:

$$g_{Na} = \frac{I_{Na}}{E_m - E_{Na}} \tag{1}$$

$$g_K = \frac{I_K}{E_m - E_K} \tag{2}$$

where the conductances are expressed in mmho/cm², the ionic currents in μA/cm², and the potentials in mV.

The total membrane current is given by the sum of the ionic currents and the current flowing into the membrane capacity.

$$I_m = C_m \frac{dE_m}{dt} + I_{Na} + I_K + I_{An}$$

In squid nerve, changes in the membrane potential have a dual effect on g_{Na}. When the membrane is suddenly depolarized there is initially a very large increase of g_{Na}, but even if the depolarization is maintained sodium conductance quickly falls again to a low value. The initial increase in g_{Na} depends on the previous value of the membrane potential. Hodgkin and Huxley (1952) defined this behaviour by proposing that g_{Na} was determined by two variables, m and h, which varied with the membrane potentials in opposite directions and with different time constants.

$$g_{Na} = m^3 h \bar{g}_{Na} \tag{3}$$

where $\bar{g}_{Na}$ is a constant (maximal value of g_{Na}) and m and h obey the equations

$$dm/dt = \alpha_m(1 - m) - \beta_m m \tag{4}$$
$$dh/dt = \alpha_h(1 - h) - \beta_h h \tag{5}$$

where the α and β factors are rate constants which are functions of E_m but not of t. The dependence of h on E_m describes the relationship between the initial membrane potential and the maximal sodium current switched on by depolarization.

In other words, depolarization "turns on" a sodium battery switch and the sodium conductance value rises to a maximum value ($\bar{g}_{Na}$); the sodium conductance at any one time could be expressed as a function m of this maximum, m having a value between 0 and 1. The fraction m is a function of voltage and time. Once the sodium switch is turned on and m increases, it begins to turn itself off, so that there is only a transient but fulminant flash of sodium current lasting a millisecond or so. This is expressed by the factor h, which also varies between 0 and 1, but in a direction oppositely related to the voltage. At the resting potential h is nearly 1, but, as m is so small, little if any sodium current flows. Depolarization increases m from

nearly zero towards 1, and the rate constants that determine the relationship between the membrane voltage and m are faster than those that diminish h. Momentarily, then, both switches (m and h) are on together, and a
large sodium current flows. Once depolarization is achieved, however, m
begins to diminish and this turns the sodium current off again.

The equations may be given a physical basis if g_{Na} is presumed to be
proportional to the number of sites on the inside of the membrane that are
occupied simultaneously by three activating molecules but are not blocked
by an inactivating molecule. m then represents the proportion of inactivating molecules on the inside and $1 - m$ the proportion on the outside.
h is the proportion of inactivating molecules on the outside and $1 - h$ the
proportion on the inside. α_m or β_h and β_m or α_h represent the transfer rate
constants in the two directions.

Measurements of changes of potassium conductance on depolarization
led Hodgkin and Huxley to infer that g_K was proportional to the fourth
power of a variable n which obeyed a first-order equation.

$$g_K = \bar{g}_K n^4 \tag{6}$$
$$dn/dt = \alpha_n(1 - n) - \beta_n n \tag{7}$$

Where $\bar{g}_K$ is a constant with the dimensions of conductance/cm^2, α_n and β_n
are rate constants that vary with voltage but not with time, and n is a
dimensionless variable that varies between 0 and 1.

Again, these equations may be given a physical basis by assuming that
potassium ions can only cross the membrane when four similar particles
occupy a certain region of the membrane. n represents the proportion of the
particles, say inside the membrane and $1 - n$ the proportion outside. α_n
determines the rate of transfer from outside inward and β_n the transfer in
the opposite direction. If the particle has a negative charge α_n should increase and β_n should decrease when the membrane is depolarized.

Both α_n and α_m have low values in the resting membrane, as have n and
m. Depolarization increases α_n and α_m and both potassium conductance
and sodium conductance rise rapidly, but because α_m is always more than
10 times larger than α_n sodium conductance increases more quickly. The β
rate constants vary in the opposite direction, becoming smaller as the
membrane depolarizes and taking higher values as the membrane potential
increases.

The rise of potassium conductance, then, lags behind that of g_{Na}, but
as it occurs, the outward movement of K$^+$, together with the inactivation

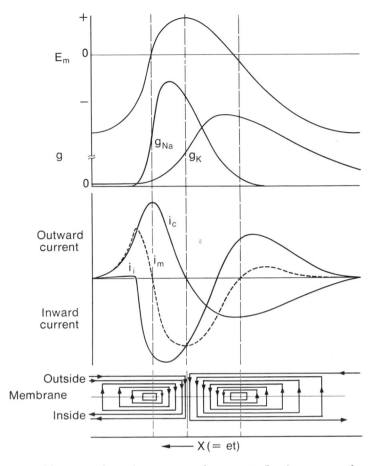

Fig. 13-2. Changes of conductance and currents flowing across the membrane during propagated action potential. Interrupted vertical lines indicate corresponding points on curves. Lowest diagram shows local circuit currents flowing between different regions of membrane. First stage of depolarization, "foot" of the action potential, occurs before any appreciable rise in g_{Na} or membrane ionic current (i_i) occurs. During this time the membrane current is generated by other areas of membrane where large conductance changes have already occurred. This local circuit depolarization then triggers changes in conductance that generate the rest of the action potential. The propagated action potential differs from the "membrane" action potential in that during a "membrane" response, the membrane current crossing from inside to outside (i_m) is zero and the membrane ionic current (i_i) and the membrane capacity current (i_c) are equal and opposite. This is true at only two points during a propagated response. Abscissa is x (distance along the fibre) and as x = et, it is proportional to time. (From Noble, 1966. By permission.)

205

of g_{Na}, helps to restore the negative resting potential (repolarization). The entire process of depolarization and repolarization in the squid axon occupies no more than 3 msec. A very useful diagram by Noble (1966) will help the reader to understand the variations in m, h, or n, and their rate constants during activity (Fig. 13-2).

Skeletal Muscle

In the main, skeletal muscle action potentials can be described in terms of the sequential movements of sodium and potassium ions across the membrane following excitation. Sodium conductance increases fulminantly on excitation but returns more slowly to its resting level. Similarly, potassium permeability increases (more slowly than does that of sodium), but the increase is short-lived. The high membrane capacity (10 μF/cm^2) for muscle compared with that of nerve (1 μF/cm^2) is a complicating factor,

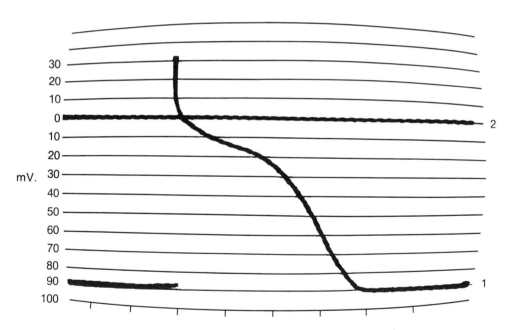

Fig. 13-3. Action potential of dog Purkinje fibre, recorded internally with fine micropipette. Ordinate: inside potential relative to value recorded by pipette in Ringer's outside fibre before penetration. Potentials above zero line are positive inside; those below zero line are negative inside. Resting potential, −90 mv. Potential at peak of activity, +31 mv. Time intervals, 0.1 sec. (From Draper and Weidmann, 1951. By permission.)

requiring as it does a much greater movement of Na^+ and K^+ per impulse to depolarize and repolarize the membrane. However, the action potential in frog skeletal muscle lasts only 12 msec or so at a temperature of 13°C.

Cardiac Muscle

Cardiac muscle action potentials differ considerably from those in nerve or skeletal muscle (Fig. 13-3). First, although they show the usual rapid reversal from a negative resting potential of -90 mV to a positive value of $+30$ mV on excitation, the "spike" achieved by this fulminant reversal is succeeded by a rapid but partial decline to a membrane potential of -10 to -20 mV, and this value is then maintained as a "plateau" for 200 to 300 msecs before rapid repolarization occurs to a diastolic level (for ref. see Woodbury, 1962; Trautwein 1963; Noble, 1966).

Second, although the membrane impedance falls during the initial spike of the action potential, it rises again during the plateau to a value equal to or greater than that during rest. Lastly, in certain fibres—notably those of the sinus venosus or sino-atrial node and those in Purkinje tissue—the termination of the "plateau" by rapid repolarization is followed by a slow depolarization (the pacemaker potential) which is responsible for initiating spontaneous action potentials.

In order to compute long-lasting action potentials from the Hodgkin-Huxley equations it is necessary to increase the time constants of the n equations or of the h equations greatly, but this is not in itself sufficient, for such manipulations yield a calculated action potential in which the membrane resistance during the plateau is several times *smaller* than the resting resistance. To account for the high plateau impedance referred to above, it is necessary to postulate a system in which g_K *falls* when the membrane is depolarized. In such a system a correspondingly lower value for g_{Na} is required during the plateau and the high impedance can then be reproduced (Noble, 1962, 1966).

Potassium Current. Hutter and Noble (1960) used the thick noncontractile Purkinje fibres to examine whether potassium conductance did decrease on depolarization. Single fibres were impaled with two closely adjacent microelectrodes and rectangular current pulses were passed through one electrode. Only limited information could be obtained on changes in membrane conductance occurring within a few milliseconds, but slow changes, such as take place during the plateau of the cardiac action potential, were recorded.

The current voltage relations were studied in sodium-deficient solutions (Fig. 13-4). In contrast to the situation in squid nerve, depolarization *decreased* potassium conductance.

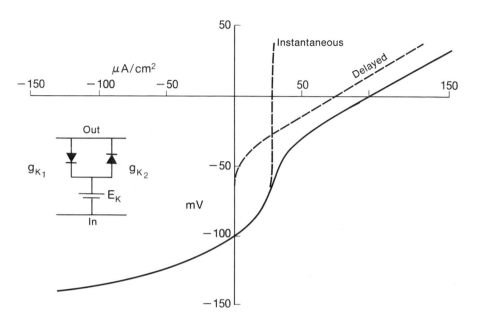

Fig. 13-4.. Current voltage relations described by K equations. Ordinate: membrane potential (mV); abscissa: potassium current (μA/cm$_2$). Interrupted curves show current-voltage relations in the two types of K channel (K$_1$ and K$_2$). The continuous curve shows total steady-state current. (From Noble, 1962. By permission.)

Noble (1966), for the purpose of describing the potassium current mathematically, supposed that K$^+$ might move through two types of channels in the membrane. In one type of channel, the potassium conductance g_{K_1} was assumed to be an instantaneous function of the membrane potential and to fall when the membrane is depolarized—showing anomalous rectification. In the other, the conductance g_{K_2} was assumed to rise slowly when the membrane is depolarized. These channels were represented in the circuit diagram (Fig. 13-5) by two parallel rectifiers, both of which are in series with the potassium battery. g_{K_1} is represented by a rectifier which

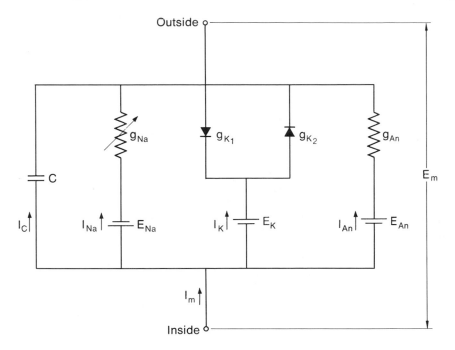

Fig. 13-5. Equivalent electrical circuit for Purkinje fibre membrane. Explanation in text. (From Noble, 1962. By permission.)

passes inward current easily and g_{K_2} by a rectifier which passes outward current easily. Noble described g_{K_1} by an empirical equation,

$$g_{K_1} = 1.2 \exp\left[\frac{(-E_m - 90)}{50}\right] + 0.015 \exp\left[\frac{(E_m + 90)}{60}\right] \qquad (8)$$

whereas he described g_{K_2} by modifying Hodgkin and Huxley's equations for potassium current. He made these two modifications: (a) the maximal value $\bar{g}_{K_2}$ of g_{K_2} was given a much smaller value than that in nerve, in order that the increase in g_{K_2}, which occurs on depolarization, should not offset the decrease in g_{K_1}; and (b) the rate constants α_n and β_n were divided by 100 to take account of the much slower onset of the effect in Purkinje fibres. The equations thus become

$$g_{K_2} = 1.2n^4 \qquad (9)$$

$$dn/dt = \alpha_n(1 - n) - \beta_n n \qquad (10)$$

$$\alpha_n = \frac{0.0001\,(-E_m - 50)}{\exp\left[\dfrac{(-E_m - 50)}{10}\right] - 1} \tag{11}$$

$$\beta_n = 0.0002 \exp\left[\frac{(-E_m - 90)}{80}\right] \tag{12}$$

The absolute values of the conductances were adjusted to give a resting conductance of about 1 mmho/cm². The potassium equilibrium potential was set at -100 mV, so that the total potassium current is given by

$$I_K = \frac{(g_{K1} + g_{K2})}{(E_m + 100)} \tag{13}$$

The current voltage relations described by equations (8) through (13) are shown in Fig. 13-4. The interrupted curve labelled "instantaneous" shows the current (i_{K_1}) flowing in the channel of the first type and the interrupted curve labelled "delayed" shows the steady-state current (i_{K_2}) flowing in the channel of the second type, given by $g_{K_2}{}^\infty\,(E_m + 100)$, where $g_{K_2}{}^\infty$ is the steady-state value of g_{K_2} at a given potential (after this potential has been held steady for a long time). Then dn/dt is zero and equations (9) and (10) give

$$g_{K_2}{}^\infty = 1.2 \left[\frac{\alpha_n}{(\alpha_n + \beta_n)}\right]^4 \tag{14}$$

The continuous curve (Fig. 13-4) shows the sum of the currents in the two channels, with a choice of constants such as to allow the curve to reproduce the experimental points determined by Hutter and Noble (1960).

The time course of the changes in g_K computed from these equations is shown in Fig. 13-6. An abrupt change of E_m causes a sudden decrease in g_K which is sustained for a hundred milliseconds or so; then g_K slowly rises over the remainder of the period of maintained depolarization. When E_m is quickly returned to the "resting" membrane potential of -90 mV, g_K increases above its own resting value and subsequently slowly falls.

Sodium Current. The Hodgkin-Huxley equations require only minor modifications in the case of the Purkinje fibre. Weidmann (1955), using a modified voltage-clamp method, studied the effect of the membrane potential on the rate of rise of the action potential in Purkinje fibres. He obtained a sigmoid relationship between the rate of rise of potential on stimulation of the cell and the "clamped" resting potential. The maximal rate of rise of the action potential occurred at a resting potential of

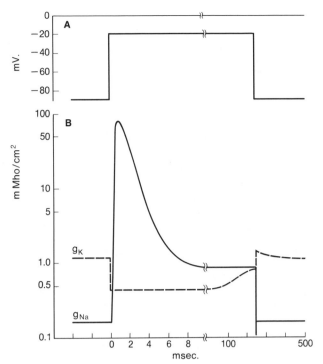

Fig. 13-6. Effect of resting potential on ion conductance in Purkinje fibres. *A* (above) shows a sudden artificial depolarization of resting potential. *B* (below) shows computed conductances (m mho/cm²) on a logarithmic scale. Continuous line: sodium conductance; interrupted line: potassium conductance. Note change of time scale after 10 msec. (From Noble, 1962. By permission.)

−90 mV. This maximum rate of rise of the action potential was thus determined by E_m and, as can be seen from Fig. 13-7, it was also dependent on the external sodium concentration. It was not affected by the external potassium concentration as long as the resting potential was maintained by voltage clamping. The only modifications required in the Hodgkin-Huxley equations for h is that the functions for α_h and β_h are displaced along the voltage axis (by about 20 mV) so as to make the relation between the membrane potential (E_m) and the steady-state value for h (h_∞) coincide with the experimental curve of Fig. 13-7.

$$h_\infty = \frac{\alpha_h}{\alpha_h + \beta_h}$$

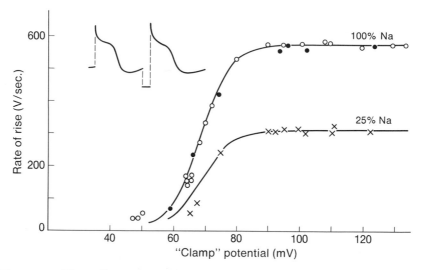

Fig. 13-7. The effect of membrane potential on the rate of rise (V/sec) of the action potential of a Purkinje fibre. The resting potential was "clamped" at various values before the fibre was stimulated. Open circles: normal Tyrode solution ("100% Na").
Crosses: solution containing 25% of the normal sodium content.
Closed circles: values obtained after restoring the normal Tyrode solution. (From Weidmann, 1955. By permission.)

Suitable equations for h (and m) were devised by Noble, and the computed effect of a long-lasting depolarization on sodium conductance is illustrated in Fig. 13-8 (see Noble, 1966). When E_m is suddenly changed from -90 mV to -20 mV it can be seen that, following the large fulminant but transient increase in g_{Na}, sodium conductance falls to a level which is thereupon steadily maintained during the depolarization and that this level of g_{Na} is appreciably higher than that at -90 mV. Repolarization rapidly restores g_{Na} to its "resting value".

Integration of Potassium and Sodium Currents. Integrating the necessary simultaneous equations by computer, Noble (1962) was able to reconstruct the action potential of the Purkinje fibre in terms of the changes in g_{Na} and g_K (Fig. 13-8), obtaining a graphic representation closely similar to those which can be experimentally recorded. The description of the conductance changes is as follows:

   1. During the spike of the action potential g_{Na} rises to a high value

because m increases much more quickly than h falls. Within a few milliseconds the fall in h causes a reduction in g_{Na}, but the inactivation is incomplete and, after a slight "undershoot", g_{Na} achieves a reasonably constant level ("plateau") at a value some 8 times that of the lowest value of g_{Na} in diastole. This fairly constant value of g_{Na} during the plateau

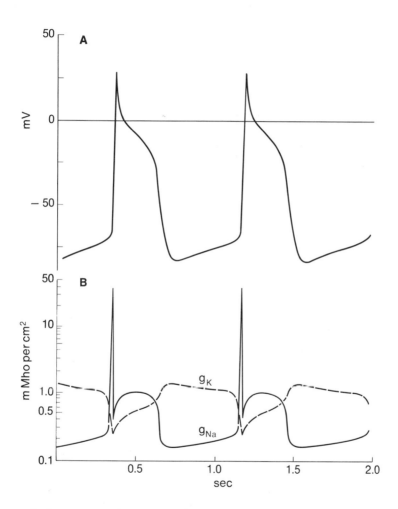

Fig. 13-8. A: computed action and pacemaker potentials.
B: time course of conductance changes on a log scale. Continuous curve, g_{Na}; interrupted curve, g_K. (From Noble, 1962. By permission.)

(despite the changes of E_m) is due to the fact that in this potential range m and h change in opposite directions so that m^3h is nearly constant. At the end of the plateau, during the final rapid phase of repolarization, the rise in h no longer fully offsets the fall in m and g_{Na} declines quickly to its diastolic value.

2. g_K (the sum of $g_{K_1} + g_{K_2}$), on the other hand, declines sharply at the onset of the action potential, owing to the fall of g_{K_1}. g_{K_1} remains at this lower value throughout the subsequent phase of depolarization, but g_K

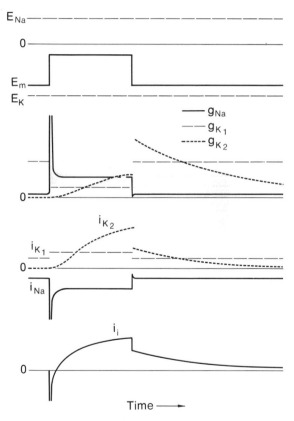

Fig. 13-9. Schematic illustration of the reconstruction of a voltage clamp current record in terms of the components of the ionic current. For the sake of clarity the capacity currents have been omitted. The reconstructed record (bottom) is similar to observed records. (From McAllister and Noble, 1966. By permission.)

again rises during the plateau owing to an increase in g_{K_2}. A further increase in g_K occurs at the end of the plateau when g_{K_1} reverts to its "resting value" on repolarization. g_{K_2} falls slowly from its increased level during diastole, so as a whole g_K exceeds its *end diastolic* value for 200 or 300 milliseconds during the pacemaker potential.

To recapitulate at this juncture, the events resulting from a sustained depolarization may be schematically illustrated (Fig. 13-9), describing the results of voltage-clamp experiments (McAllister and Noble, 1966). The step changes in E_m in relation to E_K are shown at the top. Below are shown the conductance changes (g_{Na}, g_{K_1}, and g_{K_2}). Note that g_{Na} remains quite high compared with its value at rest throughout the depolarizing clamp pulse. The sharp drop in g_{K_1}, which is sustained throughout depolarization, and the prompt reversion to the "resting" level, is shown, as is the delayed increase in g_{K_2}. Repolarization causes a further rapid rise of g_{K_2} to a high level from which it then slowly decays. The lower diagrams show the individual ionic currents and the total ionic current record.

When Noble originally computed the action potentials in 1962 (see Noble, 1962, 1966) there were very few results of voltage-clamp preparations of Purkinje fibres. Subsequent work (Deck, *et al.*, 1964; Deck and Trautwein, 1964; Vassalle, 1966; McAllister and Noble, 1966; Noble and Tsien, 1968, 1969) has furnished data which have modified Noble's original suggestions. Some of the points raised by these later papers are beyond the scope of this text, but one finding in particular requires further comment. Noble and Tsien (1968) obtained results which necessitate some modification of the interpretation given previously of the factors that govern g_{K_2}. They found not only that g_{K_2} also rectifies in the inward going direction for instantaneous changes in E_m, but also that at any specified potential, g_{K_2} is directly proportional to a first-order variable:

$$g_{K_2} \propto s^\gamma \qquad \text{where } \gamma = 1$$

(instead of $\qquad g_{K_2} \propto n^\gamma \qquad$ where $\gamma = 4$).

The new model for potassium conductance is shown in Fig. 13-10.

Changes in the magnitude of g_{K_2} at any one potential are determined by changes in s. Thus, if s increases by any given factor, g_{K_2} increases by the same factor at all potentials. The time constant τ_S for changes of s is a unique factor of Em and, as $\gamma = 1$, the time course of current change is always exponential. In this new equation the kinetic factor s is the fraction of activation and s_∞ is the steady-state fraction of activation. s kinetics

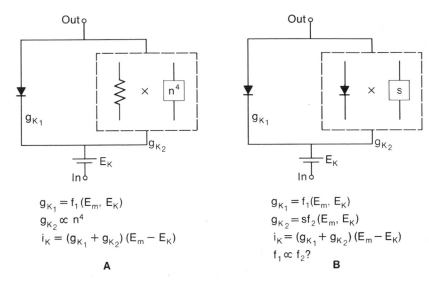

Fig. 13-10. Equivalent circuit diagrams for (a) Noble's (1962) K current equations and (b) the model obtained from the analysis of the results described by Noble and Tsien (1968). The major changes made in the new model are that g_{K_2} also shows inward-going rectification and that the exponent on the kinetic variable is reduced to 1. (From Noble and Tsien, 1968. By permission.)

are two orders of magnitude slower than are the n kinetics of nerve cells. They are very temperature-dependent ($Q_{10} = 6$ between 26° and 38°C).

The "slow potassium current" changes are very slow indeed over a wide range of potentials, as shown by Fig. 13-11, which relates τ_s^{-1} to E_m.

Determinations of the peak current change from background on return to holding potential, in voltage-clamped fibres subjected to depolarizing and hyperpolarizing clamp pulses, yielded the upper part of Fig. 13-11.

[It should be noted that

$$ds/dt = \alpha(1 - s) - \beta_s s$$

and that s_∞—the steady-state value of s—is that at which ds/dt is zero.

Hence

$$s_\infty = \frac{\alpha_s}{\alpha_s + \beta_s}$$

and

$$\tau_s^{-1} = \alpha_s + \beta_s.]$$

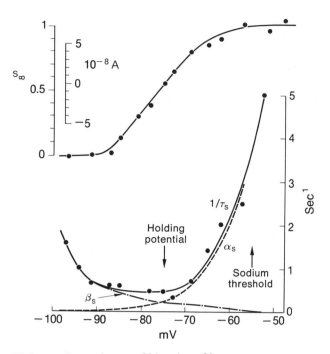

Fig. 13-11. Voltage dependence of kinetics of i_{K_2}.
Top: voltage dependence of fractional activation (s_∞) in the steady state measured as the peak current change from background on return to holding potential (-75 mV). Ordinates: peak current and s. Abscissa: membrane potential (as in bottom curves). Bottom: points show measured values of τ_s^{-1}. Interrupted lines show α_s $(----)$ and β_s $(-.-.-)$ calculated from $\tau_s^{-1} = \alpha_s t \beta_s$ and $s_\infty = \alpha_s/(\alpha_s + \beta_s)$, using continuous curves for s_∞ and τ_s^{-1}, drawn by eye through points. Arrows show position of sodium threshold and of holding potential. Temperature 36°C. (K) = 4 mM. (From Noble and Tsien, 1968. By permission.)

Pacemaker Potential

s_∞ varies from 0 to 1 over the range of potentials which characterize the slow depolarization which occurs during the *pacemaker activity* in Purkinje fibres, and this position of the $s_\infty(E_m)$ relationship is much more negative than was the slow g_{K_2} curve used by Noble in his original computations (see Noble, 1966). Noble and Tsien (1968) have calculated the changes in s, s_∞, and i_{K_2} which occur during the pacemaker potential,

using some data of Vassalle (1966). Fig. 13-12 shows that at the beginning
of the pacemaker potential E_m is so negative that s_∞ is virtually zero and
s will therefore decline slowly, for the time constants for s are longest in
this potential range. The i_{K_2} (t) curve from the calculation is in keeping
with the proposition that *this fall in i_{K_2} generates the pacemaker potential*. As a
result of a fall of i_{K_2} the inward sodium current during diastole slightly
exceeds the outward potassium current. The membrane potential slowly
but progressively becomes less negative until it reaches a critical level

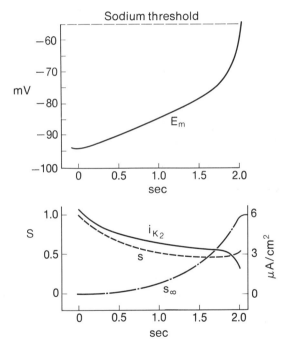

Fig. 13-12. Mechanism of pacemaker potential based on new model for K
current.
Top: variation in membrane potential during pacemaker activity, replotted
from Vassalle (1966, Fig. 1).
Bottom: s_∞ (t) relation obtained from s_∞ (E_m) relation shown in Fig. 4.
s and i_{K_2} were calculated from equations (9)–(11) using the rectifier function
for 2.7 mM (K_0) shown in Fig. 11 of Noble and Tsien. Note that, although s
does not fall below a certain value and actually increases towards the end of the
pacemaker potential, i_{K_2} falls continuously. This is a consequence of the negative
slope in the rectifier function. (From Noble and Tsien, 1968. By permission.)

(about -55 mV) at which the process becomes regenerative—g_{Na} then rises sharply and sodium ions enter quickly because $E_m - E_{Na}$ is so large.

The pacemaker potential is seen *only* in cells of nodal tissue and in the bundle of His and the Purkinje tissue. In the S-A node the rate of diastolic depolarization is 15 to 60 mV/sec and in Purkinje cells 5 to 40 mV/sec. The potential difference between the maximal diastolic membrane potential (i.e. the most negative value) and the threshold required for the next action potential to "take off" is some 15 mV in all these different spontaneously active cardiac cells. It follows (Trautwein, 1963) that the *threshold is attained earliest in the sinus* and the action potential generated there is conducted to latent pacemaker structures, arriving there before their own diastolic depolarization to threshold is reached. In this way the co-ordinated sequential rhythmic beat of the various parts of the heart is achieved. If the natural pacemaker of the S-A node is destroyed then the fastest latent pacemaker elsewhere (often the A-V node) takes over.

Cooling reduces the rate of development of the pacemaker potential and this explains the slowing of the heart beat when a cold thermode is applied to the S-A node. Stretching pacemaker tissue may have the opposite effect.

The depolarizing current in pacemaker tissue during diastole is carried by sodium ions. This current becomes increasingly effective because of the progressive fall of g_{K_2}. When the g_{Na} is largest, the effectiveness of a decrease in g_{K_2} in depolarizing the membrane is greatest, and the S-A node cells show the largest "resting" g_{Na}.

Vagal Action on Cardiac Nodal Cells

Hutter and Trautwein (1956) showed that vagal stimulation reduced the slope of the pacemaker potential recorded from a sinus venosus cell. If the vagus nerve was stimulated at a low rate the duration of the action potential and the refractory period was shortened and on regenerative repolarization the membrane potential achieved values more negative than in the control record. Stimuli delivered at 10 to 20/sec to the vagus abolished the pacemaker potential and caused hyperpolarization with cessation of the beat (Fig. 13-13A, 13-13B). The resistance across the cell membrane is markedly increased.

Acetylcholine causes similar effects on the sinus venosus and on the sinoatrial node, atrium, and atrioventricular node of the mammal, but has little effect on mammalian ventricular cells, at least in many species.

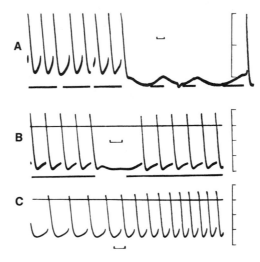

Fig. 13-13. Effect of vagal and sympathetic stimulation on pacemaker potentials in the sinus venous of the frog heart: (A and B) vagi stimulated during break in lower trace; and (C) vagosympathetic stimulation in an atropinized heart. Voltage calibration in 20 mV steps. Time: 1 second. (From Weidmann, 1957. By permission. Based on results of Hutter and Trautwein, 1956).

The effect of acetylcholine is due to an increase in g_{K_2}. This increase in potassium conductance drives the membrane potential towards the electrochemical equilibrium potential for potassium (E_K) and causes hyperpolarization whenever the membrane potential is less negative than E_K. Pacemaker cells are characterized by an appreciable resting inward sodium current which ensures that the diastolic membrane potential of these cells is always more positive than E_K. In a latent pacemaker cell, however, the diastolic membrane potential may almost equal E_K and acetylcholine therefore causes little or no detectable hyperpolarization. Trautwein and Dudel (1958) showed that acetylcholine caused a depolarization when applied to atrial cells subjected to a strong inward current (which raised their membrane potential above E_K). Furthermore, the membrane potential at which the hyperpolarizing effect of acetylcholine was reversed to a depolarizing influence became more positive when the extracellular potassium concentration was raised. Such findings prove that acetylcholine specifically increases g_K.

Hutter and Trautwein (1956) showed that vagal stimulation or acetylcholine application increased the rate of outflow of ^{42}K from the sinus venosus. The pacemaker tissue was first loaded with ^{42}K by allowing it to beat in a solution containing the radioactive potassium. It was then transferred to Ringer's solution and its rate of extrusion of ^{42}K was measured. Initially the rate of extrusion was rapid, but this soon steadied to give a predictable slope. The addition of acetylcholine to the Ringer's solution increased the extrusion rate threefold (Fig. 13-14). Atropine was then added to the bath, whereupon the loss of ^{42}K from the pacemaker tissue reverted to a rate seen before the addition of acetylcholine even though

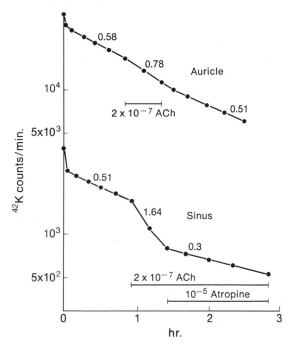

Fig. 13-14. An experiment on the isolated sinus venosus (lower graph) and right atrium (upper graph) of a tortoise heart. The tissues were loaded with ^{42}K and the rate of loss of the isotope was studied. The small figures give the rate constants in $hr.^{-1}$ at the different stages of the experiment. In the sinus venosus the action of acetylcholine was stopped by atropine. Abscissae: time (hr). Ordinates: isotope content of tissue in counts/min plotted on a logarithmic scale. (From Hutter, 1957. By permission.)

the acetycholine was still present (atropine prevents the membrane action of actylcholine). Similar experiments using atrial tissue showed an increase in g_K which was much less pronounced.

Sympathetic Action on Pacemaker Tissue

Sympathetic stimulation increases the slope of the pacemaker potential of the sinus venosus (Fig. 13-13C). It has no effect on the maximal diastolic membrane potential and does not influence the threshold voltage for regenerative polarization. As a consequence the rate of beat of the sinus cell increases (Fig. 13-13C). Adrenaline or noradrenaline added to the bath fluid likewise increases the slope of the pacemaker potential of either the S-A node or the excised Purkinje fibres of the mammal.

The mechanism of action of the catecholamines in this respect has only recently been clarified. Hauswirth *et al.* (1968) have studied the effect of adrenaline on voltage-clamp currents in Purkinje fibres. The membrane potential was voltage-clamped at -80 mV and the current changes following step depolarizations and hyperpolarizations were recorded. The current peak soon after return to -80 mV gives a measure of the degree of activation s, since $\bar{\imath}_{K_2}$ is constant when E is constant.

As $i_{K_2} = s \cdot \bar{\imath}_{K_2}$ (where $\bar{\imath}_{K_2}$ is the current when $s = 1$)

Then $i_{K_2} \propto s$.

Figure 13-15 shows the variation in s_∞ with membrane potential measured in terms of i_{K_2} at -80 mV. Adrenaline shifts the curve in the depolarizing direction by some 30 mV (*cf.* Fig. 13-11).

Figure 13-16 shows measurements of the rate of change of i_{K_2} as a function of E_m measured in terms of the reciprocal of the time constant of current change. ($\tau s^{-1} = \alpha s + \beta s$.)

Adrenaline also shifts this curve in the depolarizing direction, and at -90 mV (the beginning of the pacemaker potential) adrenaline causes a much faster change in current than occurs in the control solution.

Thus, at the beginning of the pacemaker potential, i_{K_2} drops much more quickly when adrenaline is present, and, moreover, as the steady-state relation between s and E_m is shifted in the depolarizing direction, i_{K_2} falls towards a smaller value and so accelerates depolarization of the membrane by the inward sodium current.

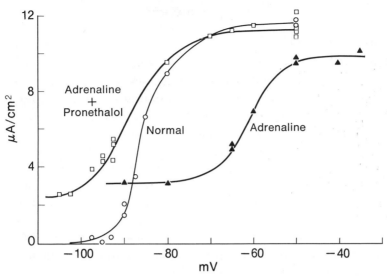

Fig. 13-15. Relations between steady-state degree of activation (s_∞) of slow K current and membrane potential, measured in terms of current immediately following return to -80 mv; O, normal Tyrode; ▲, adrenaline (5×10^{-7}g/ml); and ◻, pronethalol (10^{-6}g/ml). (From Hauswirth *et al.*, 1968. By permission.)

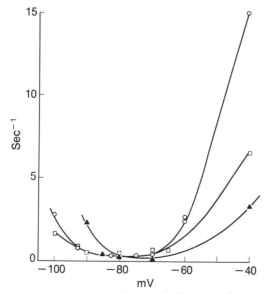

Fig. 13-16. Voltage dependence of rate of change of slow potassium current measured in terms of reciprocal of time constant (τ_s^{-1}) of current change. Symbols are the same as in Fig. 13.15. (From Hauswirth, *et al.*, 1968. By permission.)

Impulse Conduction

Although the myocardium is not a syncytium, the cells being separated from each other by the intercalated discs, these discs offer little hindrance to the intercellular conduction of the excitation process. The discs provide only slight hindrance to the diffusion of ^{42}K and their resistance is only $\frac{1}{2000}$th of that of the "regular" cell membrane.

Conduction velocity varies approximately according to the square root of the fibre diameter. In atrial and ventricular cells (average diameter $12\ \mu$) the velocity is 0.9 to 1.0 m/sec, whereas in thin fibres of the atrioventricular node (2 to $3\ \mu$) it is only 0.05 m/sec and in the thick Purkinje fibres ($40\ \mu$) it is 3 m/sec. The rapid conduction through Purkinje tissue ensures that different parts of the ventricle are excited nearly simultaneously.

The rate of rise of the action potential also modifies conduction velocity, which diminishes as this rate of rise slows.

Relationship between Electrical and Mechanical Changes

Papillary muscle preparations in which the fibres run approximately parallel have been used to study simultaneously the mechanical tension developed and the electrical changes which occur across the membrane of a cardiac fibre. Fig. 13-17 shows the typical action potential of a "non-

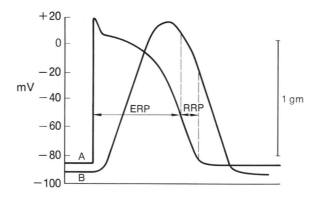

Fig. 13-17. Diagram showing relationship between membrane action potential (A) and isometric tension curve B, as recorded from a small piece of papillary muscle.

Note that peak of isometric tension curve is passed before the end of the effective refractory period (ERP) of muscle fibre membrane. RRP is relative refractory period. (From Brooks *et al.*, 1955. By permission.)

pacemaker" fibre and its isometric tension changes in response to stimulation. The figure shows that there is a considerable overlap of the action potential curve with the isometric tension record, though the peak of the tension curve is passed by the time that the membrane has repolarized to about -50 mV. Brooks *et al.* (1955) have shown that the *effective refractory period of cardiac muscle* lasts from the onset of regenerative depolarization until the muscle has depolarized to a level of about -50 mV. During this period, no matter how strong a stimulus is applied no action potential results, because there is virtually no inward sodium current. This long refractory period, which outlasts the peak of the tension curve, makes tetanization of heart muscle impossible.

Rhythmicity of the Cardiac Chambers

The results of cellular electrophysiological investigations, detailed in the preceding sections, help to explain earlier observations relating to rhythmicity of the different chambers of the heart.

None of this earlier work was more elegant than that of Stannius. By tying successively two ligatures, the first between the sinus venosus and the second between the atria and the ventricle, he proved that the heartbeat normally originates in the sinus venosus, but that after functional separation from the sinus the atria can act as pacemaker and even the ventricle possesses a latent rhythmic power when the occasion arises. Stannius's experiments cannot be performed on the mammalian heart, for the sino-atrial node—the homologue of the sinus venosus—is incorporated into the wall of the right atrium which precludes the tying of the first ligature, and the ventricles of the mammal, unlike that of the frog, are entirely dependent on a coronary blood supply. Therefore, the second Stannius ligature, tied round the atrioventricular ring, produces almost immediate ventricular fibrillation in mammals.

The Electrocardiogram

The electrocardiogram, introduced by Einthoven and developed by Lewis, gives useful information about the pattern of development of the excitation of the heart (see Schaefer and Haas, 1962). The electrical activity of the heart causes the development of small potential differences which, after suitable amplification, can be recorded from the surface of the body and displayed on a cathode ray oscilloscope or ink writing recorder. The sensitivity of the recording device is adjusted to give a 1 cm vertical deflection for 1 mV. Thick horizontal lines on the recording paper represent 0.5 mV and thin lines subdivide these, each line representing 0.1 mV. The paper moves at 25 mm/sec and broad vertical lines 5 mm apart subdivide the paper representing 0.2 sec. Thin vertical lines further subdivide the record—they are 1 mm apart and represent 0.04 sec.

Classical Bipolar Leads

The standard leads are I, II and III, respectively. Electrodes are attached to the right arm, left arm, and left leg, and these are attached in pairs across a galvanometer. Lead I is right arm and left arm, Lead II is right arm and left leg, and Lead III is left arm and left leg.

A typical ECG record shows a sequence of waves, shown diagrammatically in Fig. 13-18B. The P wave, which lasts about 0.08 to 0.1 sec, is attributable to the excitation of the atria. The record then becomes

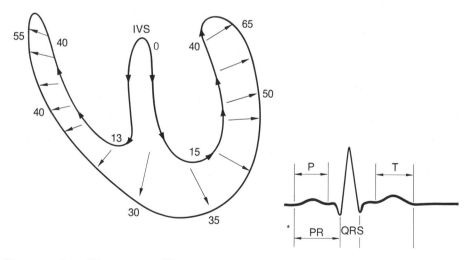

Fig. 13-18A. Diagram to illustrate the time relations of the spread of the excitation process in the ventricles of the dog. The figures show time in msec. O. represents the arrival of the excitation process at the top of the interventricular septum (IV5). (From Lewis, 1925. By permission.)

Fig. 13-18B. Electrocardiogram (diagrammatic).

"isoelectric" for 0.08 sec; this represents delay in the A-V node. There follows the QRS complex, which represents the invasion of the ventricles by the excitation process. The QRS interval lasts 0.08 sec and is followed by an isoelectric segment which lasts 0.12 sec. Finally, the T wave, which lasts about 0.4 sec, occurs; this wave is caused by the restoration of the ventricular myocardium to the resting state. The P-R interval lasts 0.13 to 0.16 sec (from the crest of the P wave to the crest of the R wave). It is indicative of the velocity of conduction of the impulse from the atria to the ventricles and in the healthy individual it should not exceed 0.2 sec. A prolongation of the P-R interval is usually due to damage to the bundle of His or its branches.

These three bipolar leads are called the *classical limb leads* and their use has led to an enormous amount of clinically important information (see e.g. Fig. 13-24). Thus, an absent P wave indicates that the sino-atrial node is no longer the site of origin of the cardiac impulse, as does an inverted P wave. In such cases the impulse originates usually in the A-V node. Atrial flutter is attended by multiple P waves, only some of which are followed by a ventricular complex. In atrial fibrillation the P waves are absent and the QRS complexes appear at irregular intervals.

Since the development of the classical bipolar limb leads, further investigations have added the use of *unipolar leads*. Here one electrode is placed on an area of the body surface and another, indifferent, electrode is maintained at zero potential by connecting all three limbs (right and left arms and left leg) to a central terminal through a 5000 ohm resistance. The unipolar lead and the central terminal are connected across a galvanometer, which records the potential changes which affect the exploring electrode only. Unipolar leads are described in Table 13-1.

Precordial Leads

One exploring electrode is placed on the chest. The indifferent electrode is kept at zero potential (Table 13-1).

Figure 13-19 shows how V_1 and V_2 represent right ventricular activity and V_5 and V_6 record left ventricular activity (the parts of the heart nearest the electrode). As the excitation process spreads towards the electrode this records an upward deflection, and, conversely, a retreating excitation wave is recorded as a downward deflection. (The wiring convention is that a downward deflection represents a state of negativity

Table 13-1

VR	Right arm
VL	Left arm
VF	Left foot
VC	Chest

Six chest positions are described:

V_1	4th intercostal space right of sternum
V_2	4th intercostal space left of sternum
V_3	Midway between left sternal border and mid-clavicular line on a line joining positions 2 and 4
V_4	5th intercostal space in midclavicular line
V_5	5th intercostal space in left anterior axillary line
V_6	5th intercostal space in left midaxillary line
V_7	5th intercostal space in left postaxillary line

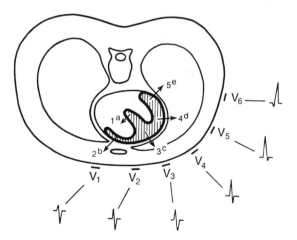

Fig. 13-19. Cross section through the chest to show the precordial leads and their relation to the heart; a, b, c, d, and e, show the order in which the electrical impulse spreads through the ventricle. Note the alteration in the configuration of the QRS complex between V_1 and V_6. (From Keele and Neil, 1965. By permission.)

relative to the indifferent electrode, and vice versa.) As the left ventricle is thicker than the right, electrical changes in the left ventricle dominate the precordial ECG. Hence, in V_1 the main QRS deflection is downward and in V_6 upward.

Unipolar Limb Leads

The unipolar limb leads represent the electrical activity of the part of the heart that faces the electrode (Fig. 13-20). VF records mainly the electrical activity of the base of the heart and the lower surfaces of the ventricles, VL the upper left side of the heart, and VR the cavity of the ventricles. The records are affected by respiratory activity. In deep inspiration the heart is vertical and VF records a QRS mainly from the left ventricle (similar to V_6). In expiration the left ventricle faces VL so the record of VL is like that of V_6.

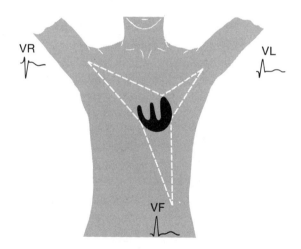

Fig. 13-20. The relation of the unipolar limb leads to the heart. The right arm lead faces the cavity of the ventricle. The foot lead faces the inferior surface of the heart; this may be formed by the right or the left ventricle or by both, depending on the position of the heart. The left arm lead may face the cavity of the ventricles or the outside of the left ventricle, depending on the position of the heart. (From Keele and Neil, 1965. By permission.)

Electrical Axis of the Heart

The standard or classical bipolar limb leads are used to calculate the instantaneous cardiac axis, or *vector*. The method employs the Einthoven triangle, which is based on the belief (an erroneous one) that the heart lies in a uniform volume conductor at the centre of an equilateral triangle with the limb electrodes at the apices of the triangle. Two standard leads must be recorded simultaneously and simultaneous points on the two complexes chosen—say the top of the R wave in Leads I and III. An upward deflection in Lead I means that the left arm is positive to the right arm, one in Lead III indicates that the left leg is positive to the left arm.

Fig. 13-21 shows an actual determination of the electrical axis. The axis is taken to indicate the *mean* direction of the wave of excitation at the particular moment chosen and its length represents the relative magnitude of the mean potential developed at that moment. If the direction of the axis lays out certain arbitrarily defined limits it is described as indicating left or right ventricular preponderance. In most normal subjects the mean electrical axis lies in the 0 to +90° range (Fig. 13-21). If the axis is more

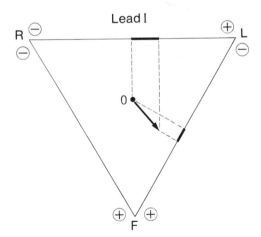

Fig. 13.21. Mean electrical axis is derived from Lead I and Lead III QRS complexes by drawing perpendiculars from the lead lines at points determined by the displacement of the point (from the isoelectric baseline) on the QRS complex determined simultaneously. The intersection of the perpendiculars gives a point which, when connected to the mid-point of the triangle (O), yields a line which gives the direction of the mean electrical axis E (its length gives the amplitude).

positive than this, then the records are deemed to betray right ventricular preponderance or right axis deviation—if more negative, left axis deviation. Many factors, however, modify the orientation of the mean axis—such as the orientation of the heart, the build of the patient, the rotation of the ventricles along a longitudinal basis. The scientific meaning of axis measurements is, to say the least, questionable, but clinicians continue to use the technique.

Vector Cardiography

This can be registered by leading the voltage from Lead I to an oscilloscope, connecting it in such a fashion that the voltage governs the horizontal deflection of the beam. Vertical deflection in turn is governed by Lead III voltage. The beam therefore describes three loops, one for the P wave, one for the QRS complex, and one for the T wave, successively. Between these loops the beam pauses because there is zero voltage in each of the leads. Such records reveal the influence of respiration on the orientation of the heart, for, although the loop moves on the face of the oscillo-

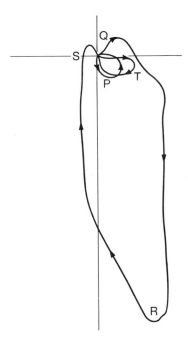

Fig. 13-22. Tracing from a normal planar vectorcardiogram.

scope, the shape of the loop is unaltered. The direction of the main or QRS loop really does give the simultaneous mean electrical axis (Fig. 13-22). Furthermore, the presence of a myocardial infarction, for instance, shows a halting of the beam track or a reversal of its direction as the QRS loop is described.

Cardiac Arrhythmias

The cardiac arrhythmias may be normal or abnormal. Normal subjects reveal sinus arrhythmia—a regular irregularity of the heart rate which is characterized by a quickening of the beat during inspiration and a slowing during expiration. This is partly central in origin; it is common in children and young adults, and less so as age advances. It is diminished in exercise tachycardia. All ECG complexes are normal in sinus arrhythmia.

Abnormal arrhythmias include *extrasystoles*, which may be atrial or ventricular, paroxysmal tachycardia, atrial flutter and fibrillation, and those of conduction defects—partial or complete atrioventricular block. Though a detailed description of these is beyond the scope of this text a brief note of each follows.

Atrial Extrasystoles

If atrial extrasystoles are occasional, they are of no consequence. They arise from irritable foci other than the sino-atrial node and give rise to a premature beat with, necessarily, an abnormal ECG complex. The ventricles respond to the atrial excitation. The P-R interval is prolonged because the rate of recovery of the A-V node and the bundle of His is longer than that of the rest of the heart.

Ventricular Extrasystoles

These may arise early in diastole, whereupon the beat is feeble and may not cause opening of the semilunar valves (Fig. 13-23). In such cases there is a deficit between the number of first heart sounds and the pulse rate palpated at the wrist. If the extrasystole occurs later in diastole the ventricular contraction may eject blood, but less than usual and the pulse beat at the wrist is small. After such an extrasystole the ventricle is refractory to the

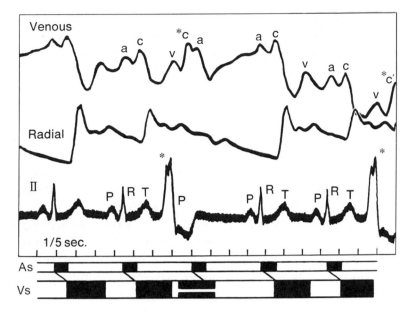

Fig. 13-23. Ventricular extrasystole. Simultaneous venous, radial, and electro-cardiographic curves from a patient, showing an extrasystole arising in the ventricle. The diagram placed below the figure illustrates the mechanism of the heart during the period of the disturbance. As, Vs = atrial and ventricular systole. The premature ventricular complex is abnormal in character; the P wave is buried in, instead of preceding, the ventricular complex. Similarly the c wave in the venous pressure curve is premature and precedes the a wave. The pause following the premature beat is longer than normal (compensatory pause); the atrial rhythm is undisturbed. (From Lewis, 1925. By permission.)

arrival of the ensuing atrial impulse, so, as no response is obtained, there is a "compensatory pause".

Paroxysmal tachycardia

This is a curious condition featured by sporadic attacks of tachycardia (150 to 200/min). It is caused by irritable ectopic foci in the atria or the ventricles. The attacks may last only a few minutes or even days. They may often be terminated by pressure on the carotid sinus, promoting thereby increased vagal tone. Such heart rates virtually cripple the circulation, for the diastolic interval for ventricular filling is grossly reduced and venous return is not boosted as is the case in skeletal muscular exercise.

Congestive heart failure may result, and in any case the attacks are liable to cause syncope. The patient becomes cyanotic and dyspnoeic. Quinidine may be required either by mouth or, in desperate cases, given intravenously.

Atrial flutter

This is due to rapid repetitive excitation from a single ectopic focus. The atria beat at 150 to 350/min and the A-V node cannot follow at this rate. Consequently a 2:1, 3:1, or 4:1 block results, the ventricle responding to every second, third, or fourth atrial beat. The regular P waves are multiple and some of them are buried in the T wave of the ECG records. The significance of atrial flutter depends essentially on the ventricular rate. If this is too fast, as in 2:1 block, diastolic filling is inadequate and the features resemble those of paroxysmal tachycardia. If 3:1 or 4:1 block is established the ventricular rate becomes regular at, say, 70 to 80/min at rest, but exercise tolerance is reduced for no further tachycardia can develop.

Atrial fibrillation

This is probably the result of the asynchronous discharge of multiple atrial ectopic foci, yielding an atrial rate of 200 to 600/min. Effective atrial contraction is eliminated and the ventricle beats completely irregularly at 100 to 150/min. The atrial P complexes on the ECG are small and irregular. Atrial fibrillation indicates organic disease unless thyrotoxicosis is present. Rheumatic myocarditis is a frequent cause. The failure of effective atrial contractile expulsion is itself of little consequence (indicating that the majority of ventricular filling is accomplished by venous return forced back to the heart by *vis a tergo*), but the effect of the irregular conduction of impulses to the ventricle by the A-V node and the bundle of His is more serious. The irregular ventricular beat may lead to congestive failure, hence it is important to institute therapeutic measures.

Digitalis provides a ready means of control of the condition. The drug actually increases the rate of atrial fibrillation, but its therapeutic action is to increase the grade of A-V block and to improve the myocardial contractility. Many patients have lived relatively normal lives for years, fibrillating continuously, under the therapeutic regime of digitalis. Quinidine also may be used, but *never* in cases of long-standing fibrillation. The reason for this lies in the fact that quinidine may convert atrial fibrillation to a normal effective rhythm of atrial contraction in about 50% of cases. This would seem to be the desired therapy, *but* long-standing cases of fibrillation often have ball thrombi in the atrial cavities, as a result of the continuous whipping action of the quivering atrial walls. If effective contraction is resumed these thrombi may be ejected into the pulmonary or systemic circuit, causing an embolus. Only fibrillation of short duration without evidence of advanced rheumatic myocarditis or history of embolic episodes and with no features of cardiac enlargement or congestive heart failure should ever be treated with quinidine.

Ventricular fibrillation

This condition is brief, for it causes immediate death. Only if it occurs on the operating table can it be recognized in time for effective treatment. A powerful electric shock delivered through cup electrodes placed on either side of the heart will often cause cessation of fibrillation and, with good fortune, a regular beat may be resumed. Modern cardiac surgery has led to full use of this technique.

Heart block

This might conceivably be due to defects at the sino-atrial node, or the A-V node, or the bundle of His. The first condition is rare, but when it occurs is usually iatrogenic and is caused by overdosage of digitalis. Atrioventricular block may be partial or complete. Partial block may appear as (1) delayed conduction with a prolonged P-R interval or as (2) dropped beats. Complete A-V block is featured by idioventricular rhythm in which the ventricles beat slowly and entirely independently of the atrial contractions. P waves and QRS complexes bear no relationship to each other, but the QRS complexes are of normal configuration.

Temporary A-V block is usually a feature of digitalis overdosage. Permanent A-V block is generally caused by a thrombosis of the coronary branch that supplies the nodal tissue.

Bundle branch block may be caused by coronary thrombosis or by diphtheritic myocarditis. The QRS complex is prolonged and there is a widening of the intervals between the pulmonary and aortic second sounds (compare Figs. 13-24A and 13-24B). This can be more easily detected when the right branch of the bundle is damaged, for the right ventricle normally contracts before the left.

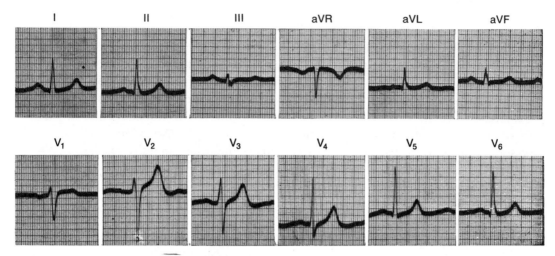

Fig. 13-24A. Electrocardiographic record of a normal man (Leads I, II, and III; unipolar limb Leads VR, VL, and VF; and unipolar precordial leads 1–6). (Courtesy of Department of Cardiology, The Middlesex Hospital; from Keele and Neil, 1965.)

to be compared with:

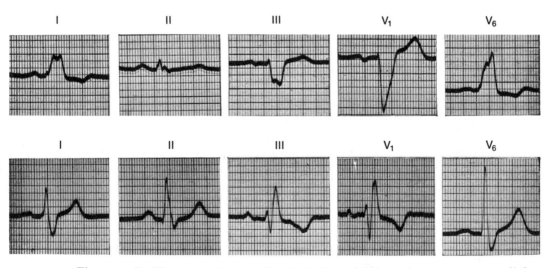

Fig. 13-24B. Electrocardiograph Leads I, II and III, and unipolar precordial Leads V_1 and V_6. Record A = patient with left bundle branch block. Record B = patient with right bundle branch block. Compare these records with those of the normal subject in Fig. 13-24A. (Courtesy of Department of Cardiology, The Middlesex Hospital; from Keele and Neil, 1965.)

References

Brooks, C. M., B. F. Hoffman, E. E. Suckling, and O. Orias (1955). *Excitability of the heart*. New York: Grune & Stratton.

Deck, K. A., and W. Trautwein (1964). "Ionic currents in cardiac excitation," *Pflügers Arch. Ges. Physiol.* **280,** 63–80.

Deck, K. A., R. Kern, and W. Trautwein (1964). "Voltage clamp technique in mammalian cardiac fibres," *Pflügers Arch. Ges. Physiol.* **280,** 50–62.

Draper, M. H., and S. Weidmann (1951). "Cardiac resting and action potentials recorded with an intracellular electrode," *J. Physiol.* **115,** 74–94.

Goldman, E. E. (1953). "Potential, impedance and rectification in membranes," *J. Gen. Physiol.* **27,** 37–60.

Hauswirth, O., D. Noble, and R. W. Tsien (1968). "Adrenaline: mechanism of action on the pacemaker potential in cardiac Purkinje fibres," *Science*, **162,** 916–17.

Hodgkin, A. L., and A. F. Huxley (1952). "A quantitative description of membrane current and its application to conduction and excitation in nerve," *J. Physiol.* **117,** 500–44.

Hodgkin, A. L., A. F. Huxley, and B. Katz (1952). "Measurement of current voltage relations in the membrane of the giant axon of Loligo," *J. Physiol.* **116,** 424–48.

Hutter, O. F. (1957). "Mode of action of autonomic transmitters on the heart," *Brit. Med. Bull.* **13,** 176–80.

Hutter, O. F., and D. Noble (1960). "Rectifying properties of heart muscle," *Nature*, **188,** 495. (London.)

Hutter, O. F., and W. Trautwein (1956). "Vagal and sympathetic effects on the pacemaker fibres in the sinus venosus of the heart," *J. Gen. Physiol.* **39,** 715–33.

Keele, C. A., and E. Neil (1965). *Applied physiology*, 11th ed. London: Oxford University Press.

Lewis, T. (1925). *Mechanism and graphic registration of the heart beat*. London: Shaw.

McAllister, R. E., and D. Noble (1966). "The time and voltage dependence of the slow outward current in cardiac Purkinje fibres," *J. Physiol.* **186,** 632–62.

Noble, D. (1962). "A modification of the Hodgkin-Huxley equations applicable to Purkinje fibre action and pacemaker potentials," *J. Physiol.* **160,** 317–52.

Noble, D. (1966). "Applications of Hodgkin-Huxley equations to excitable tissue," *Physiol. Rev.* **46,** 1–50.

Noble, D., and R. W. Tsien (1968). "The kinetics and rectifier properties of the slow potassium current in cardiac Purkinje fibres," *J. Physiol.* **195,** 185–214.

Noble, D., and R. W. Tsien (1969). "Outward membrane currents activated in the plateau range of potentials in cardiac Purkinje fibres," *J. Physiol.* **200,** 205–32.

Peachey, L. D. (1965). "The sarcoplasmic reticulum and transverse tubules of the frog's sartorius," *J. Cell. Biol.* **25,** 209–31.

Schaefer, H., and H. G. Haas (1962). "Electrocardiography," *Handbook of Physiology*, 2, Circulation **I,** 323–415.

Scher, A. M. (1962). "Excitation of the heart," *Handbook of Physiology*, 2, Circulation **I,** 287–322.

Trautwein, W. (1963). "Generation and conduction of impulses in the heart as affected by drugs," *Pharmacol. Rev.* **15,** 277–330.

Trautwein, W., and J. Dudel (1958). "Hemmende und 'erregende' Wirkungen des Acetylcholin am Warmblüterherzen. Zur Frage der spontanen Erregungsbildung," *Pflüg. Arch.*, **266,** 653–64.

Vassalle, M. (1966). "An analysis of cardiac pacemaker potential by means of a 'voltage-clamp' technique," *Am. J. Physiol.* **210,** 1335–41.

Weidmann, S. (1955). "The effect of the cardiac membrane potential on the rapid availability of the sodium-carrying system," *J. Physiol.* **127,** 213–24.

Weidmann, S. (1957). "Resting and action potentials of cardiac muscle," *Ann. N. Y. Acad. Sci.* **65,** 663–78.

Weidmann, S. (1967). "Cardiac electrophysiology in the light of recent morphological findings," *The Harvey Lectures*, Series 61, pp. 1–16. New York: Academic Press.

Woodbury, J. W. (1962). "Cellular electrophysiology of the heart," *Handbook of Physiology*, 2, Circulation **I,** 237–86.

14

Embryology of the Heart.
Foetal Circulation. Congenital and
Acquired Cardiac Abnormalities

The Development of the Heart

About the 19th day of human foetal life two cardiac primordia fuse to form a single cardiac tube which possesses an endothelial wall (endoderm) surrounded by a myoepicardial layer (mesoderm) in which differentiate the contractile myocardial cells (see Boyd, 1965). Rhythmic contraction begins on the 19th or 20th day. The heart tube grows faster than the cavity that contains it, and, as it is fixed at both ends, it bends to form a U loop. Even at this stage the tube shows three divisions—the atrium, which receives blood from the primitive veins, the ventricle, which has thicker walls, and the bulbus, which is continuous with the short ventral aortae (Fig. 14-1). A constriction of the caudal end of the tube forms the sinus venosus, which becomes then the site of confluence of the veins. From the 20th to the 42nd day the *external* appearance of the heart changes to one similar in general configuration to that of the adult. Constriction of the atrium, dorsally by the gut and ventrally by the bulbus, allows it to expand only sideways, and these lateral sacculations become the two atria. Increase in size of the bulboventricular loop is not accompanied by a parallel development of its two limbs, and as a result the wall between its two limbs

239

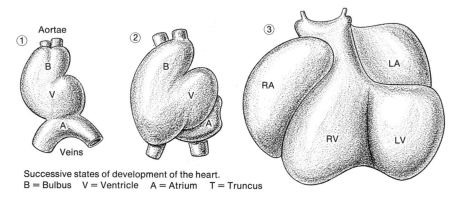

Successive states of development of the heart.
B = Bulbus V = Ventricle A = Atrium T = Truncus

Fig. 14-1. Successive states of development of the heart. B = Bulbus, V = Ventricle, A = Atrium, T = Truncus.

disappears, leaving the single primitive ventricle, separated from the two atria by the coronary sulcus. A median longitudinal groove, called the interventricular groove, is produced on the outer wall by the development of an internal interventricular septum.

Further developments include those in the interior of the heart (Fig. 14-2).

First a sickle-shaped septum primum grows down from the mid-dorsal atrial wall towards the ventricle. This fuses with two thickened parts of the endocardium which protrude, respectively, from the dorsal and ventral walls of the canal that initially existed between the atrium and ventricle. These endocardial proliferations (endocardial cushions) fuse in the middle, thus dividing the single canal into a right and left atrioventricular canal. The septum primum in turn fuses with this central partition. There are now (at 6 weeks) two atrioventricular canals separated by the structures described. The sickle-shaped septum primum is at first incomplete, for the sickle-shaped border leaves an opening, called the foramen primum, between the atria. This foramen is soon obliterated, but interatrial communication is quickly re-established by a degeneration, thinning, and perforation of the central part of the cranial end of the septum primum which forms the foramen secundum. Now an accessory interatrial partition develops, though this never reaches completion. This new septum, the septum secundum, grows down with a crescentic edge from the roof of the right of the septum primum between the upper part of this and the left

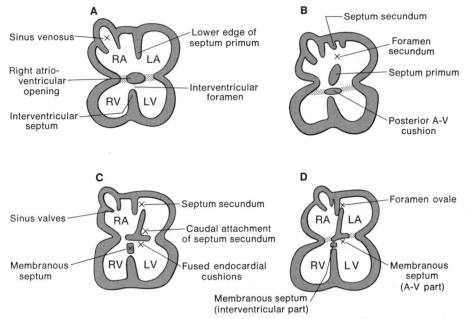

Fig. 14-2. Development of the interatrial and interventricular septa. A–D show successive sections.

venous valve. Its concave free margin forms the upper edge of the foramen ovale, which was the foramen secundum.

The foramen ovale permits blood to pass from right atrium to left atrium, and the position of the free margin of the septum secundum is such as to override the orifice of the inferior vena cava. Blood from the caudal part of the foetus and oxygenated blood from the umbilical vein enters the inferior vena cava and passes through the foramen ovale into the left atrium. Blood from the superior vena cava passes into the right atrium. This function of the septum secundum's free margin has led to its being called the crista dividens (see Fig. 14-6, page 246).

Meanwhile the sinus venosus dilates and is absorbed into the posterior wall of the right atrium. This region of the inner atrium becomes the smooth-walled part of the atrial cavity. The terminal part of the originally single pulmonary vein dilates and is absorbed into the left atrium. The primary right and left tributaries of this vein follow in this absorption to just beyond their junction with their two principal tributaries. This results

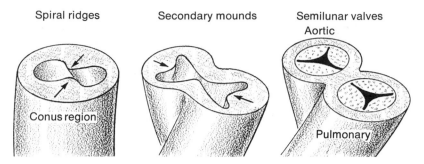

Fig. 14-3A. A. The semilunar valves develop during the separation of the truncus arteriosus by the spiral aortic pulmonary septum.
B. Pads of endocardial tissue develop at the site of the valves. These pads originate from the spiral aortic pulmonary septum and as secondary mounds on opposite sides of the channel.
C. When partitioning of the truncus is complete, three pads of endocardial tissue appear in the aorta and pulmonary artery. These pads are shaped and thinned out to form the semilunar aortic and pulmonary valves. (From Rushmer, 1961. By permission.)

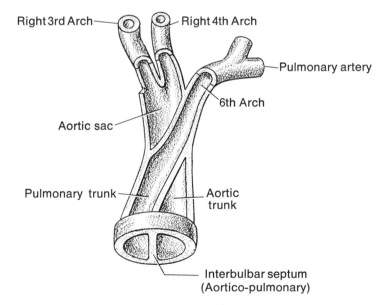

Fig. 14-3B. A scheme to show the division of the bulbus cordis by the aortico-pulmonary septum. Model is dissected and seen from its left side. (From Hamilton et al., 1945. By permission.)

in four separate pulmonary venous orifices, opening into the dorsal left atrium, which in this region is smooth walled on its inner surface.

Accompanying these atrial changes, alterations in the ventricle and bulbus occur (Fig. 14-3). The interventricular septum develops in the distal part of the truncus arteriosus to divide this channel into the *aorta*, which joins the left ventricle to the more cranial branchial aortic arch arteries (4th → 1st), and the *pulmonary trunk*, which supplies the 6th arch arteries from the right ventricle. Up to this time both ventricles are connected by the truncus arteriosus with the dorsal aorta through the six pairs of branchial aortic arches. When the truncus is divided the pulmonary trunk supplies the sixth arch (Fig. 14-3B). A remnant of the sixth arch still joining the aorta and therefore forming a communication between the aorta and pulmonary artery persists throughout foetal life; the remnant is obliterated shortly after the birth of the child (see page 247).

Subsidiary swellings of the mesenchyme eventually form the arterial valves (aortic and pulmonary, respectively; see Fig. 14-3A). The interventricular septum is not at first complete. Cranial to its free upper margin and caudal to the region of fusion of the endocardial cushions of the A-V canal a space at first remains—the interventricular foramen. Proliferation of the endocardial cushions and of the free edge of the septum close this region in such a fashion that the right A-V orifice opens only into the right ventricle and the left orifice opens only into the left ventricle (Fig. 14-2).

The right and left A-V valves arise by proliferation of mesenchyme surrounding the orifices of the A-V canals. The three cusps on the right A-V valve give the tricuspid valve its name; the two cusps on the left A-V valve resemble the mitre of a bishop, and this accounts for the nomenclature of the mitral valve.

The Foetal Circulation

The functioning lung of the foetus is the placenta, whence the umbilical vein delivers blood 80% saturated with oxygen to the foetal liver (Fig. 14-4; see also Chapter 29). At the liver some of this blood passes via the ductus venosus directly to the inferior vena cava and the remainder supplies the left two-thirds of the liver. The right third of the liver is

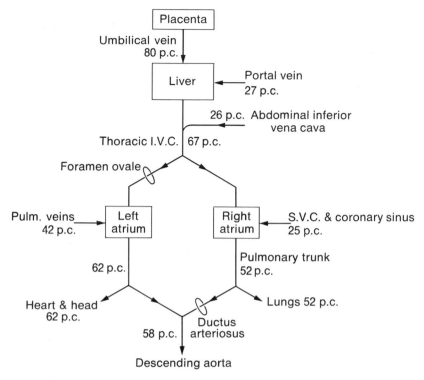

Fig. 14-4. Progressive dilution of well-oxygenated blood (derived from the placenta) by deoxygenated blood from foetal tissues, as it traverses the foetal circulation. (After Dawes; from Keele and Neil, 1965. By permission.)

supplied by the portal vein. Hepatic veins drain the liver and open into the inferior vena cava. Therefore, inferior vena caval blood reaching the right atrium is only about 67% saturated; the inferior vena cava stream is mostly directed by the crista dividens into the left atrium, while a minor component enters the right atrium. The right atrium also receives blood from the superior vena cava and the coronary sinus, and the mixture of these streams is delivered to the right ventricle, which pumps the blood into the pulmonary trunk.

Little of the right ventricular output gets to the lungs because they are collapsed and offer a very high resistance to its passage; most of it passes by the ductus arteriosus into the aorta (Fig. 14-5) as the pressure is lower here than in the pulmonary trunk of the foetus. Meanwhile the left ven-

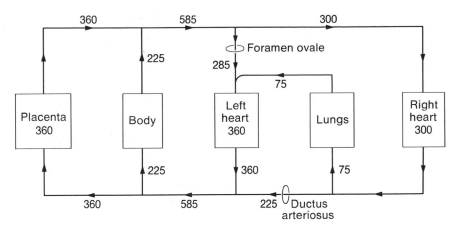

Fig. 14-5. Plan of foetal circulation in the lamb. Combined systemic output of the two ventricles is 585 ml. per minute. The left ventricle ejects 360 ml per minute and the right ventricle 300 ml per minute (of which 75 ml traverses the lungs and is finally ejected by the left heart). (After Dawes; from Keele and Neil, 1965. By permission.)

tricle expels the more oxygenated blood (60 to 65% oxygenated), directed from the inferior caval vein by the crista dividens, and most of this is delivered to the heart itself and to the head. The slightly less deoxygenated blood resulting from the mixture of right and left ventricular streams passes mainly to the descending aorta and thence to the viscera, limbs, etc., finally passing to the placenta as the umbilical artery. Umbilical capillaries are oxygenated in the placenta. Our knowledge of the details of distribution and of the state of oxygenation of the various parts of the foetal circuit largely stem from the elegant work of Dawes and his colleagues (see Dawes, 1968). Figures 14-5 and 14-6 are redrawn from his illustrations.

It will be noted that the right and left sides of the foetal heart work *in parallel*, not in series as they do in the adult. Equation of their outputs is not of paramount importance as is the case in the adult heart, and Dawes has shown that the left ventricle usually ejects about 20% more blood than does the right. Of the combined output of the two ventricles, 50% goes to the placenta and 30 to 35% to the body not including the lungs, while the lungs receive about 15%. Clearly the placenta is a low-resistance circuit, whereas the lungs provide a high resistance.

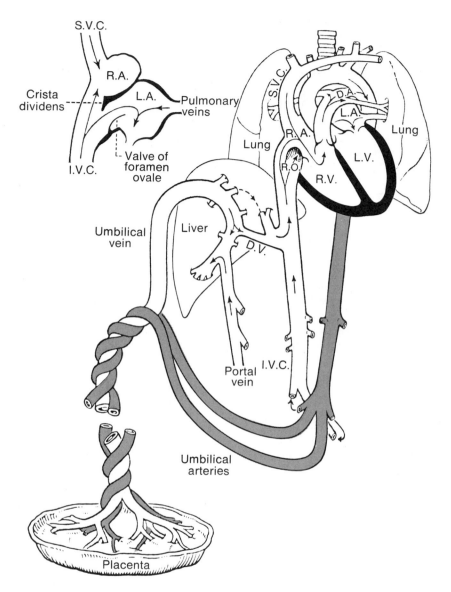

Fig. 14-6. A plan of the foetal circulation. The upper end of the inferior vena cava opens directly into the left atrium through the foramen ovale (see inset) as well as into the right atrium. (By courtesy of G. S. Dawes.)

RA and RV = Right atrium and ventricle.   DA = Ductus arteriosus.
LA and LV = Left atrium and ventricle.   DV = Ductus venosus.
SVC = Superior vena cava.   FO = Foramen ovale.
IVC = Inferior vena cava.
(From Bell, *et al.*, 1966. By permission.)

On delivery, when the umbilical cord is tied, there is a brief period of asphyxia, which ends with the first breath. Gasps give way to rhythmic breathing and the intrathoracic pressure falls during the gasps to values which may even reach 50 mm Hg below atmospheric. In 20 to 30 minutes, however, the distensibility of the respiratory apparatus has so improved that rhythmic respiration occasions an intrathoracic pressure oscillation of only 5 to 7 mm Hg, as in the adult.

Two significant alterations in the cardiovascular system occur shortly after birth. The ductus arteriosus constricts and the foramen ovale closes. These changes are of such fundamental importance as to justify their consideration in detail.

Closure of the ductus

Physiological closure of the ductus precedes its anatomical obliteration. Physiological closure is achieved by constriction of the wall which is attended by a gross diminution in the lumen of the ductus. This is achieved within 10 to 30 minutes of delivery. During this period the systemic pressure rises and the pulmonary vascular resistance and pressure fall. Consequently, the tendency is for the blood to pass from the aorta into the pulmonary artery if the ductus remains patent. Usually some degree of patency is maintained for hours or days, as evinced by phonocardiographic or stethoscopic evidence of a loud continuous murmur which reaches its peak simultaneously with the occurrence of the second heart sound heard over the left side of the chest. Commonly this murmur disappears within the first day of life in the human infant. The obliterative endarteritic process responsible for anatomical closing of the lumen requires months. The cause of constriction of the ductus is still unknown—it is not a nervous mechanism and it seems to be related to the improvement in the state of oxygenation of the blood and also the arterial pO_2. It is a thick walled vascular section and, when exposed to increasing O_2 tensions *in vitro* a shortening of outer muscle layers causes luminal obliteration (compare "critical closing", Chapter 5).

Closure of the foramen ovale

When the umbilical cord is tied there is a fall in the inferior vena caval pressure owing to the cessation of venous return from the placenta. The initiation of respiration causes a profound reduction of the resistance in the pulmonary circuit, and the increase in the left atrial pressure reverses the pressure gradient between the two atria which characterized the foetal state of the circulation. These changes cause an approximation of the valve flap of the foramen (crista dividens) to the margin of the interatrial septum. Functional closure occurs within hours, but, again, complete fusion of valve septum requires months. As many as 20% of individuals betray slight imperfections of closure of the foramen ovale, as evidenced by examination of the hearts of cadavers, which reveals that in these cases a small probe can be passed from atrium to atrium. Few of these cases are sufficiently marked to produce any functional disturbances.

Finally, it should be pointed out that the separation of the foetus from the placenta not only terminates the "venous return" of oxygenated blood via the umbilical vein, but stops the oxygen supply to the umbilical vein. This causes constriction of the umbilical vein. Once more, anatomical obliteration proceeds over the course of months.

The Diagnosis of Congenital Cardiac Disease

Cardiac catheterization

A hollow flexible catheter is passed from the antecubital or femoral vein into the right heart. The whole procedure is conducted with X-ray monitoring of the position of the catheter tip. Samples of blood are removed anaerobically from each successive section of the right atrium, right ventricle, and pulmonary artery system. Pressure measurements are also recorded at these various sites. Normally the right atrium has a mean pressure of 1 to 3 mm Hg and an oxygen saturation of 70 to 75%. The right ventricle shows a pressure swing of 20 or 25 to 3 mm Hg with each cardiac cycle and again the saturation of blood there is about 70 to 75%. When the catheter tip is pushed through the pulmonary valve to lie in the pulmonary trunk the pressure record shows a pulse of 20 to 25 systolic to about 10 diastolic. The oxygen saturation is still 70 to 75%. The technique was first used by Forssmann in 1929, in experiments on himself, and later developed for clinical use by Cournand and Richards (see Cournand *et al.*, 1949).

The left ventricle can be catheterized by the retrograde catheterization of the femoral artery: the catheter tip is gently pushed between the cusps of the aortic valve. The pressure in the aorta recorded from the catheter is 120/80, and the record changes to one showing about 120/5 when the tip enters the left ventricle. Further manipulation pushes the tip through the mitral valve into the left atrium, whereupon the pressure shows a mean value of about 5 mm Hg or so (Fig. 14-7). The state of oxygenation of

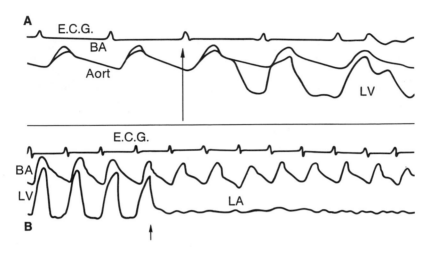

Fig. 14-7. Mitral stenosis; A = simultaneous pressure measurements in the brachial artery (BA) and in the aorta (Aort). The plastic catheter is withdrawn from the aorta into the left ventricle (LV) without change in the systolic pressure; B = the catheter is withdrawn from the left ventricle (LV) to the left atrium (LA). The mean pressure in the left atrium was 28 mm Hg. (Redrawn from Keele and Neil, 1965. By permission.)

these samples is normally the same: 95 to 100% saturated. An alternative method of recording pressures and oxygen content of the heart is to pass a bronchoscope and then pass a catheter with a needle tip into the left bronchus and manipulate this under "bronchoscopic vision" to penetrate the upper wall of the left bronchus and then the left atrium which lies immediately over it. Having reached the left atrium, the investigator can slip a further catheter through the lumen of the initial catheter and manoeuvre it into the left ventricle.

X-ray angiography

Radiopaque substances such as thorotrast can be injected through the cardiac catheter, which is initially placed in the required position, and serial X-ray films can be taken to record the passage of the radiopaque substance.

Dye Dilution Curves

When a dye is injected into a major vein its appearance on the arterial side may be recorded by either taking successive samples of arterial blood and determining the concentration of the dye in the plasma of the successive samples obtained by centrifuging, or a photocell records the alteration of light transmission across the lobe of the ear from a local light source (see Chapter 7). In this latter method the use of the dye Fox green is advisable for the sensitivity of the system to green is independent of the changes of

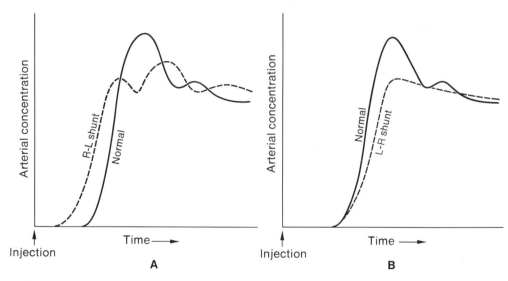

Fig. 14-8. Diagram of dye dilution curves (concentration-time) in normal subjects and in patients with either right to left shunt (a) or with left to right shunt (b). With R-L shunt some dye arrives early in the arteries having by-passed the lung; then there is a second peak. With L-R shunt some dye recirculates through the shunt; the peak is lower and disappearance is delayed.

colour of blood which may be produced by the presence of reduced haemo-globin (blue) instead of oxyhaemoglobin (red). Reduced haemoglobin is not uncommon in the arterial blood of patients who have a type of congenital heart disease associated with a shunt of venous blood from the

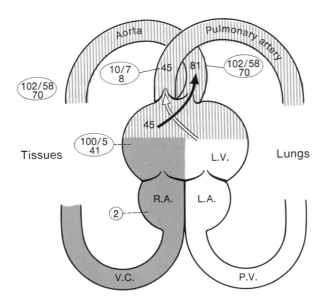

Fig. 14-9. Tetralogy of Fallot. Numerical figures *within* vessels show ml.O_2 content per litre of blood.
Circled figures indicate systolic, diastolic, and mean pressures. Dark areas—desaturated blood. White areas—saturated blood. Large systolic gradient of RV to Pulmonary Artery shows a marked pulmonary stenosis. Left to right ventricular shunt is small. Right to left ventricular shunt is large (indicated by arrows). (From Cournand *et al.*, 1949. By permission.)

right atrium (or right ventricle) into the corresponding chamber on the left side. Such blood bypasses the lungs and escapes oxygenation therein.

Normally the dye output record is as shown in Fig. 14-8. It is modified by the presence of a shunt (left to right or right to left) as shown in Fig. 14-9A and 14-9B and explained in the legend.

Clinical symptoms and signs

These are of course valuable in determining the likelihood of there being congenital heart defects and often in the accurate localization of such abnormalities. Their description in detail is beyond the scope of this text but some clinical features of each of the commoner syndromes are described below.

Developmental Abnormalities

The complicated mode of development of the foetal heart might lead us to suppose that many varieties of development defect—singly or in combination—might occur, and such is indeed the case (for ref. see Marshall *et al.*, 1962). Nevertheless, 85 to 90% of such defects fall under the headings of septal defects, patent ductus arteriosus, stenosis of the pulmonary or aortic tracts, and transposition of the major vessels.

Septal defects

These may be atrial or ventricular. *Atrial defects* are more common and can usually be detected by clinical methods, but even though such defects lend themselves to surgery it is necessary to make use of the special procedures described above to ensure that no other defects are present. Clinically the features are those ascribable to right heart hypertrophy (followed by ventricular dilation), an enlarged pulmonary artery, and the presence of a systolic murmur over the second intercostal space at the left parasternal line. The ECG may show right axis deviation and possibly signs of a partial block of the right branch of the bundle of His.

The reason for these changes should be clear. After birth pressure in the left atrium exceeds that in its right counterpart, so blood passes from left to right in an amount which essentially depends on the size of the defect. Consequently the right ventricle receives more blood than usual and ejects more blood because of its greater diastolic volume. (This is the Starling mechanism.) The right ventricle hypertrophies and the pulmonary artery responds to continued distension by enlarging and later by developing arteriolar hypertrophy. Cardiac catheterization shows that the oxygen content of the right atrium exceeds that in the inferior or superior vena cava. Surgery is required if the physical condition of the child indicates it. Fortunately, the operation now perfected carries a low mortality rate.

Ventricular septal defects are more serious, and such patients show a more rapid development of pulmonary hypertension. Initially the signs are those of a left-to-right shunt with systolic murmur, increased oxygen content of right ventricular blood, and a delay in the dye-dilution curve (Fig. 14-8), but eventually the pulmonary vascular resistance may increase so much that blood passes from right to left across the septal defect, thus causing the appearance of cyanosis. Finger clubbing and polycythaemia develop.

It is important to deal with ventricular septal defects early, for whereas their operative closure is technically feasible, once pulmonary arteriolar hypertrophy has occurred septal closure leaves the right ventricle with the enormous work of pumping the blood against this abnormally high pulmonary resistance.

Patent ductus arteriosus

As the pressure in the aorta greatly exceeds that in the pulmonary artery, if the ductus does not close, then blood passes continuously from the aorta into the pulmonary circuit, causing a continuous "machinery murmur" which reaches a crescendo in systole. Eventually pulmonary hypertension results but the condition should be diagnosed before this happens. Ligation of the ductus is surgically simple and 100% effective.

Aortic coarctation

This has been subdivided into "infantile" and "adult" types. The "infantile" type consists of the narrowing of a long segment between the origin of the left subclavian artery and the insertion of the ductus arteriosus. In the "adult" type the constriction is localized to the region of the ductus insertion. The condition is associated with the presence of a loud systolic murmur created by turbulence in the constricted region; this murmur is loudest at the base of the heart.

Coarctation throws an increased load on the left ventricle and causes left ventricular hypertrophy. The cardiac output is normal and the blood flow to the upper part of the body is normal or increased because the pressure in the vessels supplying the upper end is much higher. An extensive development of collateral vessels from the internal mammary and costocervical and thyrocervical trunks (all branches of the subclavian arteries) with the intercostal vessels which stem from the aorta below the site of the coarctation, secures a normal flow of blood to the lower part of the body. The femoral pulse is delayed and the peak of systolic pressure can be seen to be behind that in the radial artery when suitable manometric records are made. The mean pressure and the pulse pressure in the lower limbs are less than normal and are very much less than those in the carotid vessels.

Once more, early surgical treatment is important. Unfortunately many of these cases do not come to the physician's attention until some secondary complications occur.

Tetralogy of Fallot

This is characterized by four defects of development: (1) ventricular septal defect, (2) an overriding aorta with the aortic orifice overlying the interventricular septum, (3) pulmonary stenosis, and (4) right ventricular hypertrophy.

This syndrome probably results from an abnormal development of the spiral-shaped septum which is destined to divide the conus arteriosus. The septal ridges deviate to the right, thereby reducing the calibre of the pulmonary vessel and diminishing right ventricular outflow. The aortic septum fails to fuse with the developing interventricular septum, leaving a ventricular septal defect below the overriding aorta.

Pulmonary stenosis reduces the flow of blood to the lungs and causes right ventricular hypertrophy. The right ventricular systolic pressure exceeds that in the left ventricle and blood bypasses the lungs via the ventricular septal defect (Fig. 14-9).

Cyanosis and polycythaemia are consequences of the low pO_2 and increased content of reduced haemoglobin in the systemic arterial blood.

Right ventricular hypertrophy and a loud systolic murmur maximal in the third left intercostal space can be detected clinically and X-ray screening is helpful. However cardiac catheterization is always required to provide definitive confirmation of the provisional diagnosis.

Surgical treatment initially consisted of anastomosing the left subclavian artery to a pulmonary artery, thereby producing a patent ductus arteriosus.

This increases the blood flow to the lungs and hence the over-all oxygenation of the systemic arterial blood. More recently, operative repair has entailed pulmonary valvotomy or resection of the infundibular stenotic region.

Acquired Valvular Disease

Stenosis or insufficiency of the heart valves (see Werkö, 1962) are common causes of cardiac failure, being often combined with myocardial insufficiency.

Mitral stenosis

This condition is almost invariably due to rheumatic disease. When sufficiently severe (the mitral orifice being less than 1.5 cm²) the peak left atrial pressure rises and there is increased atrial dilatation. The pulmonary capillary pressure rises and may cause fluid transudation into the alveoli with attendant dyspnoea, and the production of bloodstained sputum. Haemoptysis results from the engorgement of the bronchial capillaries caused by the rise of pressure in the pulmonary veins (into which they drain).

Eventually, pulmonary congestion causes, successively, right ventricular hypertrophy, then ventricular dilatation, (perhaps tricuspid incompetence), elevated venous pressure, enlargement of the liver, oedema of the feet and legs, and ascites.

Clinically, on auscultation there is a rough, harsh, low-frequency presystolic murmur heard best in the mitral area near the apex of the heart and conducted in the direction of the left axilla. Signs vary according to the severity of stenosis and the duration of the condition. If pulmonary hypertension is present the pulmonary second sound is intensified. The ECG may show a notched P wave and evidence of a right axis deviation.

Mitral valvotomy improves the situation, but the pulmonary arterial pressure does not usually fall to normal values owing to the presence of organic structural changes of hypertrophy in the media of the pulmonary arteries which is a frequent (50%) accompaniment of long-standing mitral stenosis.

Mitral Incompetence

Again, this condition is a feature of rheumatic heart disease. It is usually accompanied by some degree of mitral stenosis. In advanced mitral incompetence, although there is little obstruction offered to ventricular filling from the atrium, the subsequent ventricular contraction ejects blood backward into the left atrium as well as forward into the aorta. The retrograde flow into the atrium causes a mitral systolic murmur which converts the first heart sound from "lub" to "lush". Pure mitral stenosis produces a "rrrrup" sound and the combination of stenosis and incompetence yields "rrrush". The forward flow of blood from the pulmonary circuit into the left atrium together with the reflux from the left ventricle results in a greater diastolic volume of the left atrium. Both the left atrium and the left ventricle respond by an increased vigour of contraction, and over months and years this leads successively to hypertrophy and dilatation of these chambers. The ECG shows left ventricular preponderance in about 50% of patients. The left atrium shows dilatation and an increase in expansile pulsation on X-ray screening. Again, the condition deteriorates with the years, causing pulmonary congestion, right ventricular hypertrophy, etc. Surgical repair may be required.

Aortic Stenosis

Aortic stenosis is usually of rheumatic origin, but may be congenital. Its effect is to reduce the rate of ejection of blood into the aorta and to cause left ventricular hypertrophy. Coronary blood flow is reduced because the intravascular pressure is reduced and the extramural pressure is increased. The prolongation of the systolic phase further jeopardizes the coronary flow. Lastly, hypertrophy increases the intercapillary distance in the myocardium and lowers the tissue pO_2. These various factors combine to endanger the supply of oxygen to the myofibrils. Myocardial ischaemia is prevalent.

   Clinically, auscultation reveals a harsh systolic murmur in the aortic area (right second intercostal space in the parasternal line). The murmur is transmitted towards the root of the neck. The aortic pulse is of a slow heaving type showing an anacrotic notch. There is a striking deficit of peak aortic systolic pressure compared with that in the left ventricle. This can be revealed by retrograde passage of a catheter (connected to an electromanometer) from the aorta through the valve into the ventricle (Fig. 14-10).

Aortic stenosis causes episodic attacks of syncope and myocardial ischaemia (angina) on exertion. Syncope results from the lowering of the mean aortic pressure head when widespread skeletal muscle vasodilatation lowers the peripheral resistance. Angina results from the lowering of the pressure head for coronary flow, the prolonged systolic phase, and the concomitant increase in myocardial oxygen usage. Attacks of left ventricular failure may occur, with backward congestion of the pulmonary capillaries and gross pulmonary oedema.

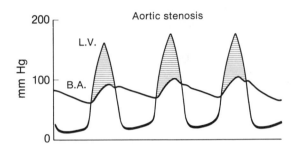

Fig. 14-10. Left ventricular (LV) and brachial artery (BA) pressure curves in aortic stenosis. Note the considerable systolic gradient. (From Keele and Neil, 1965. By permission.)

Aortic Incompetence

Aortic incompetence may be syphilitic in origin, or, sometimes, rheumatic. If rheumatic, it is accompanied by stenosis, although this stenosis is unlikely to be functionally significant.

After the cessation of the ventricular systolic ejection phase blood refluxes from the aorta into the relaxing ventricle and the volume of this blood is added to that provided by forward flow through the pulmonary circuit. Naturally the ventricle responds with an increased force of contraction and the systolic aortic or radial arterial pressure is high. The diastolic arterial pressure is low for two reasons: first, there is a reflux of blood from the aorta, and, second, there is a reflex vasodilatation of the arterioles caused by sino-aortic mechanoreceptor afferents which are unduly excited by the high systolic pressure. In the chronic condition the left ventricle hypertrophies. This throws an increasing load on the coronary supply of oxygen. The majority of coronary flow occurs in diastole, and as has been stated, the diastolic pressure is lower than normal. The coronary ostia themselves are commonly involved by the progressive syphilitic aortitis, which further reduces coronary blood flow, and lastly, the increase in intercapillary distance caused by hypertrophy (and even more so by the eventual ventricular dilatation) prejudices the myocardial pO_2.

The increased ventricular diastolic volume means that the heart must work harder to eject blood, for, by the formulation of Laplace, myocardial tension is equal to the product of the pressure times the radius. To provide a given pressure head the larger ventricle must develop a greater myocardial tension.

Clinically, auscultation reveals a loud "pistol-shot" aortic second sound which terminates with a diastolic murmur—due to turbulence at the aortic orifice as blood refluxes. The pulse is vigorous and bounding—the so-called "water-hammer" or "collapsing" pulse. This is most obvious when the radial artery is palpated when the patient's arm is raised above his head. The ECG shows left ventricular preponderance.

The most common presenting symptom of left ventricular failure is dyspnoea on exertion—the degree of exercise causing shortness of breath becomes progressively less as the condition advances. Other symptoms are those of cardiac asthma, which characteristically occurs either in the sleeping patient or simply when he is lying in bed. Urgent dyspnoea caused by acute episodic pulmonary oedema gives the patient a sensation of drowning, which indeed is the case as the fluid transudate pours into the alveoli. He struggles to sit up and let his legs dangle over the edge of the bed, thereby producing a physiological venesection and affording him relief. He coughs up clear (or perhaps blood stained) bubbly fluid in copious quantities. Cardiac asthma occurs in the recumbent patient more commonly because his thoracic blood volume is at its largest in this position (see Chapter 21) with consequent trespass on his pulmonary reserve for ventilation.

Attacks of myocardial insufficiency may occur alone on exertion or may accompany the dyspnoeic episodes.

Electromanometry shows a steeply rising systolic pressure and a steeply falling diastolic pressure with an unduly prominent dicrotic notch. The pulse pressure greatly exceeds that of the normal individual.

Surgery offers the only real hope for these patients.

It may be as well here to remind the reader that these valvular lesions would not be as clinically important of themselves if it were not for the fact that the pathological conditions which cause them affect the myocardium directly or indirectly as well. Rheumatic endocarditis *always* causes some degree of *myocardial* damage which leads to myocardial fibrosis, and successive attacks cause a progressive encroachment on the myocardial reserve. The heart is a pump, and the ability of the healthy pump to pump harder on exertion is undisputed. If the endocardial valvulitis occurred by itself it is likely that hypertrophy of the healthy myocardium could compensate for it. Artificial surgical lesions of the cardiac valves may cause little cardiovascular sequelae in experimental animals. When the myocardium itself is diseased, however, either directly by the disease process or indirectly as a consequence of narrowing of the coronary ostia (e.g. by syphilis) its powers of compensation are correspondingly reduced and a vicious circle is created.

Congestive Heart Failure

When the diseased heart can no longer provide for the range of normal physical activity which an individual requires, it is said to be failing (for ref. see Davis, 1965). Hitherto compensatory mechanisms had secured an adequate provision for such activity, but they did so by an encroachment on the cardiac reserves. The oxygen usage of the resting individual differs little whether he is healthy or not. Consequently, if the cardiac output begins to diminish, oxygen can only be provided by an increase in the extraction of oxygen from the arterial blood and the A-V difference increases. Unfortunately, even the "arterialization" of the blood begins to suffer with the advent of cardiac failure. The lungs become congested and chronic congestion leads to proliferation of the lung parenchyma with a loss of pulmonary elasticity, a thickening of the alveolar-capillary tissue, and a gross decrease in the vital capacity. Dyspnoea on exertion results, and this progresses until the patient has dyspnoea even at rest unless sitting up in bed (orthopnoea). Orthopnoea is a common presenting feature of patients with left ventricular failure. Left ventricular failure, which causes pulmonary congestion primarily, presents usually with *symptoms*, whereas right ventricular failure manifests itself usually by *signs* (Rushmer, 1961). Some clinical texts differentiate between left ventricular failure and congestive heart failure; they use the latter term to describe the results of right heart failure. This is of course permissible, because the overt signs of congestion are so clear in the case of right heart failure. It should be clearly understood, however, that the failure of either ventricle leads to congestion of the part of the circuit which feeds blood into it.

There was a period in which an attempt was made to differentiate between forward failure and backward failure. As Burton (1965) has written: "apparently the protagonists in the arguments about this understood what they meant by the terms, but not what their opponents meant and no one else understood any of them". Mercifully, these two terms have disappeared from the literature.

Finally, heart failure occurs when the heart cannot fulfil its function— that of supplying the body as a whole. An individual with an arteriovenous shunt or with Paget's disease of bone requires a higher output than does the normal man—when the heart can no longer provide this the signs and symptoms of failure may occur even though the resting cardiac output may still be well above normal—the so-called *high output failure*. Most cases of heart failure, however, are, as might be expected, *low output failure*.

Left Ventricular Failure

Syphilitic aortitis, essential hypertension, and coronary thrombosis are common causes of left ventricular failure. Coronary thrombosis causes features which are described on page 258. The chronic course of syphilis and hypertension causes left ventricular hypertrophy, and the attacks of left ventricular failure are episodic. Orthopnoea is the situation in which the patient can only breathe with ease when sitting up (or erect)—a position which favours pooling of the blood below the thoracic cavity. Cardiac asthma occurs characteristically in the recumbent patient with his increased thoracic blood volume. Pulmonary oedema is much more common in cases with acute left ventricular failure than in mitral stenosis. Repeated attacks of cardiac asthma necessitate not only the assumption of the orthopnoeic position for the bedridden patient but also the administration of digoxin to improve myocardial contractile force and diuretics to reduce the blood volume.

Right Heart Failure

Right heart failure is most commonly caused by mitral stenosis or by left ventricular failure. Additional causes are primary lung disease with pulmonary hypertension and pulmonary valvular stenosis.

The signs include:

1. Hepatic enlargement due to congestion which in turn causes proliferation of fibrous tissue. There may be signs of liver dysfunction—even overt jaundice may be present.

2. Splanchnic engorgement (kidneys, gut, spleen, etc.) and ascites (free fluid containing as much as 5% of protein in the peritoneal cavity).

3. Peripheral oedema of the dependent parts and particularly of loose tissue—e.g. scrotum or vulva. The protein content of the fluid is only 0.5%.

4. Cyanosis—although this is variable.

5. Distension of the superficial veins. The jugular vein may remain distended even when the head is erect as in sitting or standing. Normally the veins on the back of the hand collapse when the hand is held slightly above heart level, for the intravenous pressure is only 5 to 10 cm of saline. In congestive failure it remains distended with further elevation of the arm, and the height at which the veins collapse is a rough measure of the peripheral venous pressure. Similarly, the head may be raised passively (the patient being recumbent) and the height at which the jugular vein collapses can be observed.

McMichael (1952) has emphasized that patients with heart failure may manifest marked peripheral vasoconstriction—gangrene of fingers and/or the nose have occurred. The exact background of this is obscure, but autonomic blockade may alleviate the constriction and prevent gangrene. Howard and Leathart (1951) noted that venesection alleviated the peripheral vasoconstriction of cardiac heart failure and they hypothesized that cardiac receptors excited by the raised central venous pressure were reflexly responsible for it. Two arguments may be levelled against this suggestion: first, no cardiac or venous receptor causes reflex systemic vasoconstriction, and second, venesection reduces the diastolic load of the ventricles and thereby probably improves the length/force-of-contraction relationship (Starling mechanism) of the myocardial fibres. In the overdilated heart the response to further stretch may even be a further reduction of myocardial force. The smaller heart may in such a situation improve its stroke volume and by increasing the pulse pressure increases cardiac and systemic baroreceptor reflex inhibition of sympathetic vasoconstrictor tone.

Both the red cell mass and the plasma volume are increased in heart failure (but not in heart disease where there has been no failure). The renal blood flow has been shown to be invariably reduced—sometimes very considerably—and this has two important effects. First, the output of erythropoietin rises—hence the increase in red cell mass—and second, the output of renin from the juxtaglomerular apparatus increases, with the secondary production of increased amounts of aldosterone as a consequence (see Chapter 20). Cardiac heart failure is characterized by hyperaldosteronaemia, and experimentally induced cardiac heart failure in animals (aortic-caval fistulae) is attended by elevated levels of aldosterone and, on post mortem, evidence of hypertrophy of the zona glomerulosa of the adrenal cortex. Some of the increase in aldosterone concentration may be due to the reduction in the metabolism of the steroid by the congested liver. The hepatic blood flow is grossly reduced to values of only 20% of normal even when minor physical activity is undertaken.

Nevertheless, the evidence available indicates that there is an increase in the *output* of aldosterone which is mainly responsible for the hyperaldosteronaemia. The sequelae of a raised plasma concentration of aldosterone are sodium retention, and, secondarily, water retention; these factors are responsible for the increase in plasma volume and extracellular fluid volume. Inadequate distal tubular reabsorption of sodium results in sodium retention; this feature provides a hindrance to the effective treatment of cardiac heart failure by cardiac glycosides and mercurial diuretics without further precautions. The growing understanding of the importance of the secondary hyperaldosteronaemia of cardiac heart failure in holding back sodium and therefore water in the body has led to the use of "aldosterone-competitors" as an adjuvant therapeutic measure. Spirolactones competitively inhibit the action of aldosterone on the distal tubules and overcome its salt-retaining activity, thereby causing diuresis.

From the account of secondary hyperaldosteronaemia of cardiac heart failure it follows that the diet of such patients should be salt-free when they are in gross failure, and that subsequently a low-salt diet must be used.

Total body water and extracellular fluid volume are raised in cardiac heart failure, which presents the question of, first, whether this water retention is simply a consequence of sodium retention, or, second, whether it can be correlated with either an increased output of ADH, or, if this output is normal, a deficient metabolism of ADH by the liver. This is not yet settled, partly because of the difficulty of measuring ADH concentration in the plasma. It is possible that the feebler pulsations of the left atrium of the cardiac heart failure patient may cause a lower impulse traffic of left atrial vagal afferents from the mechanoreceptors of this region and this *may* lead to an "escape" of the hypothalamic neurones of the supra-optic area and hence a release of ADH from them. It is not proven, however, and meanwhile it is sufficient to consider water retention as a secondary consequence of sodium retention.

References

Bell, G. H., J. N. Davidson, and H. Scarborough (1966). *Textbook of Physiology and Biochemistry*, 7th ed. Edinburgh: Livingstone.

Boyd, J. D. (1965). "Development of the heart," *Handbook of Physiology*, 2, Circulation **III,** 2511–44.

Burton, A. C. (1965). *Physiology and biophysics of the circulation*. Chicago: Year Book Med. Publ.

Cournand, A., J. S. Baldwin, and A. Himmelstein (1949). *Cardiac catheterization in congenital heart disease*. New York: Commonwealth Fund.

Davis, J. O. (1965). "The physiology of congestive heart failure," *Handbook of Physiology*, 2, Circulation **III,** 2071–2122.

Dawes, G. S. (1965). "Oxygen supply and consumption in late fetal life," *Handbook of Physiology*, 3, Respiration, **II,** 1313–28.

Dawes, G. S. (1968). *Foetal and neonatal physiology*. Chicago: Year Book Med. Publ.

Hamilton, W. J., J. D. Boyd, and H. W. Mossman (1945). *Human embryology*. Cambridge: Heffer.

Howard, P., and G. L. Leathart (1951). "Changes of pulse pressure and heart rate induced by changes of posture in subjects with normal and failing hearts," *Clin. Sci.* **10,** 521–26.

McMichael, J. (1952). *In Peripheral circulation* (Ciba Symposium) ed. by G. E. W. Wolstenholme, p. 235. London: Churchill.

Marshall, H. W., H. F. Helmholz, Jr., and E. H. Wood (1962). "Physiologic consequences of congenital heart disease," *Handbook of Physiology*, **2,** Circulation, **I,** 417–87.

Rushmer, R. F. (1961). *Cardiovascular dynamics*, 2nd ed. London: Saunders.

Werkö, L. (1962). "The dynamics and consequences of stenosis or insufficiency of the cardiac valves," *Handbook of Physiology*, 2, Circulation **I,** 645–80.

15

The Vascular Effector Cells

General Considerations

Bozler (1948) defined two types of smooth muscle cells: (1) *single unit*; and (2) *multiunit*. Single unit, or *visceral* smooth muscles occur, for example, in the ureter, the uterus, and the intestine. They resemble those constituting the syncytial cardiac pacemaker cells in exhibiting automatic myogenic activity. The resting membrane potential is only 40 to 50 mV, on which are superimposed rhythmic oscillations which build up local potentials. When these become sufficiently pronounced they evoke a total depolarization, a spike potential, and contraction. Though there is no morphological continuity between such "visceral" smooth muscle cells, a characteristic cell-to-cell propagation of an excitation process from pacemaker cells occurs. In addition, the inherent activity is usually enhanced even by a stretch of slight degree.

Multiunit smooth muscles, on the other hand, resemble skeletal muscle in being dominated by motor nerves. They show little evidence of inherent myogenic activity or of extensive cell-to-cell propagation of excitation; further, they are usually not excited by stretch, except when it is severe. The intrinsic ocular muscles exemplify the multiunit type particularly well.

Although Bozler's classification is useful, it should hardly be taken to imply that there is any sharp demarcation between two distinct types of smooth muscle. It is more rational to consider the "single unit" (visceral) and "multiunit" variants as representing the extreme ends of a continuous spectrum of functional differentiation. As will be outlined below, vascular muscle indeed displays a wide range of smooth muscle types, some vascular sections featuring mainly multiunit characteristics, others betraying more typical "visceral" properties, apparently as a consequence of the highly specialized vascular functions (see Chapter 1). The literature concerning vascular smooth muscles was recently surveyed in an excellent review (Somlyo and Somlyo, 1968).

Morphological Features

Cell design

In large vessels the smooth muscle cells are 50 to 60 μ long and about 2 μ wide and are arranged helically. The smallest arteries and arterioles manifest a more circular arrangement of the muscle cells which are usually only some 25 μ long in these vessels (Fig. 15-1).

As in all muscle cells, the sarcolemma encloses myofilaments. These filaments, about 50 to 80 Å wide, are of unknown length, for they appear to twist around each other and are lost when one attempts to follow successive electron microscopic sections (Rhodin, 1962). It seems likely that the myofilaments comprise some type of sliding arrangement, with two components, actin and myosin, as muscle cells do elsewhere. However, so far it has not been possible to demonstrate more than one type of filament and this seems to be composed of *actin*; the state and location of the myosin component is not as yet known.

Moreover, the contraction unit is not limited by any Z bands, which might explain why some smooth muscle *in vitro* can shorten up to as much as to some 25% of resting length. On the other hand, even maximal neurogenic activation of vascular smooth muscles *in vivo* only exceptionally results in their shortening below some 70% of initial length (see Chapter 5). It is possible—even probable—that the obvious differences between smooth and skeletal muscles in the extent and speed of contraction and relaxation which they evince may be related to the differences in the myofibrillar arrangement between the two.

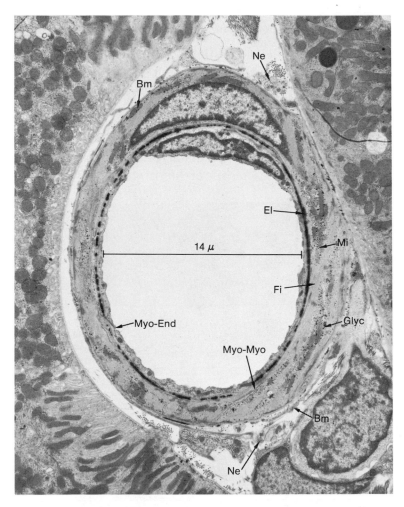

Fig. 15-1. Cross-section from an arteriole (aff. arteriole of the rat kidney) with the muscle layer composed of several smooth muscles, the nucleus of one seen at top. The muscle layer is surrounded by a basement membrane (Bm) and just outside this, non-myelinated sympathetic nerves (Ne) are seen. A thin elastic membrane (El) separates the smooth muscle layer from the endothelial cells, the nucleus of one seen at upper margin of endothelium.

Membraneous contacts are seen between muscle cells (Myo-Myo) and between muscle cells and the endothelium (Myo-End; "myoendothelial junctions"). In the smooth muscle cells mitochondria (Mi) and particulate glycogen (Glyc) are scattered throughout the cytoplasm which is largely dominated by the myofilaments (Fi). (Courtesy of Dr. J. Rhodin, New York Medical College.)

Intercellular relationships

Electron microscope studies of intestinal—and, more recently, vascular—smooth muscle show that the membranes of adjacent cells are often very closely approximated over short distances. Dewey and Barr (1964) refer to the site of such a close approximation as a *nexus*, where a true fusion of the outer lamellae of the cell membranes occurs but where complete continuity of the intracellular spaces nevertheless does not (Fig. 15-2). A spread of excitation probably occurs across such nexuses, which thus would be preferentially characteristic of the visceral type of smooth muscle.

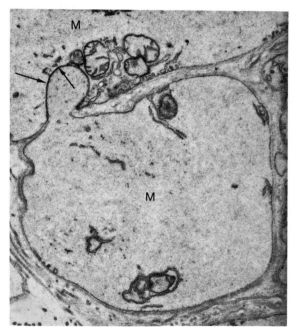

Fig. 15-2. Nexus between two vascular smooth muscles (M). (Courtesy of Dr. L. Barr, Department of Physiol. and Biophysics, Woman's Medical College of Pa., Phila.)

Connections with other wall elements

In most vessels stiff collagen fibrils form an outer "jacket", and they provide wall rigidity when ultimately stretched. Burton (1954) suggested that even during smooth muscle contraction these collagen fibrils might keep the wall rigid, if they are tightened round the vessel by means of a special anchoring to the smooth muscles. Thus, force may be gained by a lever arrangement if the connection of the collagenous to the muscular elements is such as to produce, say, a threefold increase of tightening force by allowing the muscles to shorten three times more than do the collagen fibrils. In fact, Bader (1963) has suggested that some of the "windkessel" vessels (aorta) evince such arrangements, where the muscles seem to act rather by stiffening the wall than by causing reduction of the lumen (see Chapter 6).

In the small resistance vessels, on the other hand, the muscle cells and collagen fibrils are arranged largely in parallel, and here muscle contraction causes marked luminal reduction. This parallel arrangement suggests that the muscle contraction slackens the collagen jacket. In such a situation, resistance to distension would depend mainly on the contracted muscle cells. Accordingly, as contracted smooth muscle is to some extent distensible, so are the resistance vessels—even when they are contracted, although the *extent* of such distensibility varies with the wall/lumen ratio (see Chapter 5).

Functional Differentiation

Large arteries and veins usually possess muscles which are more related to the multiunit than to the visceral type, insofar as they exhibit only little evidence of automaticity and cell-to-cell propagation, and are relatively insensitive to stretch stimuli. As most detailed studies of *isolated* vascular smooth muscle have been performed on vessels belonging to this category, some investigators have been loath to accept the proposition that visceral smooth muscle is represented in the vascular bed.

However, there is now abundant evidence that all the characteristics of visceral smooth muscle are indeed found in the all-important precapillary resistance and sphincter sections especially, but also in some systemic venular sections and in the portal-mesenteric veins.

1. Microcirculation studies indicate that many independent pacemakers exist in the precapillary vessels, resulting in "vasomotion" and rhythmic closure of the precapillary sphincters; when several pacemaker

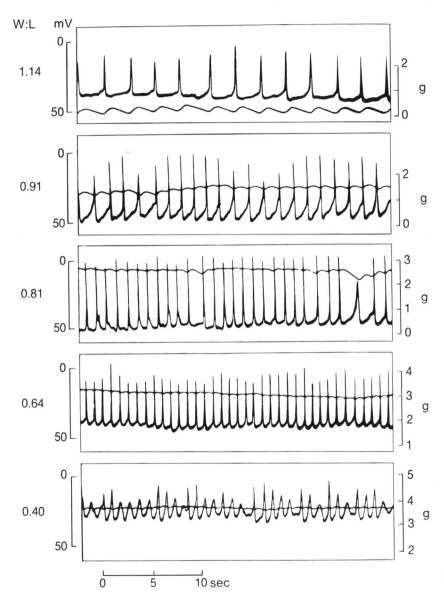

Fig. 15-3. Intracellular records showing the effect of stretch on intestinal smooth muscle with respect to membrane potential, rate of spontaneous discharge and tension. (After Bueding and Bülbring; from Bülbring, 1964. By permission.)

sources fuse the over-all activity of the media cells, they may generate a more steady tone (see Chapter 16).

2. In tissues under "resting" conditions the precapillary vessels often show a striking "basal tone" (see Chapter 16), which is not due to specific extrinsic influences of blood or tissue fluids (Folkow and Öberg, 1961; Uchida and Bohr, 1968). Neither cutaneous A-V shunts nor most veins show much basal tone; these vascular segments largely possess multiunit smooth muscles which are dominated by extrinsic neural control.

3. An increase in the transmural pressure in precapillary vessels generally increases their tone, though powerful extrinsic influences of excitatory or inhibitory nature may obscure or even abolish such local responses to light stretch (see Folkow, 1964). The smallest of such vessels possess a discontinuous muscle coat, and stretch increases the *rate* of the inherent rhythmic activity (Wiedeman, 1957). This is also the case in isolated strips of the small precapillary vessels (Fig. 15-4), analogous with the electrophysiological and mechanical behaviour of intestinal smooth muscle when stretched (Fig. 15-3). As a contrast, very strong mechanical stimuli (such as pinching) are usually needed to excite the multiunit type of vascular smooth muscle.

4. The precapillary vessels yield evidence of a considerable cell-to-cell propagation of activity. Thus, strips from small arteries show a clear-cut rhythmicity, as does the portal vein, due to such intercellular propagation

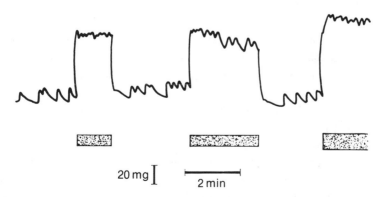

20 mg I   2 min

Fig. 15-4. Effect of passive stretch on the frequency of phasic contractions of strip from a small subcutaneous artery of the dog. (From Johansson and Bohr, 1966. By permission.)

of pacemaker activity (Fig. 15-4). Most large artery or vein preparations
show little or no such co-ordinated rhythmicity.

5. Microelectrode studies of precapillary smooth muscles *in situ* reveal
typical "pacemaker" characteristics in many cells (Fig. 15-5), with low
oscillating membrane potentials from which rhythmically developed local
potentials and excitation propagation ensue (Funaki, 1961). Sucrose-gap
studies of isolated portal veins, for example, reveal similar characteristics
(Axelsson *et al.*, 1967), possibly as a remnant of the "portal heart" in
primitive animals. Therefore the portal and mesenteric veins may be used
as a suitable experimental "model" of the all-important arterioles and
other small vessels, at least with respect to studies of pacemaker activity
and cell-to-cell spread of excitation.

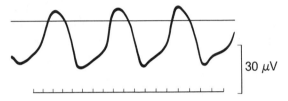

Fig. 15-5. Intracellular recording from vascular smooth muscle in the frog
showing spontaneous discharge with initial slow potentials leading to spike
discharge. (From Funaki, 1961. By permission.)

In summary, then, there is good evidence from modern experimental
techniques that *the visceral type of vascular effectors* abounds in the precapillary resistance and sphincter sections (and in some systemic venular
sections as well as in the portal-mesenteric veins). It seems that the sodium
permeability is relatively high and fluctuating in this type of smooth
muscle. This higher permeability may be due to the poorer calcium
fixation which the membrane exhibits compared with that of nerve or
skeletal muscle (Bohr, 1965). Factors which reduce the membrane potential—thereby decreasing its stability (e.g. light stretch, or membrane
distension by cell swelling)—increase the *rate* of "spontaneous" discharge
and contractions, perhaps by further increasing the sodium permeability.
Conversely, hyperpolarization stabilizes the membrane and the "spontaneous" spikes and contractions then disappear.

This type of vascular effectors seems ideally suited for executing the *local* control of flow and flow distribution by their influence on these fundamentally important vascular segments (Fig. 15-6). Such muscle cells act as a sort of *spontaneously active mechanoreceptor with a built-in contraction system*. Metabolites produced by the tissues provide a powerful *negative* feedback in limiting these "single cell receptor-effector units". Thus, if the precapillary sphincteric activity becomes predominant, capillary flow is reduced, tissue metabolite concentration rises and exerts a vasodilator influence on the sphincter mechanisms, etc. (see Chapter 16).

The *multiunit type of vascular effectors*, which is present in most veins, and large arteries, and which possibly also constitutes the *outer* sheath of smooth muscle in at least the larger precapillary resistance vessels, is primarily under the influence of *extrinsic* neural and humoral mechanisms and therefore executes the central and reflex adjustments of the vascular bed. As the regional sympathetic discharge increases, the outer, predominantly "multiunit" muscles either recruit (by cell-to-cell propagation; Johansson and Ljung, 1968) and /or unload the inner layers, in both cases "centralizing" control of the resistance vessels (see below). Conversely, in the absence of sympathetic discharge, relaxation of the outer sheath might transfer the control of the local circulation to the predominantly "visceral" components of the media which, because of their inherent activity, display a considerable "basal tone". These "visceral" characteristics seemingly become increasingly dominant the closer the arterial smooth muscles are to the capillary site. Some morphological and functional characteristics favour this adumbration of the activity of precapillary smooth muscles (Folkow *et al.*, 1964).

The role of the veins as important capacitance vessels would seem to require a dominant nervous control and a differentiation of their muscle into a predominantly multiunit type. Such is the case at least in mammals, whose venous smooth muscle (with some notable exceptions) show little sign of automaticity and cell-to-cell propagation, and which manifest a relative insensitivity to stretch. The muscular elements of the A-V shunt vessels, strictly subordinated to the thermoregulatory nervous control, likewise evince mainly multiunit type properties.

Vascular smooth muscle also show considerable differences in speed of contraction and relaxation. Those of large arteries and most veins are sluggish, while those of the precapillary resistance vessels and cutaneous A-V shunts, for example, are far more rapid, and may respond with a

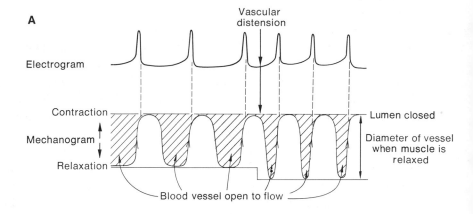

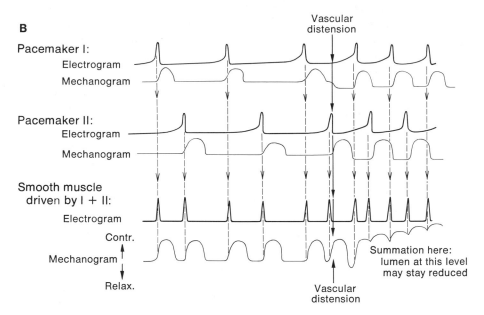

Fig. 15-6. A. Schematic illustration of haemodynamic events expected when a precapillary "sphincter" smooth muscle is exposed to increased transmural pressure.
B. Schematic illustration of expected effects of true pacemaker smooth muscles on nearby muscle cells when the "pacemaker" activity is facilitated by distension. If the "driven" smooth muscles are simultaneously affected by several unsynchronized "pacemakers," tetanic contractions might be accomplished. (From Folkow, 1964. By permission.)

brief "twitch" to a single impulse in their adrenergic fibres. Further, the myogenically active venules in the bat's wing contract rhythmically at some 60/min (Wiedeman, 1957).

Generally speaking, the vascular bed seems to exhibit a whole spectrum of smooth muscle differentiation, from distinct multiunit types over to typical visceral types. However, even though differences between them can be so marked as to preclude far-reaching generalizations of any certainty, such differences are probably to be looked upon as *quantitative* rather than qualitative. Thus, the more stable and polarized the membrane, the more the cells will exhibit multiunit properties, being excited first when exposed to distinct extrinsic stimuli such as by adrenergic nerve excitation. It is not unlikely that one and the same cell may sometimes exhibit multiunit behaviour, sometimes visceral behaviour depending, for example, on local factors affecting membrane excitability; thus, denervation may reveal "latent" myogenic activity, etc.

Neuroeffector Arrangement

Here also a considerable range of differentiation exists among the vascular effector cells. Thus the post-ganglionic adrenergic supply to different vascular circuits varies between that of the brain, which is sparse, and that of muscles and skin, which is generous (see Chapter 16). Large arteries are poorly innervated in most species, save those of the diving animals. Arterioles are densely innervated in most circuits, while usually relatively few adrenergic ramifications reach the precapillary "sphincters". Veins show an innervation whose density again varies in different regional circuits. No ganglia exist in the vascular walls, though the synapses between preganglionic and postganglionic neurons may occasionally be displaced from the sympathetic ganglia towards the periphery along the vessels.

The histochemical method of Falck and Hillarp has shown that ramifications of the adrenergic nerves make contact only with the adventitial surface of the *outermost* muscle layer of the media in most vessels (Fig. 15-7). However, in the larger veins the adrenergic fibres may penetrate to reach the deeper parts of the media as well (Falck, 1962; Norberg and Hamberger, 1964).

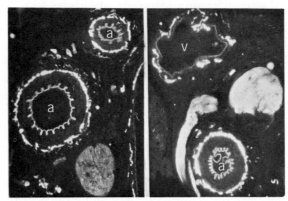

Fig. 15-7. Highly fluorescent adrenergic terminals on the outside of the media in arterioles (a) and venules (v) in the submaxillary gland of the rat. Note that no terminals penetrate the media of the vessels. The internal elastic membranes display marked autofluorescence. (From Norberg and Hamberger, 1964. By permission.)

Even though only the outer sheath of muscle cells is thus directly excited by the vasoconstrictor fibres in most vessels, the frequent presence of nexus connections between the vascular smooth muscles may imply a cell-to-cell propagation and hence a secondary "recruitment" of the inner layers which thus participate in the primary neurogenic excitation of the outer layer. Such a recruitment—though presumably not complete—clearly takes place in the portal vein (Fig. 15-8). However, such a "recruitment" is not necessarily present throughout, because in small mesenteric arteries only a restricted wall section is contracted by the microapplication of catechol-amines from the outside (Van Citters et al., 1962). Such small vessels, placed just upstream of the myogenically active arterioles and metar-terioles, thus behave as if cell-to-cell propagation were limited; in other words, the smooth muscles may here exhibit multiunit rather than visceral properties.

The adrenergic axons, which show a considerable convergence arrangement, especially in the richly innervated vascular sections, branch up strikingly and thus also display the divergence principle of innervation. The ramifications show pearl-string varicosities in close contact with the smooth muscles, establishing "en passage" synapses (see Iversen, 1967). Richly innervated vascular smooth muscles of the outer wall layer are

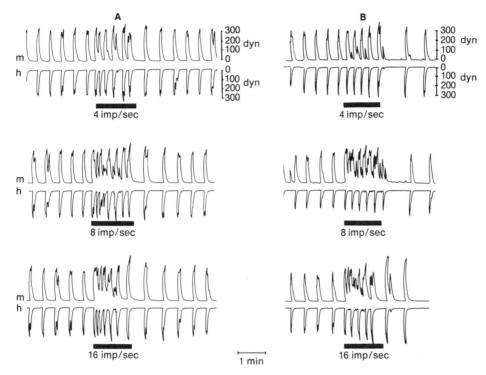

Fig. 15-8. The response of the rat portal vein to gradual vasoconstrictor fibre stimulation before (A) and after (B) its hepatic end (constrictions recorded downwards; "h") had been made insensitive to the adrenergic transmitter by means of phenoxybenzamine 10^{-8}. Note that the neurogenic stimulation of the mesenteric end of the vein ("m") is still in part propagated to "h" after nerve blockade which must be ascribed to myogenic cell-to-cell propagation. (From Johansson and Ljung, 1968. By permission.)

probably in contact with several such synapses. The adrenergic transmitter, noradrenaline (NA), is released from these varicosities (1 to 2 μ long, containing about 500 to 800 NA granules), which are in rather close contact with the muscle membrane, the gap varying between perhaps 500 Å to 2000 Å in vessels, occasionally more. Most of the transmitter—an average of some 400 to 500 NA molecules appear to be released per varicosity and impulse—is taken back into the varicosity, so that its direct vascular action is usually strictly limited to the cell(s) in contact with the varicosity (Folkow et al., 1967).

The cholinergic sympathetic vasodilator nerves affect the precapillary resistance vessels of skeletal muscle. They appear to be distributed only to a limited section of these precapillary resistance vessels, where the muscle cells exhibit features of the "visceral type" of activity. This limited fibre distribution is nevertheless efficient in producing a powerful precapillary vasodilatation, possibly by supressing peripheral pacemaker activity and/or centripetal spread of excitation from such pacemakers (see Chapter 16). Such an arrangement would resemble that of the vagal innervation of the heart, where the effect of these nerves is mainly confined to the nodal tissue and the conduction system but may nevertheless stop the ventricular beat.

Access of Humoral Agents

Vascular structure must greatly influence the routes by which blood-borne and tissue-produced agents reach the contractile elements. Blood-borne factors can to some extent directly traverse the arterial-arteriolar endothelium (which thus appears to contain at least a few pores) because luminal perfusion of isolated small arteries with vasoactive, water-soluble substances does induce smooth muscle effects (Uchida *et al.*, 1967). No doubt such agents also reach the interstitial fluid via the capillary pores and thus affect the vessels from their outside as well, and this is perhaps the more important route of access. Lipid-soluble substances such as oxygen and carbon dioxide must still more easily reach the smooth muscles of small vessels directly from the bloodstream, as they freely pass the entire endothelial lining. This of course does not deny that the interstitial tensions of O_2 and CO_2 *outside* the vessels, in the tissue interstitium, are of great importance in vascular smooth muscle control.

Thus, the contractile elements of the pre- and post-capillary vessels are affected by blood-borne agents both from the bloodstream directly, and—like ordinary tissue cells—from the interstitial space as well; after that such agents reach this space via transcapillary diffusion. The smooth muscles of larger vessels, which have their own vasa vasorum, will naturally to a great extent depend on them for their supply, but probably only in the outer part of the wall (Woerner, 1959).

All substances produced by the tissue cells affect the regional vessels mainly from their *outside*. Such substances will first reach the interstitial fluid, which is in turn in immediate contact with all smooth muscles of the vessels that are situated within the tissue. This seems self-evident, but nevertheless it has sometimes been assumed that dilatation of the "upstream" arterioles in activated tissues should require specific ascending dilator mechanisms. Clearly, ascending dilatation (Chapter 16) occurs and contributes, but it is a true prerequisite only for such precapillary vessels as are placed definitely *outside* the metabolite-producing tissue.

Mode of Action of Humoral Agents

Most vasoactive substances exert their action on vascular smooth muscle by coupling to specific membrane "receptors", while changes in, for example, the ionic or osmotic environment by a more generalized action seem to influence the membrane properties, the contractile machinery, etc. Whenever vascular smooth muscle is activated at least four processes are involved, as is the case in muscle in general: (1) membrane excitation, (2) excitation-contraction coupling, (3) myofibril shortening, and (4) energy metabolism (Bohr, 1965). However, the fact that these four processes are common to all muscles does not mean that their arrangement is necessarily the same throughout (see Somlyo and Somlyo, 1968).

For example, the action potentials of mammalian smooth muscle are little dependent on external $[Na^+]$ and they are not abolished by tetrodotoxin. It has even been suggested that Ca^{++} is mainly responsible for the action potentials in smooth muscle. Further, in some situations electrical membrane events might not be involved at all in vascular smooth muscle activation. As to the excitation-contraction coupling, Ca^{++} is no doubt all-important, but the sarcotubular system is poorly developed in smooth muscle compared with skeletal muscle. The peculiarities of the contractile proteins have been mentioned above.

Many of the chemical substances that affect vascular smooth muscles may act on more than one of the four basic processes mentioned above. The over-all effect and the point of action of such chemical agents may even be varied by their local concentration. Thus, noradrenaline (NA) is bound to α-receptors in the membrane and causes depolarization and contraction of the muscle, perhaps by releasing calcium ions from the membrane itself. This seems to be the most important effect of NA *in vivo*.

However, NA may, at least *in vitro*, cause smooth muscle contraction even when the membrane is initially depolarized (Waugh, 1962), suggesting that there is also a direct NA effect on some other link in the contraction events.

The relaxation of *intestinal* smooth muscle by adrenaline via β-receptors may be mainly due to a facilitation of energy processes (Bülbring, 1962, 1964), which hyperpolarizes the membrane. Such events would block the membrane-induced "spontaneous" activation of the contractile process and thereby cause muscle relaxation.

In the vascular smooth muscle the nature of the β-receptor-induced relaxation may be entirely different. For instance, in the myogenically active portal vein β-receptor stimulation *increases* the frequency of the "spontaneous" membrane depolarizations but weakens so markedly the ensuing contractions as to produce a net relaxation. In other words, β-receptor stimulation produces here positive chronotropic and negative inotropic effects (Fig. 15-9). Moreover, it is possible that the relaxation of vascular smooth muscle, produced by catecholamines *in vivo*, is sometimes in part *indirect* and due to the stimulation of metabolic events in the tissue cells surrounding the vessels (Lundholm *et al.*, 1966).

Further, when potassium is added to multiunit smooth muscle, e.g. from large arteries, depolarization and contraction are produced. However, "physiological" increases in potassium cause *relaxation* of small arteries and arterioles, both *in vivo* and *in vitro*, probably by supressing myogenic activity and/or cell-to-cell propagation in these visceral types of smooth muscle (Johansson and Bohr, 1966). This is a quite different membrane effect from that on the multiunit type of smooth muscle; it resembles the potassium effect on the cardiac pacemaker cells.

Lastly, vascular smooth muscle from different vascular sites exhibits considerable differentiation with respect to sensitivity to hormones and local chemical factors, which is one of the prerequisites for normal vascular control (see Mellander and Johansson, 1968). While the adrenergic α-receptors show a fairly general distribution, the β-receptors are mostly but not solely confined to some precapillary resistance sections, such as in skeletal muscle, myocardium, etc. Similarly, angiotensin, serotonin, and "vasopressin" (ADH) receptors are largely restricted to precapillary smooth muscle sites. Some relaxants of vascular muscle seem to affect predominantly the precapillary sections, e.g. K^+ and hyperosmolarity (which both seem to be of importance in exercise hyperaemia, see Chapter 22), as

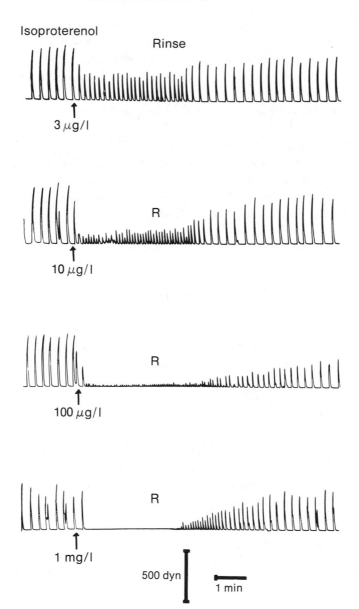

Fig. 15-9. Effects of β receptor stimulation by increasing isoproterenol concentrations on mechanical activity of portal vein. Note the increased rate but decreased amplitude of the spontaneous rhythmic contractions. (From Johansson *et al.*, 1967. By permission.)

do histamine and the drug hydralazine. Others relax both pre- and post-capillary smooth muscle—e.g. acetylcholine, adenosine compounds, bradykinin—while a few, such as nitrites, predominantly affect postcapillary smooth muscle as well as those of large arteries. The smooth muscle of the pulmonary vessels react differently in many respects (Chapter 21). Thus, K^+, bradykinin, kallidin, ATP, and histamine all produce constriction in this circuit, as indeed does oxygen lack.

These examples illustrate the considerable differences that exist between vascular smooth muscle of various origins with respect to basic characteristics, innervation, responsiveness to hormones, drugs, and local chemical factors, and with respect to how such extrinsic influences may in different ways affect the basic processes involved in cell activation.

References

Axelsson, J., B. Wahlström, B. Johansson, and O. Jonsson (1967). "Influence of the ionic environment on spontaneous electrical and mechanical activity of the rat portal vein," *Circ. Res.*, **21,** 609–18.

Bader, H. (1963). "The anatomy and physiology of the vascular wall," *Handbook of Physiology*, 2, Circulation **II,** 865–89.

Bohr, D. F. (1965). "Individualities among vascular smooth muscles," in *Electrolytes and cardiovascular diseases* (ed. E. Bajusz), pp. 342–55. Basel/New York: Karger.

Bozler, E. (1948). "Conduction, automaticity, and tonus of visceral muscle," *Experientia*, **4,** 213–18.

Bülbring, E. (1962) "Electrical activity in intestinal smooth muscle," *Physiol. Rev.* **II,** Suppl., 5, 160–74.

Bülbring, E. (1964). *Pharmacology of smooth muscle*, Czechoslovak Medical Press. Prague: Pergamon.

Burton, A. C. (1954). "Relation of structure to function of tissues of the wall of blood vessels," *Physiol. Rev.*, **34,** 619–42.

Dewey, M. M., and L. Barr (1964). "A study of the structure and distribution of the nexus," *J. Cell. Biol.* **23,** 553–85.

Falck, B. (1962). "Observations on the possibilities of the cellular localization of monoamines by a fluorescence method," *Acta Physiol. Scand.* **56**, Suppl., 197.

Folkow, B. (1964). "Description of the myogenic hypothesis," *Circ. Res.* **14–15**, Suppl., I, 279–87.

Folkow, B., and B. Öberg (1961). "Autoregulation and basal tone in consecutive vascular sections of the skeletal muscles in reserpine-treated cats," *Acta Physiol. Scand.*, **53**, 105–13.

Folkow, B., B. Öberg, and E. H. Rubinstein (1964). "A proposed differentiated neuro-effector organization in muscle resistance vessels," *Angiologica*, **1**, 197–208.

Folkow, B., J. Häggendal, and B. Lisander (1967). "Extent of release and elimination of noradrenaline at peripheral adrenergic nerve terminals," *Acta Physiol. Scand.*, Suppl., 307.

Funaki, S. (1961). "Spontaneous spike-discharges of vascular smooth muscle," *Nature*, **191**, 1102–3.

Iversen, L. L. (1967). *The uptake and storage of noradrenaline in sympathetic nerves.* Cambridge University Press.

Johansson, B., and D. F. Bohr (1966). "Rhythmic activity in smooth muscle from small subcutaneous arteries," *Am. J. Physiol.* **210**, 801–6.

Johansson, B., and B. Ljung (1968). "Role of myogenic propagation in vascular smooth muscle response to vasomotor nerve stimulation, "*Acta Physiol. Scand.* **73**, 501–10.

Lundholm, L., E. Mohme-Lundholm, and N. Svedmyr (1966). "Introductory remarks," in *Second symposium on catecholamines* (ed. G. H. Acheson), *Pharmacol. Rev.* **18**, 255–72.

Johansson, B., O. Jonsson, J. Axelson, and B. Wahlström (1967). "Electrical and mechanical characteristics of vascular smooth muscle response to norepinephrine and isoproterenol," *Circ. Res.* **21**, 619–33.

Mellander, S., and B. Johansson (1968). "Control of resistance, exchange, and capacitance functions in the peripheral circulation," *Pharmacol. Rev.* **20**, 117–96.

Norberg, K.-A., and B. Hamberger (1964). "The sympathetic adrenergic neuron," *Acta Physiol. Scand.* **63**, Suppl., 238.

Rhodin, J. A. G. (1962). "Fine structure of vascular walls in mammals with special reference to smooth muscle component," *Physiol. Rev.* **42,** 48–87.

Somlyo, A. P., and A. V. Somlyo (1968). "Vascular smooth muscle," *Pharmacol. Rev.* **20,** 197–272.

Uchida, E., and D. F. Bohr (1969). "Myogenic tone in isolated perfused resistance vessels from rats," *Am. J. Physiol.* **216,** 1343–50.

Uchida, E., D. F. Bohr, and S. W. Hoobler (1967). "A method of studying isolated resistance vessels from rabbit mesentery and brain and their response to drugs," *Circ. Res.* **21,** 525–36.

Van Citters, R. L., B. M. Wagner, and R. F. Rushmer (1962). "Architecture of small arteries during vasoconstriction," *Circ. Res.* **10,** 668–75.

Waugh, W. H. (1962). "Adrenergic stimulation of depolarized arterial muscle," *Circ. Res.* **11,** 264–76.

Wiedeman, M. P. (1957). "Effect of venous flow on frequency of venous vasomotion in the bat wing," *Circ. Res.,* **5,** 641–44.

Woerner, C. A. (1959). "Vaso vasorum of arteries, their demonstration and distribution," in *The arterial wall* (ed. A. I. Lansing), pp. 1–14. Baltimore: Williams & Wilkins.

16

The Principles of Vascular Control

The general characteristics of the control mechanisms that govern the vascular bed may be listed under basal vascular tone and its local control, neurogenic influences, and hormonal influences. A recent review (Mellander and Johansson, 1968) should be consulted for details.

Basal Vascular Tone and its Local Control

Establishment of Basal Vascular Tone

Inherent myogenic activity, particularly pronounced in "single-unit" (visceral) smooth muscles in the precapillary resistance vessels and sphincters, is responsible for a basal vascular tone which keeps these vessels in a state of partial constriction. This basal activity of the smooth muscle of these vascular sections is manifest even in the absence of extrinsic nervous influences or of blood borne excitatory agents.

In contrast, the venous capacitance vessels manifest little basal myogenic activity and their tone is determined mainly by the influence of sympathetic vasoconstrictor activity of extrinsic origin. Such vessels contain smooth muscles which are predominantly of the "multiunit" type.

285

Portal and mesenteric veins (and many venular sections), however, contain "single-unit" muscles and manifest a considerable inherent activity; it is possible that such behaviour reflects the function of the "portal heart" seen in more primitive organisms (Chapter 15).

Myogenic activity, though a primary consequence of an *intrinsic* membrane instability in "single-unit" (visceral) muscles, may of course be facilitated or even dominated by extrinsic neurogenic or humoral factors in certain circumstances. Vascular distension, occasioned by a rise in the arterial pressure, provides a positive feedback (Bayliss, 1902) which may at first sight suggest a source of instability of the system. Thus, stretching of the cell membranes increases the rate of spontaneous activity of the smooth muscles and the functional effect of vasoconstriction to such a rise of intravascular pressure would seem to create a vicious circle. However, the response to such distension is only featured by a moderate increase in the rate of "single twitches" of individual muscle cells, for it appears to be limited by the relative refractory period of these cells. Moreover, if there should be any tendency for the development of a tetanic contraction, this itself would automatically eliminate the stretch stimulus, for a maintained shortening of the muscles would then result. Additionally, the accumulation of tissue metabolites—which occurs when the blood flow lessens—exerts a local vasodilator influence on the precapillary vessels, and this mechanism provides a powerful negative feedback (Fig. 16-1).

The muscle cells of the metarterioles and precapillary sphincters often lack direct contact with each other and, consequently, cell-to-cell propagation of activity cannot be effected. Such vessels manifest a rhythmic unsynchronized vasomotion due to the activity of independent pacemaker cells. Tissue activity increases the production of "vasodilator metabolites" which, suppressing the inherent myogenic activity of metarterioles and sphincters, allow a more continuous perfusion of the entire capillary network.

The larger arterioles with continuous smooth muscle coats usually exhibit a more synchronized pattern of myogenic activity. Pacemaker cells, whose site may vary from time to time, initiate myogenic activity by cell-to-cell propagation in either direction. Spread in a proximal direction, however, might lead to a fusion of the effects of independent rhythmic activity (initiated from several arteriolar sites) when the larger parent arterial branches are reached. Sometimes the fusion of such independently

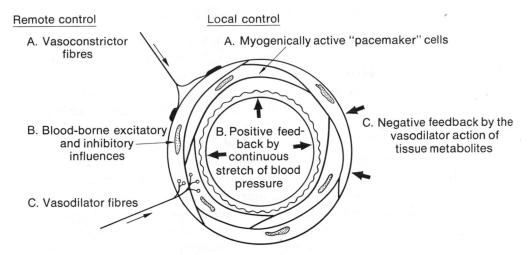

Fig. 16-1. Basic machinery of local vascular control: myogenic "pacemaker" activity, reinforced by the continuous stretch offered by the blood pressure, constitutes, *via* cell-to-cell excitation spread, the *basal vascular tone*, being steadily counteracted by the continuously produced tissue metabolites. Extrinsic excitatory and inhibitory factors, in the form of nervous and blood-borne influences modulate, and sometimes dominate, the local control system.

initiated rhythms may secure a tetanus-like contraction of the arterial branches, which then would manifest a steady "basal" vascular tone. This hypothesis (Folkow, 1964), which seeks to explain the features of a steady basal tone in the larger vessels that co-exists with the unsynchronized vasomotor tone of the peripheral resistance vessels, requires more documentation, but is itself attractive. It further provides a reasonable explanation of the phenomenon of *ascending dilatation*, in which—following a vasodilatation of the peripheral resistance vessels (induced by tissue activity, by a regional pressure drop, or by the peripheral injection of vasodilator drugs)—there occurs sequentially a reduction of tone in vessels situated successively more proximally. This ascending vasodilatation spreads centripetally at a rate consonant with that of cell-to-cell propagation; it is independent of nerves (Hilton, 1962). It seems likely that the primary loss of peripheral pacemaker activity leads secondarily to the relaxation of larger vessels whose tone may largely depend on centripetally propagated myogenic activity.

Extent and Localization of Basal Vascular Tone

If the regional sympathetic vasoconstrictor nerves are cut and the source of blood-borne constrictor substances, such as catecholamines, is eliminated, the extent of basal vascular tone of the various regional circuits can be examined. The ratio between the flow resistance encountered in resting conditions and in maximal vasodilatation, induced by supra-maximal doses of a suitable drug injected intra-arterially, reflects the level of the *basal vascular tone* if the pressure head and transmural pressure are kept constant in the two conditions. This technique reveals only the basal tone of the resistance vessels. However, the changes in pre/post capillary resistance ratio, in CFC or PS product may be measured simultaneously, as may the regional blood content (see Chapters 7 and 8). From changes in these parameters the alteration in pre- and post-capillary resistances, in precapillary sphincter activity and in capacitance vessels may be deduced.

Muscle, skin, and intestine vessels have been subjected to rigorous investigations of this type as detailed elsewhere (see Chapters 22, 25, 26). In general, these studies have revealed that the marked tone of systemic precapillary vessels in resting tissues is primarily due to inherent myogenic activity and not to sympathetic vasoconstrictor influences. Sympathetic discharge is so low in resting conditions as to provide only a minor contribution to precapillary vascular tone. For example, sympathetic blockade lowers the flow resistance in resting muscle of man only from the normal 20 to 30 PRU_{100} down to 10 to 15 PRU_{100}, whereas in maximal vasodilatation the resistance drops to 1.5 to 2 PRU; sympathetic vasoconstriction thus only provides 15 to 20% of the vascular tone at rest.

When maximally dilated—a circumstance in which flow resistance of any individual vascular circuit is dictated by its dimensional structure—the fall of pressure along the circuit may become almost linear. In sharp contrast, the pressure drop along a vascular circuit in resting tissue shows a reversed S shape (Fig. 6-1), being in several tissues, like muscle, further accentuated by constrictor fibre activity. The lumina of the larger arteries and the majority of the venous compartments are much less affected by the changes which occur during maximal vasodilatation and thus contribute relatively much more to the total resistance offered to maximal blood flow. In muscle, the pre/post capillary ratio is only between 2 and 3 to 1 and the mean capillary pressure 25 to 30 mm Hg, when the circuit is maximally dilated. At rest with normal basal tone, the resistance ratio is between 4 and 5 to 1 and the mean capillary pressure is approximately 15 to 20 mm Hg, showing that the resting basal tone of the precapillary vessels exceeds that of the postcapillary vessels.

Tissues that evince a wide range of metabolic activity, such as muscles, and salivary glands, manifest an especially high basal vascular tone which is correspondingly reduced when the tissue does work. In contrast, in the kidney, which works steadily, basal vascular tone is low. The relationship between maximal blood flow and resting blood flow in a number of tissues is schematically illustrated in Fig. 16-2.

When an acutely sympathectomised vascular circuit is dilated maximally the regional blood volume only increases by 10 to 20%, which indicates that the basal tone of the venous capacitance vessels is low in

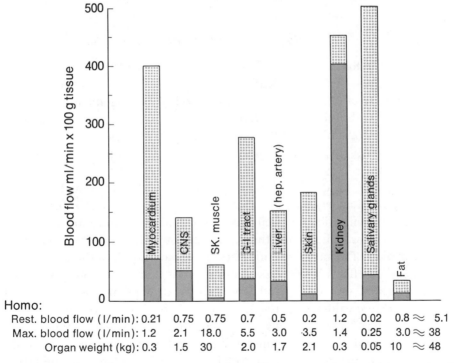

Homo:										
Rest. blood flow (l/min):	0.21	0.75	0.75	0.7	0.5	0.2	1.2	0.02	0.8	≈ 5.1
Max. blood flow (l/min):	1.2	2.1	18.0	5.5	3.0	3.5	1.4	0.25	3.0	≈ 38
Organ weight (kg):	0.3	1.5	30	2.0	1.7	2.1	0.3	0.05	10	≈ 48

Fig. 16-2. Diagram illustrating regional blood flows at "rest" and at maximal dilatation, adapted to fit approximately the situation in a 70 kg man. The flow figures are given both for 100g of tissue and for the entire organs. (From Mellander and Johansson, 1968. By permission.)

resting conditions. Sympathetic vasoconstrictor discharge, when superimposed, causes marked changes in this situation and these are particularly vivid in the skin.

The precapillary vessels possess a higher wall/lumen ratio than the others (Chapter 5) and this favours the establishment of strong luminal reduction in resting conditions, as a given degree of shortening of the muscle fibres causes a more marked reduction in the lumen (see Fig. 5-6, page 48). Approximate calculations suggest that the entire range of change in the luminal dimensions, which occurs between maximal vasoconstriction and maximal vasodilatation, may be achieved by only some 30% alteration in the length of the circular smooth muscle of the arterioles. Venules and veins (capacitance vessels) appear to undergo an active change in smooth muscle length of 20 to 30% over their full range of physiological adjustment (see Mellander, 1960).

Basal Vascular Tone and Control of Local Flow

Control of the local blood supply is achieved by the algebraic summation of two factors—the mechanically reinforced myogenic activity and the vasodilator effect of the local metabolites. When neurogenic and humoral influences are abolished, then blood flow (and capillary pressure) tend to remain fairly constant when the arterial pressure is artificially varied. This "autoregulation" of capillary flow and pressure is important in several respects.

Suppose that the arterial pressure is raised. Then the transmural pressure increases, particularly in the precapillary sections, and this provides a mechanical facilitation of their myogenic activity. Simultaneously, the increase in flow, caused by the raised pressure head, lowers the local concentration of metabolites and raises the tissue pO_2. Both the mechanical and chemical effects thus serve to increase basal vascular tone, especially in the precapillary vessels, and flow and mean capillary pressure revert towards normal values (Fig. 16-3).

When arterial pressure falls, decreased inherent myogenic tone and a greater accumulation of tissue metabolites combine to secure a re-establishment of the status quo. If blood flow is abolished by clamping the artery of supply, then the subsequent re-establishment of flow is attended by the features of "reactive hyperaemia", in which the negligible transmural pressure and the profound vasodilatation due to metabolites initially

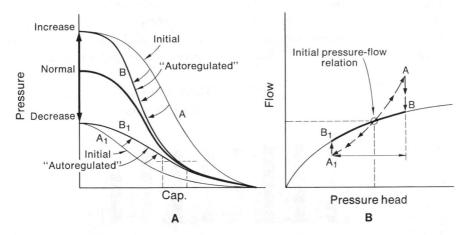

Fig. 16-3. Diagrams illustrating by means of (A) the pressure drop profile and (B) the pressure-flow curve the initial, physical consequences of a change in arterial pressure and the secondary, smooth muscle "*autoregulatory*" adjustments in the precapillary sections, which tend to return both flow and capillary pressure to the normal "control" level.

allows maximal flow, which subsides as these two factors alter in their quantitative importance.

If only the *venous* pressure is raised, the pressure head is lowered while the transmural pressure is increased. In this situation, the local chemical influence and the mechanical influence on smooth muscle activity *oppose* each other. At least if the change is pronounced the local chemical influence usually "wins" this competition and the vessels tend to relax. Thus, the control exerted by local chemical factors appears to be more powerful than that due to the mechanical factor, that is, the negative feedback overrules the positive one, which is reasonable enough. However, in the usual type of autoregulation of flow the two factors *co-operate*, as outlined earlier (see also Folkow, 1962).

The simultaneous and equal increase of arterial and venous pressures does not alter the pressure head, but obviously it increases the transmural pressure, which of itself causes an initial improvement of flow by causing some distension of the circuit. However, this stretching of the vessel wall causes a secondary increase in the precapillary resistance and sphincteric tone, thereby counteracting the distension and reducing the fraction of the capillary bed which is patent, thus minimizing the tendency to oedema (Fig. 16-4). Little interference with tissue nutrition results, and if any accumulation of metabolites does occur, then its local effect would offset the mechanically induced exacerbation of precapillary sphincteric activity.

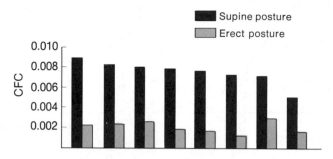

Fig. 16-4. Average change of capillary filtration coefficient (CFC; reflecting the number of perfused capillaries per unit time) in the feet of eight human subjects, on shifting from the supine to the erect posture. Such effects are locally induced as they also occur in denervated vascular beds. (From Mellander *et al.*, 1964. By permission.)

The mode of action of chemical factors

Obviously the chemical factors that influence myogenic tone include not only the metabolites, which are produced locally and cause vasodilatation, but also the substances delivered by the blood itself. Blood-borne oxygen and carbon dioxide and hydrogen ions influence the activity level of the vascular smooth muscle cells, and in the *systemic* vascular bed the *local* effects of a fall in the arterial pO_2 or a rise in the arterial pCO_2 and hydrogen ion concentration causes vasodilatation. The *pulmonary* circuit, however, *constricts* when exposed to hypoxia (Euler and Liljestrand, 1946; Duke, 1957)—an interesting difference which is important functionally in distributing blood properly to the various parts of the lung (see Chapter 21).

The local concentration of metabolites will clearly depend on the balance between tissue activity and the flow (and composition) of the blood provided. These metabolites particularly affect the precapillary vessels—resistance and sphincter sections (Fig. 16-5)—and have relatively little influence on the postcapillary vessels which remain predominantly under the control of sympathetic nervous influences.

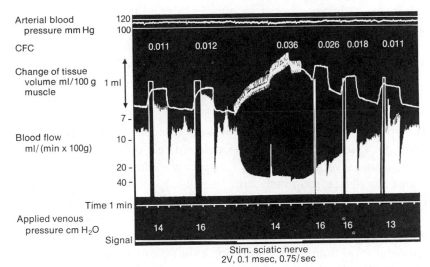

Fig. 16-5. The effect of light muscle exercise on blood flow and perfused capillary surface area, estimated in terms of CFC. Note considerable increase of flow as well as of CFC. The volume increase during exercise is only to a minor degree due to increased blood content; it is mainly a consequence of increased tissue fluid volume, due to increased filtration and osmotic fluid transfer when capillary pressure increases upon the precapillary relaxation and tissue osmolarity increases due to the exercise. (From Kjellmer, 1965. By permission.)

The Nature of the Vasodilator Metabolites

Although the notable role of chemical factors in securing local vasodilatation has been fully realised for many years, argument has raged as to which metabolites or chemical influences are of importance. Low pO_2, high pCO_2 and/or $[H^+]$, adenosine compounds, and lactic acid have all been shown to exercise dilator properties, but none singly is adequate to simulate, in *all* tissues, the chemical effects of increased tissue metabolism in inducing hyperaemia. Recently, the local release of potassium ions, the effects of local hyperosmolality, and the effects of low pO_2 have engaged attention as possible causative agents for functional hyperaemia in skeletal muscle (Chapter 22). Each factor exerts a strong relaxant effect on the precapillary resistance vessels and "sphincters" and causes a vascular response that closely stimulates that of exercise hyperaemia. It is not yet known, however, whether these influences can mimic the features of the hyper-

aemia seen in tissues other than muscle in conditions of increased metabolism. Probably the importance of the individual factors varies from one
tissue to the other; perhaps this is the case even in the same tissue from
one time to the next, depending on the actual situation. Thus, adenosine
(Katory and Berne, 1966) and low pO_2 have powerful effects on the
coronaries (Chapter 23), and [H$^+$] appears to be the main regulator of the
cerebral vessels (Chapter 24).

It appears that the long search for a *key* vasodilator metabolite has been
in vain, for it seems likely that no single entirely dominating factor exists;
in most tissues several factors may co-operate so that one may be "blocked"
without interfering too much with the all-important adjustment of blood
supply to local demands. A possible exception in this respect may be
kallidin, the polypeptide liberated in salivary glands, the pancreas
(Chapter 26), and sweat glands—all tissues which sporadically secrete
large volumes of fluid, which secretion calls for an especially large delivery
of blood. This specific vasodilator factor seems to be particularly dominating in its action. Kallidin, like bradykinin, not only causes precapillary
vasodilatation; it also increases capillary permeability (Chapter 26).

Neurogenic Mechanisms

Although the level of basal vascular tone in a local circuit is determined by
the interplay of local mechanical and chemical factors, neurogenic mechanisms exert a "remote" control of the over-all situation, which permits
optimal distribution of the circulating blood in emergency states and
which serves to adjust the circulation to the requirements of the body as a
whole. Far and away the most important influence in this respect is
furnished by the activity of the sympathetic adrenergic vasoconstrictor
nerves.

Vasoconstrictor Fibres

The adrenergic vasoconstrictor fibres act by releasing noradrenaline (NA)
(Euler, 1956) in direct contact with the outer sheath only (in most vessels)
of the vascular media (Fig. 16-6). NA couples with α-receptors in the
membrane of the muscle cell and causes contraction of the muscle. Only

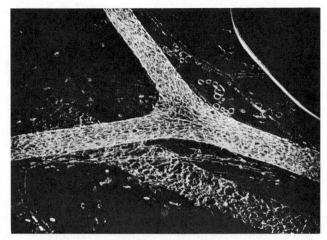

Fig. 16-6. Microphotograph of an arteriole and a small vein with the Falck-Hillarp fluorescence method, illustrating the very dense network of adrenergic axon ramifications, making "en passant" synaptic connections with the outer sheath of smooth muscle. (From Falck, 1962. By permission.)

the placental vessels lack noradrenergic vasoconstrictor innervation entirely; all other circuits possess this innervation—some sparsely supplied, such as the cerebral or coronary vessels, others densely, such as the cutaneous vessels. Modulation of the discharge over such nerves achieves the central and reflex control of the vascular bed in all but a few instances.

Adjustment of regional flow by sympathetic constrictor nerves depends on several factors.

Density of Regional Fibre Distribution

This varies between the sparse innervation of cerebral vessels, supplying a tissue which can ill afford ischaemia, and the dense innervation of skin vessels. Skin does not indulge in much metabolic activity, but it does furnish the most important site of regulation of heat loss. Maximal vasoconstrictor discharge may almost completely stop cutaneous blood flow and thereby ensure heat conservation; conversely, the inhibition of cutaneous vasoconstriction by hypothalamic mechanisms, which operate in circumstances of hyperthermia, markedly increases heat loss from the body. Between the extremes represented by these two vascular circuits, sympathetic effects vary quantitatively in the different regional circuits and these circuits are correspondingly rationed thereby.

The various *consecutive* components of the series-coupled vessels comprising each vascular circuit may receive different numbers of vasoconstrictor fibres. Usually, large arteries and veins and the precapillary sphincters are relatively sparsely innervated. It would appear that the patency of the sphincter sections, and hence of the capillary bed which they command, is more affected by local factors, such as are provided by the interstitial concentrations of tissue metabolites.

It seems that three major effects may be produced by variations of vasomotor supply and/or discharge to a regional circuit. First, there is the adjustment of total regional flow resistance. Second, there is the adjustment of the pre/postcapillary resistance ratio, which secures a mobilization of tissue fluid when such is required. The huge mass of the muscles is the most important site of such fluid transfer. In this particular tissue constrictor fibre activity produces a more profound change in the precapillary resistance than in that of the postcapillary vessels, and an exacerbation of the vasomotor discharge thus lowers the mean capillary pressure and favours fluid imbibition from the tissues—*a mobilization of extravascular fluid*. Third, there is the adjustment of venous capacitance *in toto*, so as to secure appropriate priming of the cardiac pump by the venous return (*intravascular fluid mobilization*).

Differences in Effector Sensitivity

Differences in sensitivity among the vascular smooth muscle of the various regional circuits to the vasomotor transmitter and/or to local metabolites may provide further differentiation of vascular responses. Thus, stimulation of the sympathetic nerves to the vessels in resting skeletal muscle causes a vasoconstriction which is fairly well sustained, despite the concomitant accumulation of tissue metabolites (Chapter 22), whereas some of the precapillary vessels in the intestinal circuit, despite the maintenance of sympathetic stimulation (Chapter 26), show only a transient vasoconstriction before flow returns towards normal.

Postcapillary vessels, less sensitive to metabolites than those in the precapillary sections, characteristically display well-sustained responses to vasoconstrictor nerve discharge. Thus, the control of venous capacitance by nervous influences is still manifest in the vascular bed of exercising muscle even though the vasodilator influence of the tissue metabolites has almost entirely overcome the effects of vasoconstrictor discharge on the precapillary vessels (Chapter 22). (It is important to remember, however, that the diving species provide a notable exception to this last statement, for in such creatures vasomotor discharge can maintain complete muscle

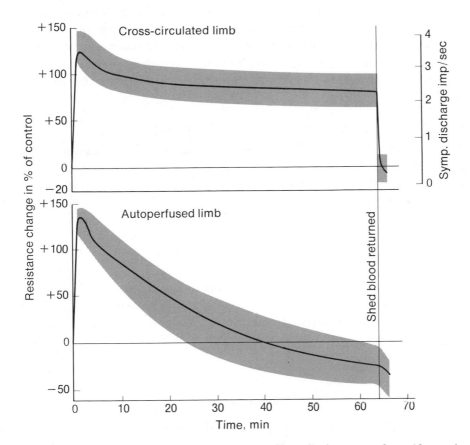

Fig. 16-7. Reflex increase in vasoconstrictor fibre discharge to the calf muscle vessels in a cat, produced by blood loss. The constriction is well maintained in one of the limbs which is provided with a satisfactory blood supply by cross-circulation. In the autoperfused limb, where the lowered pressure head implies a poor flow and a relative ischaemia, the neurogenic constriction gradually fails, predominantly on the precapillary side. Ultimately the resistance may become *lower* than control and the initial decrease of capillary pressure (with tissue fluid absorption) may derange into an increased capillary pressure with filtration losses as a consequence. (From Lundgren *et al.*, 1964. By permission.)

ischaemia during prolonged submersion. To.a great extent this is due to an extensive vasoconstrictor fibre influence also in larger arteries.)

In pathophysiological situations, such as shock, neurogenic precapillary resistance—initially intense—fades as the ischaemic situation is long sustained, yielding to the vasodilator influence of the accumulated metabolites; while postcapillary resistance, exacerbated by the vasoconstrictor discharge and more impervious to the effects of the tissue metabolites, remains raised. A situation results which favours an increase in capillary pressure, thereby minimizing fluid absorption from the tissues, or perhaps even promulgating fluid loss from the intravascular compartment (Fig. 16-7).

Variations in Vasoconstrictor Discharge Frequency

These variations may be achieved either by reactions involving the higher centres of the central neuraxis (as exemplified by the cortico-hypothalamic discharge which characterises the "defence reaction" or the activity of hypothalamic heat regulating centres) or by reflex influences exerted mainly at bulbar levels, stemming from alterations of the afferent activity in cardiovascular mechanoreceptor fibres or chemoreceptor fibres. Such problems are discussed in detail in Chapters 17, 18, and 19. It is worth mentioning here, however, that the range of discharge frequency in the tonically active vasoconstrictor fibres is narrow, varying from less than 1 impulse to about 8 impulses/sec. Nevertheless, this narrow range of discharge will virtually cover almost the full range of obtainable effector responses, especially on the postcapillary side (Fig. 16-8; see also Mellander and Johansson, 1968).

Vasodilator Fibres

The vasodilator fibres are not ubiquitous and are not tonically active. They comprise:

Cholinergic Sympathetic Vasodilator Nerves

These supply only the larger precapillary resistance vessels of skeletal muscle. They are activated only during the "defence reaction" which occurs when the animal is "alerted" and which is most manifest during intense fear or rage (see Chapter 19). The barrage of vasodilator impulses to the muscle vascular bed is accompanied by intense discharge of the other

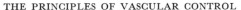

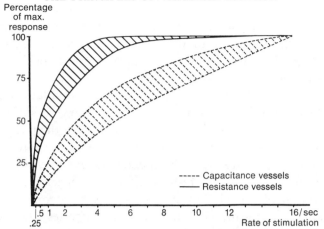

Fig. 16-8. The frequency-response relationship for the resistance and capacitance vessels of the cat's hindquarters. The rate of fibre stimulation is varied from 0-16/sec, and the responses are expressed as *per cent* of the maximal ones. It should be noted that in *absolute* values the resistance changes are by far the most powerful ones: the constrictor fibres can accomplish about an 8-fold resistance increase, but will only expel about 40% of the venous blood content. (From Mellander, 1960. By permission.)

sympathetic nerves, which increase the rate and force of the heart and which secure vasoconstriction of virtually all other regional vascular circuits except that of the brain and the myocardium. The muscles may thereby be provided with a nearly maximal blood supply.

Parasympathetic Vasodilator Nerves

These supply the salivary and some gastrointestinal glands and the external genitalia. Thus stimulation of the chorda tympani causes vasodilatation of the submaxillary gland and vagal stimulation evokes gastric mucosal hyperaemia. However, these effects are probably only to some extent, and perhaps not at all in some tissues, the result of specific vasodilator fibres. For example, in the salivary glands a specific enzyme, kallikrein, is liberated from the gland cells and this splits off a vasodilator polypeptide from globulin (Hilton and Lewis, 1956). The peptide, earlier thought to be bradykinin (nine amino acids) but now known to be kallidin (ten amino acids) (Webster and Pierce, 1963), is not only a potent vasodilator but also increases capillary permeability. Aminopeptidases can rapidly transform kallidin into bradykinin. However, it appears that, besides the kallidin-bradykinin mechanism, the vessels of the salivary glands, at least the larger vessels, are supplied with specific vasodilator fibres as well (see Chapter 26).

The pial vessels of the brain are supplied with vasodilator fibres emerging from the facial nerve; their functional significance is still unknown.

Engorgement of genital erectile tissue occurs when the parasympathetic component of the second and third sacral roots are excited. The exact haemodynamic events are not fully understood but they no doubt are of paramount importance for the preservation of the species. Evidently, profound dilatation of the "inflow channels" leads to rapid filling of the erectile tissue at a pressure close to that in the arteries; therefore it must be assumed that the "outflow channels" in this situation offer the main resistance to flow by far, without being primarily constricted. Restoration of tone of the inflow channels normalizes the pressure drop curve along this specific circuit by increasing inflow resistance well beyond the outflow resistance, so that the erectile tissue is again emptied (Dorr and Brody, 1967).

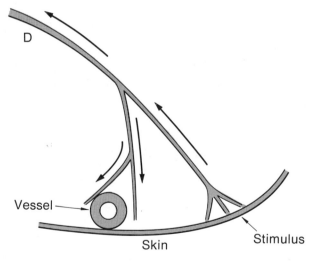

Fig. 16-9. D is a sensory fibre destined for the dorsal root cell body and thence the spinal cord. It is an unmyelinated fibre and its peripheral branches furnish the pathways of the axon reflex. An injurious stimulus not only arouses impulses which travel to the spinal cord but also by the axon reflex pathway to the arterioles of the skin in the vicinity, producing vasodilatation and flare.

Dorsal root dilator fibres cause a vasodilatation of significant magnitude only in skin and superficial mucous membranes. They are demonstrated by stimulation of the peripheral end of the cut dorsal root. In this case there is an antidromic conduction of the impulse to the periphery; the same situation occurs naturally when the dorsal root ganglion is infected by the virus of herpes zoster (shingles) which causes the well-known manifestation of vasodilatation and vesicles in the skin supplied by that root. Nevertheless their physiological role is to secure cutaneous arteriolar dilatation as a response to local injury or infection. The C fibres, which supply the skin and which convey nociceptive information therefrom to the neuraxis, branch peripherally and excitation of these fibres causes impulses to pass both centrally and, by the peripheral branch, to arterioles in the vicinity (Fig. 16-9). These dilate and their response causes the "flare" which appears as part of the triple response noted by Lewis (1927). The transmitter that they liberate is not known but it causes a much more prolonged vasodilatation than that of other known agents.

Hormonal Influences

Several hormones influence vascular calibre.

The adrenal medulla secretes either mainly adrenaline (A), e.g. in man; or mainly noradrenaline (NA), e.g. in diving species and in the human foetus; or a mixture of the two, e.g. in cats and dogs.

Noradrenaline exerts pure vasoconstrictor effects essentially everywhere (except possibly in the coronary vessels) by coupling with α-receptors in the smooth muscle membranes. Adrenaline combines both with α-receptors, causing constriction, and β-receptors, causing dilatation. In the vascular beds of skeletal and cardiac muscle, the liver, and the adrenal glands themselves, the precapillary sections possess either so many β-receptors or, alternatively, such an affinity of their β-receptors for adrenaline that adrenaline in "physiological" concentrations causes a pure resistance decrease in these circuits. Thus adrenaline causes a redistribution of blood flow, myocardium, muscle, and liver receiving more blood at the expense of other circuits (kidney, skin, gastrointestinal tract) which suffer constriction (see Euler, 1956). Nevertheless the cardiovascular influence of the catecholamines liberated naturally from the adrenal medulla is usually trivial compared with that evoked by sympathetic nervous discharge to the heart and most systemic circuits (Celander, 1954). However, adrenaline also causes important metabolic effects in the liver, in muscles and in fat (manifest e.g. by the hyperglycaemia which results from increased glycogenolysis) and these represent perhaps the most important physiological actions of adrenaline.

It is not known why the medulla of diving creatures secrete only NA. It is interesting to note that the adrenal glands of the human foetus contain only NA, and, after all, the foetus lives submerged *in utero* exposed to oxygen pressures lower than that supplying the adult; the foetus also displays cardiovascular adjustments similar to those of the diving reflex (see Chapter 19). These adjustments are utilized when the maternal blood supply is hampered during labour. Clearly the diving species are adapted for profound vasoconstriction of their skeletal muscle beds while swimming underwater and NA, with its vasoconstrictor effect on muscle vessels, is "more appropriate".

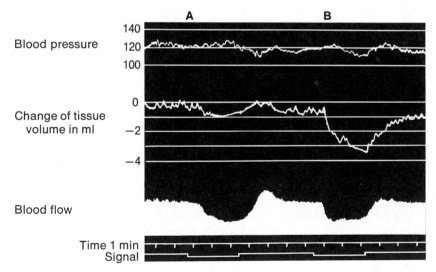

Fig. 16-10. Comparison between the effects of angiotensin (A) and noradrenaline (B), when given as intra-arterial infusions in concentrations that produce equally pronounced resistance responses. Note that noradrenaline produces a marked reduction of *tissue volume*—due to constriction of the venous capacitance vessels—while angiotensin in this respect induces only trivial effects. (From Folkow *et al.*, 1961. By permission.)

Vasopressin was so christened when an extract of the posterior pituitary gland was shown to cause a marked sustained rise of blood pressure when injected into an experimental animal. "Antidiuretin", or "ADH", should replace the name "vasopressin", since it is now known that the substance is an octapeptide which exerts profound antidiuretic effects at plasma concentrations usually well below those required for vascular changes, except perhaps in the cutaneous circuit. Thus, it has been suggested that the prolonged skin pallor in connection with fainting may be due to the excessive secretion of this octapeptide, known to occur in this situation.

Angiotensin B (see Page and McCubbin, 1968) is an octapeptide which is formed from the globulin preangiotensin by the enzyme renin, formed and liberated by the myoepithelial cells of the renal juxtaglomerular apparatus in circumstances of reduced flow and/or reduced pulsatile pressure. Angiotensin, the most powerful biological vasoconstrictor known, with respect to some vascular circuits at least, exerts its action mainly on the systemic *resistance* vessels (Fig. 16-10). Recent findings suggest that angiotensin may not achieve plasma concentrations in the intact resting organism that would affect vascular tone significantly *by a direct action*. Nevertheless, angiotensin plasma concentrations appear to be sufficient to stimulate aldosterone production by the zona glomerulosa of the adrenal cortex and this in turn modifies renal sodium excretion and hence contributes to the retention of sodium and thus water in the body. Salt/water equilibrium profoundly affects the activity of vascular smooth muscles.

In blood loss, exercise, and other situations involving neurogenic reduction of renal blood flow, plasma angiotensin concentration rises and may then exert a more marked influence on precapillary tone. Further, there is evidence that angiotensin reinforces the effect of sympathetic vasoconstriction on the vascular system (McCubbin *et al.*, 1965), but it is unknown whether it does this by a central action or whether it exerts a peripheral influence (see Chapter 31).

Adrenal corticoids influence vascular tone by affecting the salt-water environment of the smooth muscle cells, and seem to be "permissive" in action rather than being immediately involved in the regulation of vascular tone.

Serotonin (5-HT) was once thought to be important in normal vascular control mechanisms. However, it is not primarily involved in systemic control, although it undoubtedly exerts a local influence in vascular damage, being liberated from the thrombocytes when these aggregate either in the vicinity of endothelial lesions or in circumstances of embolism or thrombosis. Serotonin powerfully constricts the small resistance vessels and contributes to haemostasis. Otherwise serotonin is of interest with respect to cardiovascular pathophysiology in carcinoid of the intestine, a tumour which secretes and liberates this compound (see Page, 1968).

Prostaglandins exert powerful vasodilator effects, but it is as yet not known whether they are primarily involved in the control of vascular tone (see Bergström and Samuelsson, 1967).

Histamine dilates precapillary vessels and increases capillary permeability. It is released from local mast cells in tissue injury and in some allergic manifestations and causes the red reaction, flare and wheal in the cutaneous "triple response", probably in co-operation with locally formed *"plasma kinins"*, such as bradykinin. There is no evidence that histamine participates in any other specific vascular control mechanisms, with the possible exception of the gastric mucosal vessels during acid secretion.

Bohr has recently found that normal plasma contains a chemical agent (or agents) which reinforces vascular myogenic tone and may even initiate such activity when it is latent. The nature of this agent is unknown but it might prove to be of considerable importance for "setting" the level of myogenic activity throughout the vascular bed (see Bohr and Johansson, 1966). However, small arterial-arteriolar vessels display myogenic activity even when perfused with Krebs solution, where specific vasoactive substances are absent (Chapter 15), illustrating the inherent nature of basal vascular tone.

References

Bayliss, W. M. (1902). "On the local reactions of the arterial wall to changes in internal pressure," *J. Physiol.* **28,** 220–31. (London.)

Bergström, S., and B. Samuelsson (1967). *Prostaglandins.* Stockholm: Almqvist and Wiksell.

Bohr, D. F., and B. Johansson (1966). "Contraction of vascular smooth muscle in response to plasma". *Circ. Res.* **XIX,** 593–601.

Celander, O. (1954). "The range of control exercised by the 'sympathico-adrenal system', " *Acta Physiol. Scand.*, **32,** Suppl. 116.

Dorr, L. D., and M. J. Brody (1967). "Hemodynamic mechanisms of erection in the canine penis," *Am. J. Physiol.* **213,** 1526–31.

Duke, H. (1957). "Observations on the effects of hypoxia on the pulmonary vascular bed," *J. Physiol.* **135,** 45–51. (London.)

Euler, U. S. von (1956). *Noradrenaline.* Springfield, Ill.: Charles C. Thomas.

Euler, U. S. von, and G. Liljestrand (1946). "Observations on the pulmonary arterial blood pressure in the cat," *Acta Physiol. Scand.* **12,** 301–20.

Falck, B. (1962). "Observations on the possibilities of the cellular localization of monoamines by a fluorescence method," *Acta Physiol. Scand.*, **56,** Suppl., 197, 1–25.

Folkow, B. (1962). "Transmural pressure and vascular tone—some aspects of an old controversy," *Arch. Int. Pharmacodyn.* **139,** 455–69.

Folkow, B. (1964). "Description of the myogenic hypothesis," *Circ. Res.* **XIV, XV,** Suppl., 1, 279–85.

Folkow, B., B. Johansson, and S. Mellander (1961). "The comparative effects of angiotensin and noradrenaline on consecutive vascular sections," *Acta Physiol. Scand.* **53,** 99–104.

Hilton, S. M. (1962). "Local mechanisms regulating peripheral blood flow," *Physiol. Rev* **42,** Suppl., 5, 265–75.

Hilton, S. M., and G. P. Lewis (1956). "The relationship between glandular activity, bradykinin formation and functional vasodilatation in the sub-mandibular salivary gland," *J. Physiol.* **134,** 471–83. (London.)

Katori, M., and R. M. Berne (1966). "Release of adenosine from anoxic hearts". *Circ. Res,* **XIX,** 720–25.

Kjellmer, I. (1965). "Studies of exercise hyperaemia," *Acta Physiol. Scand.* **64,** Suppl., 244, 1–27.

Lewis, T. (1927). *The blood vessels of the human skin and their responses.* London: Shaw & Sons Ltd.

Lundgren, O., J. Lundvall, and S. Mellander (1964). "Range of sympathetic discharge, and reflex vascular adjustments in skeletal muscle during hemorrhagic hypotension," *Acta Physiol. Scand.,* **62,** 380–90.

McCubbin, J. W., and I. H. Page (1963). "Neurogenic component of chronic renal hypertension," *Science*, **139**, No. 3551, 210–15.

McCubbin, J. W., R. Soares De Moura, I. H. Page, and F. Olmsted (1965). "Arterial hypertension elicited by subpressor amounts of angiotensin," *Science*, **149**, No. 3690, 1394–95.

Mellander, S. (1960). "Comparative studies on the adrenergic neuro-hormonal control of resistance and capacitance blood vessels in the cat," *Acta Physiol. Scand.* **50**, Suppl., 176, 1–86.

Mellander, S., and B. Johansson (1968). "Control of resistance, exchange and capacitance functions in the peripheral circulation," *Pharmacol. Rev.* **20**, 117–96.

Mellander, S., B. Öberg, and H. Odelram (1964). "Vascular adjustments to increased transmural pressure in cat and man with special reference to shifts in capillary fluid transfer," *Acta Physiol. Scand.* **61**, 34–48.

Page, I. H. (1968). *Serotonin.* Chicago: Year Book Med. Publ.

Page, I. H., and J. W. McCubbin (1968). *Renal Hypertension.* Chicago: Year Book Med. Publ.

Webster, M. E., and J. V. Pierce (1963). "The nature of the kallidins released from human plasma by kallikreins and other enzymes," *Ann. N. Y. Acad. Sci.* **104**, 91–107.

17

Nervous Control of the Circulation:
1   The Medullary Cardiovascular Centre

Historical Landmarks

Physiologists were slow in analysing the influence of the central nervous system on cardiovascular performance, despite the fact that blanching and blushing of the face and changed beating of the heart have, since the dawn of literature, been colourfully described as the mirror of man's joy and distress. Even though scattered experimental observations were made in the eighteenth century (for ref. see Heymans and Folkow, 1964) it was only towards the middle of the nineteenth century that the first real progress was made. Experimental workers at this time had recently enjoyed the advantages of three important new technical methods: the mercury manometer of Poiseuille, the kymograph of Ludwig, and the induction coil of du Bois-Reymond. Continuous graphic registration of blood pressure, heart rate, etc., permitted an evaluation of the effects of electrical stimulation of efferent and afferent nerves.

Thus, Claude Bernard, Brown-Séquard, Budge, and Waller in Paris, almost simultaneously between 1851 and 1853 defined the vasoconstrictor function of the sympathetic nerves supplying the peripheral blood vessels. Shortly afterward, Bernard made the important observation that section

307

of the spinal cord in the lower cervical region caused a profound fall of blood pressure. This suggested a tonic sympathetic discharge causing arteriolar constriction with the activity emerging somewhere in the brain stem. It was further shown that afferent stimulation of "somatic" nerves caused pressor responses, due to the activation of all the sensory fibres, with the effects of the nociceptive C fibres predominating.

Then, in 1866, Cyon and Ludwig found that the stimulation of the central end of a nerve emerging from the cardiovascular system itself, lying parallel to but separate from the cervical vagus and sympathetic trunks, caused marked bradycardia and hypotension. This discovery of the "depressor nerves" was a great landmark in the history of servocontrol. Ludwig suggested that these sensory nerves arose from the heart itself, reporting overloading of the cardiac chambers to the neuraxis and inducing reflex changes in cardiac force and rate of contraction and in arteriolar resistance which would lessen the work done by the heart. It was shown during the next forty years that the depressor nerves in fact arose from the aortic arch and right subclavian arteries rather than the heart, but the brilliance of the idea remains.

In the 1870's, directed by Ludwig, Dittmar and Owsjannikow delineated the site of the "vasomotor" centre by several different techniques. First, successive transections of the brain stem caused no change in the arterial blood pressure until the transection involved that part of the medulla below the level of the facial colliculus. At and below that level, transections caused an increasing slump of arterial pressure so that cutting at the level of the obex caused a fall of pressure to 40 mm Hg—a level similar to that produced by transection of the cervical spinal cord. Second, stimulation of the floor of the IVth ventricle at certain sites—between the facial colliculus and the obex—caused marked vascular pressor effects. Third, the pressor responses to stimulation of the central end of the sciatic nerve were progressively abolished by such transections at increasingly lower levels of the medulla.

As a consequence of these findings there was a clear understanding in the 1870's that the medulla contained a vasomotor, or, more correctly, a cardiovascular centre which tonically excited the sympathetic system, thereby causing vasoconstriction and cardiac acceleration. The main interest, however, was on the effects of the vasoconstriction on the arterioles, rather than on the veins, although Goltz had shown in 1864 that paralysis of the abdominal sympathetics produced marked dilatation of the splanchnic veins and a bloodless heart. This observation received little further attention for another fifty years.

Later work, e.g. by Ranson and his colleagues some fifty years ago, showed that the "pressor" afferents of the sciatic nerve were transmitted by fibres which coursed dorsolaterally in the spinal cord in the tract of Lissauer. If these tracts were cut bilaterally at the level of the first thoracic segment, the systemic blood pressure did not fall, but the pressor responses evoked by afferent sciatic stimulation were abolished. It follows that the activity of the medullary vasomotor centre is not normally dependent upon such afferent impulses, and that its descending fibres run elsewhere, notably in ventrolateral parts of the cord.

Section of the spinal cord at L3 of an otherwise intact anaesthetized animal does not cause a fall of blood pressure. Hence the spinal neurones responsible for "keeping the blood pressure up" must lie between these two spinal segmental levels. The relevant cell bodies—the "final common path" for central and reflex effects on the cardiovascular system—are found in the intermediolateral horn of the grey matter of the thoraco-lumbar segments T1–L2. They and their axons form the *preganglionic* neurones of the sympathetic outflow. With considerable convergence and divergence they form synapses with the *postganglionic* neurones in the sympathetic ganglia, but no reflex integration occurs at this level. The axons of the postganglionic neurones ramify extensively and—again with considerable convergence and divergence—they make *en passant* synaptic contacts with cardiac and vascular effectors, as described in Chapter 15.

Thus, the basic principles of nervous cardiovascular control were established almost 100 years ago: Tonically active neurones in the oblongate medulla, adjusted in their activity by the afferent input from cardiovascular receptors, control the heart and blood vessels via vagal and sympathetic fibres. Modern research has, however, greatly expanded our knowledge about the operation of this servocontrol and has additionally focused our attention on the importance of cortico-hypothalamic influences, which were unknown up to some fifty years ago. Present-day concepts are summarized below, starting with the functional organization of the tonically active cardiovascular centre in the oblongate medulla. There is also an extensive literature in this field, and many reviews that present various aspects of reflex and central nervous control of the circulation (e.g. Heymans and Neil, 1958; Uvnäs, 1960; Eichna and McQuarrie, 1960; Lindgren, 1961; Folkow *et al.*, 1965; Peiss, 1965).

Function of the Medullary and Spinal Cardiovascular Centres

Organization

Present knowledge of the medullary control is mainly based on the studies by Wang and Ranson (1939), Monnier (1939), and Alexander (1946), who explored the effects of topical stimulations and of transections on the blood pressure and heart rate and on the impulse activity in cardiac sympathetic and cervical sympathetic nerves. Stimulation of the bulbo-pontine region caused either pressor or depressor effects depending upon the site of the stimulating electrode. Figure 17-1 shows the respective sites from which pressor or depressor responses could be induced. The pressor areas extended slightly more rostrally and were more laterally situated than those of the depressor areas.

Ablation experiments gave additional information. Transection at the level of the facial genu detached some of the rostral pressor region whilst leaving all of the depressor region intact (Level I). The blood pressure fell appreciably and the impulse activity in the cardiovascular sympathetic nerves lessened. The reflex increase of systemic blood pressure and cardiac sympathetic impulse activity in response to central sciatic nerve stimulation was also diminished. Stimulation of the medial reticular area—the "medullary depressor point"—then caused a further fall of arterial pressure and a reduction in such sympathetic impulse activity as was still present. Section at level II (Fig. 17-1), immediately above the obex, abolished sympathetic impulse activity completely and caused a maximal fall of blood pressure. This second section abolished nearly all of the lateral "pressure area" while the major part of the medial depressor area was still in contact with the spinal cord. However, section at level III restored some slight tonic discharge in the sympathetic fibres. This latter finding is of interest for two reasons. First, it may suggest that the spinal preganglionic neurones are also capable of some tonic activity (at least during the current experimental situation) and, second, that the medial depressor area exerts a *tonic inhibitory* influence via direct descending pathways converging on the autonomic "final common path" in the spinal cord.

Lateral parts of the bulbar reticulum thus contain pools of "spontaneously" active neurones, which, via descending excitatory fibres, "drive" the pre- and post-ganglionic sympathetic neurones to exert a tonic excitatory influence on both heart and blood vessels. Presumably these neurone pools in the lateral pressor area are in mutual contact with the inhibitory ones in the medial depressor area with reciprocal interaction between them, at the same time as they both send descending fibres— with excitatory and inhibitory actions, respectively—to the spinal "final common paths", their net effect being in most situations an *excitatory* one.

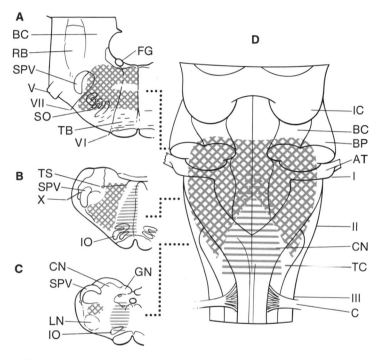

Fig. 17-1. Localization of pressor (crosshatching) and depressor (horizontal ruling) centres in the brain stem of the cat. A-C: cross sections through medulla at levels indicated by guide lines to D; D: semidiagrammatic projection of pressor and depressor regions onto the dorsal surface of the brain stem viewed with the cerebellar peduncles cut across and the cerebellum removed. AT: auditory tubercle; BC: brachium conjunctiva; BP: brachium pontis; C_1: first cervical nerve; CN: cuneate nucleus; FG: facial genu; GN: gracile nucleus; IC: inferior colliculus: IO; inferior olivary nucleus; LN: lateral reticular nucleus; RB: restiform body; SO: superior olivary nucleus; SPV: spinal trigeminal tract; TB: trapezoid body; TC: tuberculum cinerum; TS: tractus solitarius. V, VI, VII: corresponding cranial nerves; I, II, III: levels of transection. (From Alexander, 1946. By permission.)

This medullary complex of tonically active neurone pools, which exert a net excitatory drive on the cardiovascular system via the adrenergic sympathetic pathways, is often called the *"vasomotor centre"* (VMC). This name is hardly adequate, however, since the sympathetic control of the heart is involved as well, and this control is structurally so interwoven with the vascular control that a separation in terms is hardly justified. Furthermore, these neurone pools function in close association with the "cardio-inhibitory centre" in the dorsal motor nucleus of the vagus, which exerts a tonic restraining influence on the heart via the cholinergic vagal neurones. The whole complex is, perhaps, best defined as the *medullary cardiovascular centre*, in which three subdivisions—the vasomotor "centre" and the reciprocally active cardio-excitatory and cardio-inhibitory "centres"—may be distinguished.

Together, these medullary "centres"—receiving the all-important information derived from the cardiovascular "proprioreceptors" (see Chapter 18)—form the key to cardiovascular homeostasis, exposing the heart to the reciprocal tonic control of vagal inhibitory and sympathetic excitatory fibres, while the steady control of the vascular bed is exercised by the sympathetic constrictor fibres only (see Folkow, 1955). As mentioned in Chapter 16, the dilator fibres are distributed to a few tissues only and their activation is restricted to particular situations.

The medullary cardiovascular centre is, thanks to its servocontrol, capable of regulating the blood pressure, the cardiac output, and the flow distribution, and of displaying a considerable range of adjustments appropriate for these purposes even when it is disconnected from higher nervous structures. In *this* sense it functions as a true "centre" of considerable independence. This does not, of course, deny that it normally works in such intimate and steady association with higher autonomic integration centres (see Chapter 19) that they should be considered together as a *functional unit* rather than as independent control levels (see Peiss, 1965). For instance, the cardiovascular proprioreceptors—as well as other receptors affecting cardiovascular control—also establish reflex connections with autonomic structures at higher levels of the neuraxis. By means of descending excitatory and inhibitory pathways such higher autonomic structures may modulate, or, in some situations, even over-sway, the tonically active medullary centre. Beautiful examples of this are given in the studies made by Khayutin *et al.* (see Fedina *et al.*, 1966) and in the analysis of the reflex adjustments to hypoxia made by Korner and his group (1969). In addition, such descending pathways may also affect the "final common path" directly, i.e. the preganglionic sympathetic neurones. This system for control of the autonomic "final common path" is hardly inferior in complexity to that directing the somatomotor "final common path", the motoneurones. It is certainly not a simple system for diffuse excitation-inhibition, as was often assumed earlier; it is characterized by adjustments of great subtlety, as will be seen below.

Background of the Tonic Activity

It should be stressed that the medullary neurone pools, responsible for tonic sympathetic activity, are normally exposed to a considerable *restraining* influence from the cardiovascular mechanoreceptors (see Chapter 18). Even when the bulb is entirely isolated from all afferent impulses, a considerable tonic discharge prevails, similar to that emanating from the primary respiratory centres. The local chemical environment is highly important for this "spontaneous" neuronal activity, especially perhaps the local pH, but also pCO_2 and pO_2 (compare respiration; Pappenheimer, 1967). This local environment, again, is dependent on the current balance between metabolism, blood supply, and blood composition. Therefore, these neurone pools—at least their "pacemakers"—might in a sense be considered as sensitive chemoreceptors, which at normal $[H^+]$, etc., are sufficiently active to provide a considerable neurogenic "drive" for the cardiovascular system. In resting organism equilibrium, under the restraining effect of the cardiovascular mechanoreceptors, this "drive" corresponds to a discharge below or around 1 to 2 impulses/sec, though it is not always uniform throughout the system (Folkow, 1955, 1960). The importance of the local chemical environment is perhaps best illustrated by the reduction and ultimate cessation of tonic sympathetic discharge if $[H^+]$ and pCO_2 are lowered enough, e.g. by hyperventilation.

The vagal cardio-inhibitory "centre", in contrast to the sympathetic ones, is tonically active, mainly owing to the input from the cardiovascular mechanoreceptors, and it has little or no "inherent" activity. Thus section of the carotid sinus and aortic nerves virtually abolishes cardiac vagal tone.

The powerful negative feedback provided by the cardiovascular mechanoreceptors is relayed in the medial depressor area of the medulla. These inhibitory neurones are excited thereby and presumably damp both the medullary tonic activity and the spinal preganglionic neurones directly. While the cardiovascular mechanoreceptors thus form a *negative* feedback for the medullary drive on the sympathetic activity, the arterial chemoreceptors exert a *positive* drive, but essentially only on the "vaso-motor" and cardio-inhibitory "centres". In other words, a chemoreceptor excitation has basically opposite effects on heart and blood vessels, pro-ducing reflex bradycardia but systemic vasoconstriction. Such a primary chemoreceptor reflex bradycardia is seen only during enforced apnea and

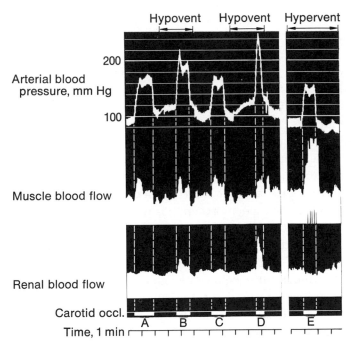

Fig. 17-2. Curarised, anaesthetized, and atropinised cat; vagal nerves cut in the neck and adrenal glands denervated. Effect of bilateral occlusion of the common carotid arteries on blood pressure, muscle, and renal blood flows under dif-ferent respiratory conditions. The muscle vessels are considerably affected by carotid occlusion irrespective of the respiratory state, whereas the renal vessels are markedly affected only during hypoventilation. In hyperventilation renal blood flow is merely passively increased in connection with the reflex blood-pressure rise following carotid occlusion. The ordinates in the blood-flow tracings are inversely proportional to the rate of flow. (From Folkow *et al.*, 1961. By permission.)

is the key to the diving response (see Chapter 19). Whenever hyperpnea can normally occur as a result of chemoreceptor stimulation, reflex tachycardia ensues instead, as a result of the secondary afferent discharge from pulmonary stretch receptors that masks the "primary" bradycardia. In the resting animal, chemoreceptor reflex circulatory effects are insignificant, in contrast to the effects of the mechanoreceptors.

To complicate matters further, it appears that the various neurone pools of the medulla, which control the sympathetic fibres to the heart and various vascular circuits, may differ somewhat in excitability and hence in basic activity rate (Löfving, 1961; Folkow et al., 1961). For instance, elimination of the restraining influence exerted by the cardiovascular mechanoreceptors causes a bigger sympathetic vasoconstriction of the muscle resistance vessels, more pronounced than in those of the renal and cutaneous circuits or in the veins. However, when further excitation is added (e.g. by increasing $[H^+]$ and pCO_2) all the neurone pools become increasingly involved, until an over-all, massive discharge results (Fig. 17-2). Such features are reminiscent of those involving the organization of the respiratory centres. Here again the excitability level of the different neurone pools controlling normal and accessory respiratory muscle certainly differs, but a sufficiently intense drive will recruit them all and ultimately will excite them maximally.

Lastly, other afferents can also influence the discharge of the medullary neurone pools variably. As an example, somatic pressor fibres (mainly unmyelinated nociceptive fibres) cause a greater constrictor response in the kidney than in the muscle vascular bed (Fig. 17-3). The hypothalamic thermoregulatory centres are fairly selective; they engage only the neurone pools that control the cutaneous vasoconstrictor fibres. The hypothalamic defence area (see Chapter 19) engages virtually all the vasoconstrictor fibres save those to the muscle resistance vessels. Whether these differentiated effects are induced at medullary or spinal levels, or both, is not known, but these examples illustrate the degree of differentiation of the medullo-spinal control of the circulation. As seen in Chapter 16, however, differentiation of the neurogenic cardiovascular control is not only a matter of different discharge *rates* (where only minor differences are of great consequence for the effector responses); fibre distribution, effector sensitivity, etc., contribute as well.

Be this as it may, these regional differences in discharge indicate that the seemingly extensive convergence and divergence principle of the sympathetic innervation must be delimited to take place within well-defined "functional units" of the cardiovascular system such as the pre- and post-ganglionic compartments of individual vascular circuits, or the rate- and power-controlling parts of the heart. It would otherwise be difficult to explain that the "resistance" and "capacitance" sections of the muscle circuits are involved to a different extent in baroreceptor reflexes (Chapter 20), or that chronotropic and inotropic effects on the heart can be quantitatively different (Fang and Wang, 1962).

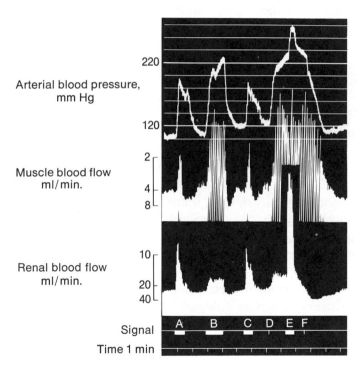

Fig. 17-3. Curarised, anaesthetized, and atropinised cat, vagal nerves cut in the neck. Effects of stimulation of "somatic pressor afferents" and of carotid artery occlusion on blood pressure, muscle and renal blood flows in the cat. A, C, and E: afferent "pressor" fibre stimulation; B and D-F: carotid occlusion. The muscle vessels, markedly constricted by unloading of the baroreceptors, show only moderate, transient responses to somatic pressor fibre stimulation. The renal vessels, on the other hand, are relatively more engaged in the latter reflex. (From Johansson, 1962. By permission.)

The Spinal Autonomic "Centres"

The medullary cardiovascular centre exerts a tonic excitatory influence on the preganglionic sympathetic neurones in the thoracolumbar sections of the spinal cord. However, these descending connections are probably not the only ones converging upon the spinal autonomic neurones. Thus, it is likely that still higher autonomic structures have direct excitatory pathways (via the pyramids?) and in all likelihood there are also descending inhibitory pathways, probably all relayed in, and hence emerging from, the medullary depressor area in medial parts of the oblongate medulla (see Löfving, 1961).

A variety of somatic and visceral afferents (with the exception of the cardiovascular "proprioreceptors") also make sequential spinal connections with the autonomic "final common path" in the thoracolumbar sections of the spinal cord. Normally, however, the activity of these spinal autonomic neurones is so dependent on the excitatory drive exerted from the bulbar centres that their activity is entirely dominated by this descending influence. Thus, even if segmental spinal reflexes affecting the blood vessels can be traced as the result, for example, of pain stimulation (such as segmental blanching of the skin over an intra-abdominal inflammatory reaction; Adams-Ray and Norlén, 1951), the *major* reflex impact of somatic and visceral afferents on the circulation is normally relayed at the bulbar level, or still higher levels, as was shown by Ranson and Billingsley (1916).

Nevertheless, the spinal autonomic reflexes may be very powerful after spinal transverse lesions (Whitteridge, 1960). Spinal autonomic neurones also appear to exert an increased tonic discharge in chronic spinal man, and their activity can, moreover, be enhanced by increased $[H^+]$ or pCO_2, and vice versa. Thus, although the isolated spinal autonomic neurones lack the fine integrative powers of the medullary structures, these neurones can still display similar but less powerful activity, but they are deprived of the all-important modulating influence exerted by the cardiovascular "proprioreceptors". Therefore, in spinal patients, because of this lack of reflex buffering, pain fibre stimulation ("pressor" afferents) may produce such violent vasoconstriction that dangerous pressure rises ensue (see Whitteridge, 1960).

References

Adams-Ray, J., and G. Norlén (1951). "Bladder distension reflex with vaso-constriction in cutaneous venous capillaries," *Acta Physiol. Scand.* **23,** 95–109.

Alexander, R. S. (1946). "Tonic and reflex functions of medullary sympathetic cardiovascular centres," *J. Neurophysiol.* **9,** 205–17.

Cyon, E. de, and C. Ludwig (1966). *Ber. sächs. Ges. (Akad.), Wiss.* **18,** 307.

Eichna, L. W., and D. G. McQuarrie (1960). "Symposium on nervous control of circulation," *Physiol. Rev.,* **40,** Suppl., 4.

Fang, H. S., and S. C. Wang (1962). "Cardioaccelerator and cardioaugmentor points in hypothalamus of the dog," *Am. J. Physiol.* **203,** 147–50.

Fedina, L., Y. Katunskii, V. M. Khayutin, and A. Mitsányi (1966). "Responses of renal sympathetic nerves to stimulation of afferent A and C fibres of tibial and mesenterial nerves," *Acta Physiol. Acad. Scient. Hung.* **29,** 157–76.

Folkow, B. (1955). "Nervous control of the blood vessels," *Physiol. Rev.* **35,** 629–63.

Folkow, B. (1960). "Range of control of the cardiovascular system by the central nervous system," *Physiol. Rev.* **40,** Suppl., 4, 93–99.

Folkow, B., B. Johansson, and B. Löfving (1961). "Aspects of functional differentiation of the sympatho-adrenergic control of the cardiovascular system," *Med. Exp.* **4,** 321–28.

Folkow, B., C. Heymans, and E. Neil (1965). "Integrated aspects of cardiovascular regulation," *Handbook of Physiology,* 2, Circulation **III,** 1787–1823.

Heymans, C. J. F., and B. Folkow (1964). "Vasomotor control and the regulation of blood pressure," in *Circulation of the Blood* (ed. A. P. Fishman and D. W. Richards), pp. 407–86. New York: Oxford University Press.

Heymans, C. J. F., and E. Neil (1958). *Reflexogenic areas of the cardiovascular system.* London: Churchill.

Johansson, B. (1962). "Circulatory responses to stimulation of somatic afferents," *Acta Physiol. Scand.* **57,** Suppl., 198.

Korner, P. I., J. B. Uther, and S. W. White (1969). "Central nervous integration of the circulatory and respiratory responses to arterial hypoxemia in the rabbit," *Circ. Res.* **24,** 757–76.

Lindgren, P. (1961). "The central regulation of the autonomic nervous system with special regard to the vasomotor control," in *Biochemistry, Pharmacology and Physiology*, pp. 103–16. Great Britain: Pergamon.

Löfving, B. (1961). "Cardiovascular adjustments induced from the rostral cingulate gyrus," *Acta Physiol. Scand.* **53,** Suppl., 184.

Monnier, M. (1939). "Les centres végétatifs bulbaires," *Arch. Int. Physiol.* **49,** 455–63.

Pappenheimer, J. R. (1967). "The ionic composition of cerebral extracellular fluid and its relation to control of breathing," from *The Harvey Lectures*, Series 61. New York and London: Academic Press.

Peiss, C. N. (1965). "Concepts of cardiovascular regulation: past, present and future," in *Nervous control of the heart*. Baltimore: Williams & Wilkins.

Ranson, S. W., and P. R. Billingsley (1961). "Vasomotor reactions from stimulation of the floor of the fourth ventricle," *Am. J. Physiol.* **41,** 85–91.

Uvnäs, B. (1960). "Central cardiovascular control," in *Handbook of Physiology*, 1, Neurophysiology **II,** 1131–62.

Wang, S. C., and S. W. Ranson (1939). "Autonomic responses to electrical stimulation of the lower brain stem," *J. Comp. Neurol.* **71,** 437–55.

Whitteridge, D. (1960). "Cardiovascular reflexes initiated from afferent sites other than the cardiovascular system itself," *Physiol. Rev.* **40,** Suppl., 4, 198–200.

18

Nervous Control of the Circulation:
11   Reflex Influences on the
Cardiovascular System

The Cardiovascular "Proprioceptors"

The main tonic influence exerted on the medullary cardiovascular centre emanates from *stretch receptors*, situated in the so-called reflexogenic zones. In addition there are *chemoreceptors* with only faint tonic activity during rest but of the utmost importance in some situations. For reviews of the literature see Heymans and Neil (1958), Paintal (1963), and Kezdi (1967).

The reflexogenic zones include the carotid sinus, the aortic arch, the thyrocarotid junction, and the cardiopulmonary area. With one notable exception (see below), the stimulation of the stretch receptors inhibits sympathetic discharge, chemoreceptor activation enhances sympathetic discharge, and both of them excite the vagal cardio-inhibitory "centre".

The stretch receptors, placed both at strategic "low-pressure" and at "high-pressure" sites of the cardiovascular system, inform the medullary cardiovascular centre about the degree of filling, the pressure level, etc., at the various sites, thus allowing for appropriate neurogenic adjustments for the maintenance of cardiovascular homeostasis. It seems reasonable that the reflex patterns from the various receptor sites—though usually similar in *direction*—are not quantitatively identical throughout (see below).

The Stretch Receptors

The Carotid Sinus

Because of its site, the carotid sinus is the most easily studied of the reflexogenic zones. As a dilatation at the origin of the internal carotid artery, it receives a sensory innervation via the carotid sinus nerve, which itself is a branch of the glossopharyngeal nerve. There are several hundred myelinated afferent fibres in each carotid sinus nerve and a much greater number of unmyelinated fibres, a fact which suggests some type of functional differentiation between them (Landgren, 1952).

These afferents are commonly called baroreceptors, although their nerve endings, arborizing in the adventitia of the sinus, are not excited by pressure per se, but by the expansion of the arterial wall which the pressure rise occasions. In other words, they are *mechanoreceptors* or *stretch receptors*. Thus, if such expansion is prevented by surrounding the arterial wall with a plaster of Paris cast, as the intraluminal pressure is artificially raised, the discharge of the nerve endings is no longer increased. Removal of the rigid cast restores their responsiveness. If the pressure is gradually lowered, their activity of course decreases, and it vanishes at the slight wall distension present at pressures around 40 to 60 mm Hg. If arterial pressure is further lowered, so that the vessel collapses, some of the nerves again become active, owing to the deformation of the vascular wall. This again illustrates that they are mechanoreceptors, not baroreceptors.

Furthermore, infiltration of the sinus wall with constrictor drugs causes powerful discharge, predominantly by thin fibres, despite the fact that pressure is not increased. Here the contracting smooth muscles have so deformed the wall that the mechanoreceptors become excited. On the basis of this observation, it has been much debated whether a specific servocontrol is established by an efferent sympathetic innervation of the smooth muscles in the sinus wall. Increased sympathetic discharge would then excite the mechanoreceptors via the muscle contraction and in such a way "amplify" the damping effect of the baroreceptor activity on tonic sympathetic discharge. However, no unequivocal evidence of such a mechanism exists so far, though the sinus region has a rich supply of adrenergic nerve fibres in some species (Reis and Fuxe, 1968).

Wherever these stretch receptors are situated, pressure is *pulsatile*. In the carotid sinus, each heart beat causes a pulsatile expansion of the sinus wall, which excites the receptors to discharge. Nerve impulse activity can be recorded from the cut sinus nerve (Fig. 18-1). At a normal mean arterial pressure the impulse activity is phasic, showing an outburst with each rise of pressure during systole, then being reduced or falling silent after the dicrotic notch in the carotid sinus arterial pressure tracing. When the pressure rises, each unit discharges at a greater frequency during systole and the discharge may persist (at a reduced frequency) during the whole of diastole. Conversely, if the arterial pressure falls, impulse activity of any one unit decreases and may even disappear.

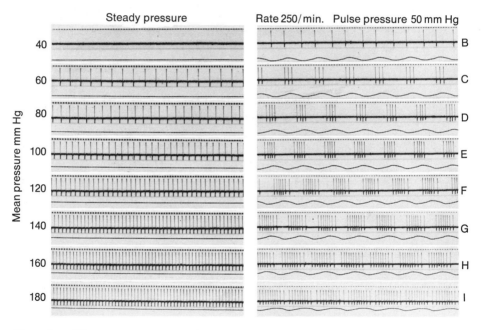

Fig. 18-1. Electroneurograms of a single baroreceptor fibre from the junction of the thyroid artery with the common carotid artery—a twig of the "common carotid nerve." The segment of the carotid artery was isolated and submitted to rises of static pressure. On the left, the pressures were maintained steadily at each level. On the right pulsations were delivered by a pump. Each record shows from above downwards, time (50c/s) electroneurogram and hydrostatic pressure (mm Hg) in the segment. (From Green, 1954. By permission.)

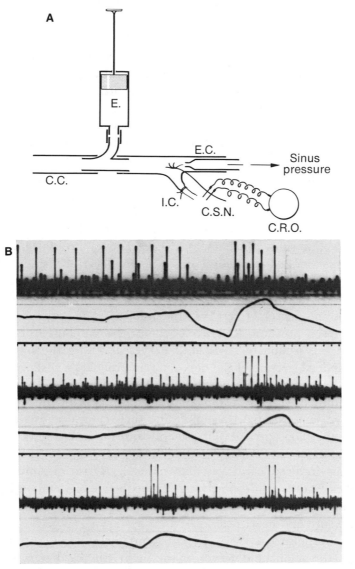

Fig. 18-2A. Upper diagram shows arrangement of a T-tube in the common carotid artery (CC). The stem of the T-tube can be connected to an elasticity reservoir (E) which then damps the pulsations delivered to the internal carotid (IC) and external carotid (EC). Sinus pressure is recorded by an electromanometer. Carotid sinus nerve (CSN) is laid on electrodes and baroreceptor impulse activity recorded on the cathode ray oscillograph (CRO).

Fig. 18-2B. Shows the alteration of afferent discharge in the baroreceptor units when the damped pulsation changes to the full carotid pulse. Three different pulsations are shown.

It is important to realize that these various units usually discharge with each pulse, although their *thresholds* may differ. A rise of pressure not only causes an increase in the discharge frequency of any one unit, but also provokes activity in a greater number of units (*recruitment*). Moreover, the frequency of discharge per unit time of any one unit is higher when it is exposed to a pulsatile pressure than to a steady pressure, even when the *mean* pressures are identical (Fig. 18-2). It follows that the afferent discharge, because it emanates from the pulsatile arterial pressure, has a more powerful inhibitory influence on tonic sympathetic discharge than if the the pressure had been non-pulsatile (Fig. 18-3).

These electroneurographic features can be correlated with evidence obtained from other experiments. Thus, clipping the common carotid arteries on both sides provokes a striking rise of arterial pressure—a response once ascribed to cerebral anaemia. However, it is simple to show that the application of clips on the efferent branches of the carotid bifurcation (internal and external carotid and occipital arteries), which causes the same degree of cerebral anaemia, does not provoke a rise of systemic arterial pressure. Moreover, when the common carotid arteries are clipped the section of both sinus nerves abolishes the hypertensive response—indeed, section of the nerves alone provokes a sustained hypertension, indicating that the nerves have been hitherto exerting a tonic inhibitory influence on the cardiovascular system. Their influence may be dramatically demonstrated by stimulating their central ends electrically, whereupon the blood pressure falls steeply and the heart slows.

Heymans and others showed that perfusion of the isolated innervated carotid sinus induced cardiovascular reflexes. A rise of sinus pressure caused reflex bradycardia—partly as a consequence of vagal excitation—and systemic hypotension; a fall of sinus pressure led to a reflex rise of arterial pressure and heart rate.

When the impulse activity of efferent sympathetic nerves supplying the vessels (e.g. the splanchnic nerve) or the heart (the cardiac sympathetic nerves) is recorded, it is readily shown that a rise of pressure in the isolated innervated sinus region reflexly induces an inhibition of sympathetic impulse activity and, conversely, that sinus hypotension provokes an exacerbation of sympathetic discharge. With respect to the vascular bed, these nerves appear to modulate especially sensitively the tone of the muscle resistance vessels, a fact that has important consequences for the reflex control of the plasma volume (Chapter 20).

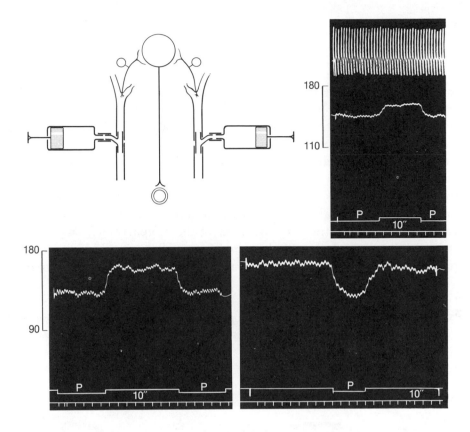

Fig. 18-3. A: Both common carotid arteries were cannulated and the cannulae attached to syringes containing air. When the syringes were excluded by clips the blood flow through the carotid sinuses was pulsatile. Removal of the clips converted the sinus blood flow to a non-pulsatile flow. Both sinus nerves were intact and exerted afferent inhibition of vasomotor discharge. Changes of peripheral resistance thereby induced caused changes of systemic blood pressure. B: Both aortic nerves cut, vagi intact. Common carotid arteries cannulated as shown in A. Records from above downwards: respiration, systemic blood pressure, signal marker and time in 10 sec intervals. Note that the systemic blood pressure is maintained at a higher level when sinus flow is non-pulsatile (as shown by signal marker) than when it is pulsatile (P). Respiration is unaffected. C: Aortic nerves and vagi cut. Arrangements as in A. Note that the systemic blood pressure is higher during non-pulsatile sinus flow (shown by signal marker) than that during pulsatile flow (P).
D: Obtained from the same preparation, 30 min later. During this period the carotid sinuses were exposed to non-pulsatile flow. The high level of systemic pressure was maintained (cf. C), but conversion to pulsatile sinus flow (P) lowered the systemic pressure. (From Ead et al., 1952. By permission.)

325

The Aortic Arch

In the mammal, the transverse part of the aortic arch represents the fourth left branchial gill arch, and its homologue (the fourth right arch) is represented by the root of the right subclavian artery. Each of these regions is innervated by vagal sensory branches whose endings are situated in the adventitia. The afferent fibres themselves course in the right (from the subclavian) and left aortic nerves. In the rabbit, these aortic (depressor) nerves are separate; in the cat, they may be discerned to be separate from the main vagal trunks. They join the central end of the superior laryngeal nerves and run centrally to their cell bodies in the nodose ganglia of the vagi, whence the central afferent fibres of these bipolar neurones run to the medulla. Stimulation of the central end of the aortic nerve causes reflex bradycardia and systemic hypotension. Atropinization greatly diminishes the bradycardia but not the hypotension, suggesting that the

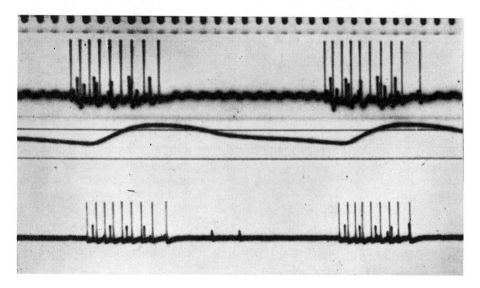

Fig. 18-4. Baroreceptor afferent discharge. Records from above downwards: time 50 c/s, "single" fibre of left aortic nerve, femoral arterial pressure, "single" fibre of right sinus nerve. Note that only two cardiac cycles are shown. Note that the aortic nerve ending discharges before the sinus nerve ending and that both discharge before the rise of pressure in the femoral artery (which is delayed). It must be remembered that each nerve contains several hundred such baroreceptors as are recorded singly here. (From Green and Neil, 1953. By permission.)

aortic afferents reflexly inhibit the sympathetic activity and excite the vagal heart fibres.

Selective section of the aortic nerves causes only a slight rise in systemic pressure because the remaining baroreceptor afferents (carotid sinus, pulmonary arterial, and cardiac) compensate for the loss of the tonic inhibitory influence of the aortic baroreceptors on the medullary cardio-vascular centre.

Impulse activity in the aortic nerves resembles that in the sinus nerves. The impulse bursts slightly precede those of the sinus nerve in each cardiac cycle (Fig. 18-4) because, of course, with each systolic ejection of the heart the expansion of the aorta occurs before that of the more peripherally placed carotid sinus.

Hering recognized that the sino-aortic nerves, being "high-pressure" receptors, act as a functional entity, and they are often known as the "buffer nerves". Whenever the blood pressure tends to fall their impulse activity is reduced. This reduction of their inhibitory effect on the medullary cardiovascular centre allows an escape of sympathetic adrenergic discharge which consequently increases. This helps to minimize the fall of pressure and may even restore the blood pressure to its original level. Conversely, a primary rise of blood pressure is buffered by an increase in baroreceptor afferent activity. This buffering effect is clearly shown in Fig. 18-5, in which the response of the systemic blood pressure to a rise in the pressure in both isolated carotid sinuses is shown to be considerably increased after cutting the vagi (which, in the dog, contain the aortic and cardiac receptor afferents). Prior to vagal section the intact aortic and other vagal afferents served to minimize the effect of sinus hypertension on the systemic blood pressure.

The Pulmonary Artery

This artery and its branches contain receptors of vagal fibres which subserve a reflex function, in principle identical with that of the sino-aortic afferents so far as the *systemic* blood pressure is concerned (Coleridge and Kidd, 1960). It is still not clear whether they influence *pulmonary* arterial resistance itself.

Cardiac Vagal Receptors

The cardiac vagal receptors are found at the junction of the atria with their corresponding veins and also in the ventricles (see Paintal, 1953;

Coleridge *et al.*, 1957). On the right side they are distributed at the atrio-caval junction and on the left side at the junction of the pulmonary veins with the left atrium. They can be artificially excited by the drug veratridine. It is preferable to administer veratridine via the coronary arteries, for these vessels supply the myocardium and adjacent structures. When given by this route, a dose of 2 μg suffices to excite the atrial and ventricular receptors, and powerful reflex effects of bradycardia, hypotension, and apnea result. This response was first noted a hundred years ago by Bezold, but was not proved to be due to a cardiac vagal reflex until the work of

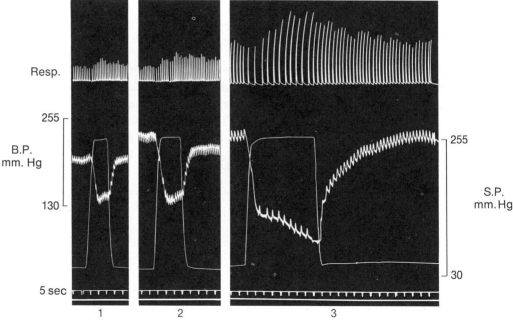

Fig. 18-5. Dog 13.7 kg. Bilateral preparation of carotid sinuses. Moissejeff "blind sac" technique. Records from above downwards: respiration systemic blood pressure, static sinus pressure.

(1) Rise of pressure in both sinuses from 40 mm Hg to 230 mm Hg. Between (1) and (2) left vagus cut. Systemic pressure increases.

(2) Repeat rise of pressure in both sinuses—fall of systemic blood pressure is greater. Between (2) and (3) right vagus cut. Systemic blood pressure again rises.

(3) Repeat rise of pressure in both sinuses. Note profound fall of blood pressure, with no evidence of "compensation" during sustained sinus hypertension. Note also marked slowing of breathing during sinus hypertension.

Jarisch in 1930–1948 (see Heymans and Neil, 1958). The veratridine effect, which is known as the Bezold-Jarisch reflex, is an artificial example of the role of these cardiac mechanoreceptors in the cardiovascular system. Afferent fibres from these cardiac proprioceptors all course in the vagal trunks (the cardiac sympathetic nerves carry the cardiac nociceptive fibres alongside the efferent adrenergic fibres). Cardiac vagal mechano-receptor fibres are best identified by recording their activity simultaneously with the ECG and the right or left ventricular pressure (Fig. 18-6).

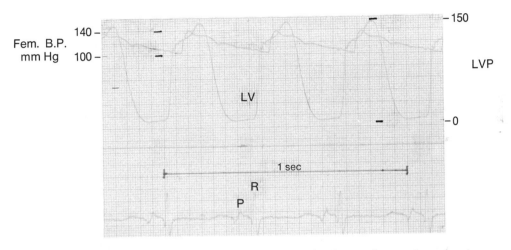

Fig. 18-6. Cat; chloralose anaesthesia. Records from above downwards: femoral arterial pressure, left ventricular pressure, electroneurogram of single left atrial vagal receptor, electrocardiogram. Note discharge in P-R interval, preceding isometric phase of ventricular pressure ("A" type discharge). Femoral pulse pressure delayed compared with systolic rise of left ventricular pressure. Left hand scale: femoral BP. Right hand scale: LVP.

Atrial Receptors

These are of two types (Paintal, 1953). "A" type receptors discharge in the P-R interval of the ECG, just before the rise of intraventricular pressure. They may show a secondary discharge during venous filling of the atrium. "B" type receptors show only a "venous filling" discharge (Fig. 18-7).

Both of these types of receptors are found in the subendothelial layer of the junctions of the cavae with the right atrium or the junctions of the pulmonary veins with the left atrium.

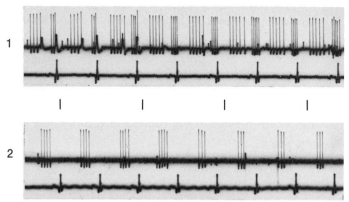

Fig. 18-7. Cat; right atrial vagal receptors.
Record 1 shows neurogram of type A receptor and e.c.g.
Record 2 shows neurogram of type B receptor and e.c.g.
Time marks at one-second interval between (1) and (2). (From Neil and Joels, 1961. By permission.)

The majority of these "low-pressure" (volume) receptors (Chapter 20) produce reflex inhibition of sympathetic tone and reflex accentuation of vagal tone, just as do the arterial "high-pressure" receptors. However, the balance of their reflex pattern appears to be quantitatively somewhat different, with a more pronounced inhibitory effect on the heart and, for example, on the renal circuit as compared with the effect on the muscle vessels (compare Fig. 20-3, page 372). Moreover, they may reflexly affect ADH and aldosterone secretion, hence influencing salt/water equilibrium of the organism and therefore also the blood volume (Chapter 20). One group of the left atrial receptors form a striking exception from other cardiovascular mechanoreceptors insofar as they produce reflex *acceleration* of the heart (Ledsome and Linden, 1967). The functional significance of these receptors is not known, but they might form the background of the classical Bainbridge reflex. Earlier investigators thought that this made an important contribution to the acceleration of the heart in exercise.

Ventricular Receptors

These receptors are also vagal, and they are sparsely distributed, mainly around the apex of the left ventricle. Their impulse activity is a characteristically brief discharge of only a few impulses (or even a single impulse)

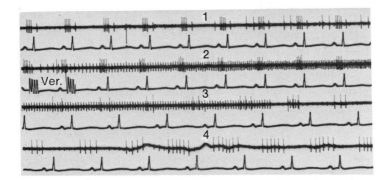

Fig. 18-8. Cat; pentobarbitone anaesthesia. Four successive film strips showing electroneurogram of a right cardiac vagal; preparation filmed simultaneously with the e.c.g.

Record 1. control. Note that the electroneurogram shows the discharge of an atrial receptor (in the P-R interval) and a small spike single discharge after the QRS (ventricular receptor).

Record 2. 15 seconds after 100 μg veratrine given i.v. The two signal marks (ver) show the injection of 1 ml saline into the femoral cannula to wash in the remainder of the veratrine solution. Note that the small ventricular spike fires with a steadily increasing frequency. Records (2) and (4) were photographed at 30-second intervals subsequently. Note that this right atrial receptor showed no evidence of excitation and changes its pattern of discharge. (From Neil and Joels, 1961. By permission.)

shortly after the QRS wave of the ECG (Fig. 18-8); this burst precedes that in the aortic nerve, as might be expected. Normally these receptors appear to be only faintly active, but strong ventricular distension excites them, as does a minute dose (0.5 μg) of veratridine injected into the left coronary artery. Striking reflex vagal bradycardia and over-all sympathetic inhibition result. It has been suggested that such ventricular receptor activation, when the heart "pumps empty" under strong sympathetic drive in connection with failing venous return (blood loss, peripheral pooling, etc.), might provoke a fainting attack (vasovagal syncope) (Pearce and Henry, 1955); this interesting proposal deserves further study.

The Systemic Arterial Chemoreceptors

These important reflexogenic areas are found in the carotid body on each side of the neck immediately rostral to the carotid bifurcation and in the so-called aortic bodies, which are scattered in the tissue between the aorta and the pulmonary artery. They subserve a function which is entirely different from that of the stretch receptors. Again, the anatomical position of the carotid body favours studies of its reflex influence on circulation and respiration because it can be isolated and perfused much more easily than can the aortic bodies, without extensive operative interference in the chest.

The carotid body, or glomus, is a highly vascular structure composed of groups of epithelioid cells virtually interlaced with sinusoids. Although it weighs only 2 mg or so, its blood flow (Daly *et al.*, 1954) is 40 μl/min, which yields the extraordinary figure of 2000 ml/100 g/min. Its oxygen usage expressed in similar terms is 9 ml/100 g/min, which indicates that it has a high rate of metabolism. The carotid body veins, which are supplied by branches of the occipital and ascending pharyngeal arteries, drain into the internal jugular. The structure receives an afferent innervation from the sinus nerve and these afferent nerve endings are admirably situated to "sample" the chemical composition of the arterial blood and to serve therefore as chemoreceptors. The chemoreceptors are sensitive

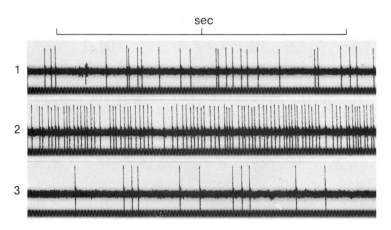

Fig. 18-9. Cat: spontaneous breathing (air). Blood pressure 120 mm Hg. Chemoreceptor activity from thin fibre preparation of carotid sinus nerve.
1. Before clipping corresponding common carotid artery.
2. Common carotid artery clipped—"stagnant" anoxia of carotid body.
3. After releasing clip.
No change of blood pressure on clipping carotid, because the relevant sinus nerve is cut. (From Neil and Joels, 1963. By permission.)

to hypoxia and their impulse activity is increased in circumstances of oxygen lack. Oxygen lack is of four types: (1) hypoxic (low arterial pO_2), (2) anaemic (low HbO_2 content), (3) stagnant (low oxygen flow) and (4) histotoxic (paralysis of cellular enzymes). Of these, all but anaemic anoxia stimulate chemoreceptor impulse activity powerfully (e.g. "stagnant anoxia"—see Fig. 18-9) and thereby cause important reflex effects on the circulation and respiration. Sodium cyanide (which causes histotoxic hypoxia), when injected intra-arterially close to the carotid body, causes reflex vasoconstriction, hypertension, and hyperpnoea, together with increased heart rate. These effects are abolished on cutting the appropriate sinus nerve.

Although a raised pCO_2 or $[H^+]$ of the arterial blood does stimulate chemoreceptor discharge and thereby provokes chemoreceptor reflexes, the *central* action of these chemical factors is more important unless the rise of pCO_2 and $[H^+]$ is accompanied by hypoxia. Hypercapnia plus hypoxia exert together a more powerful chemoreceptor effect than would be expected from "adding" the results of either acting alone.

The efferent response pattern produced by the chemoreceptors is characteristic (see also Chapters 17 and 19): The primary effect on the circulation is bradycardia, a diminution of cardiac output, and peripheral vasoconstriction (Daly and Scott, 1963). However, this primary response is greatly modified by the reflex hyperpnoea simultaneously induced in the spontaneously breathing animal. The increased lung movements cause reflex tachycardia with some reflex inhibition of the vasoconstrictor fibre discharge as well (Daly and Robinson, 1968). In addition, whenever general hypoxia is the primary stimulus the cardiovascular system is also exposed to the peripheral effects of such hypoxia, and to the catecholamine release from the adrenal glands. The net cardiovascular changes are therefore complex (see Korner *et al.*, 1967). In most species the "secondary" reflex cardiovascular response to chemoreceptor stimulation, when the reflex hyperpnoea is allowed to occur, is characterized by an increased cardiac output and heart rate and by a peripheral flow pattern which depends on the balance between constrictor fibre distribution and discharge and the local dilator effect of hypoxia itself, as modified by the blood-borne catecholamines. Both cerebral and coronary blood flow increase while gastrointestinal and renal blood flows, for example, usually decrease.

Haemorrhage sufficient to lower the systemic blood pressure causes a striking discharge of chemoreceptor impulses, partly because the perfusion

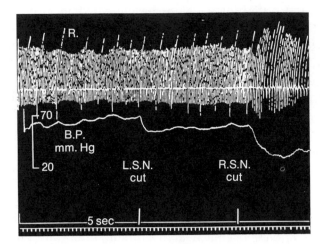

Fig. 18-10. Cat: 3.1 kg, chloralose anaesthesia. Both vagi cut. Previously bled 45 ml. The effects of successive section of the right and left sinus nerves are shown. (From Kenney and Neil, 1951. By permission.)

pressure for the carotid and aortic bodies is lowered, partly because the arteries supplying the carotid body become constricted. This strikingly enhanced chemoreceptor discharge in turn provokes powerful reflex vasoconstriction, an interesting type of positive feedback. This response is important in helping to sustain the mean blood pressure, as can be shown by a simple experiment illustrated in Fig. 18-10. After bleeding the animal to secure a fairly stable mean arterial pressure of 65 mm Hg, the carotid sinus nerves (previously isolated) are cut, whereupon the blood pressure falls to a much lower level. It must be stressed that, in animals with a normal blood pressure, when the sinus nerves are cut the systemic arterial blood pressure *rises* owing to section of the baroreceptor fibre components of the nerves with elimination of their tonic inhibitory action on the medullary centre. However, after bleeding an animal to yield a low mean pressure, baroreceptor activity is relatively feeble but chemoreceptor activity is now intense due to stagnant hypoxia. *In such conditions*, section of the sinus nerves causes a fall of blood pressure which may then have grave consequences. The administration of oxygen may, by reducing the enhanced chemoreceptor discharge, sometimes cause the same untoward effect on the blood pressure level and perhaps trigger cardiovascular collapse.

The carotid body chemoreceptors discharge only sparsely in an anaesthetized animal, breathing air spontaneously, which is in "good condition". Whereas it is arguable whether such impulses influence the *breathing*
of the eupnoeic animal (see Biscoe and Purves, 1967; Torrance, 1968),
there is general agreement that the chemoreceptors exert little if any reflex
influence on the cardiovascular system in such circumstances. Their
emergency role is important in hypoxia and/or asphyxia and is particularly
important in hemorrhagic hypotension.

Other Reflex Influences on the Cardiovascular System

Pain Fibres

Afferent stimulation of somatic or abdominal visceral nerves may reflexly
cause either an increase or a decrease of blood pressure ("somatic pressor"
and "depressor" fibres). It is common experience that pain may cause
tachycardia, vasoconstriction, and hypertension, and there is little doubt
that the major part of the "somatic pressor fibres" is constituted of unmyelinated nociceptive fibres.

Deep pain, such as is induced by testicular trauma, by distension of
abdominal organs, by distortion of joints, or by severe trauma to skeletal
muscle, commonly produces feelings of weakness, nausea, accompanied
by bradycardia, cold sweat, and even fainting. The "somatic depressor
fibres"—mainly thin myelinated fibres from the deep tissues—are probably identical with those mediating deep pain. A closer analysis of the
cardiovascular effects of these two types of nociceptive fibres (see Johansson, 1962) reveals that in the anaesthetized or decerebrated animal the
"pressor" type produces, via the cardiovascular centre, a characteristic
pattern of reflex sympathetic stimulation accompanied by reflex inhibition
of cardiac vagal tone—a pattern which closely resembles that of the
"defence reaction" even though the cholinergic muscle vasodilatation
(which requires hypothalamic engagement) is lacking (see Chapter 19).
However, in conscious or lightly anaesthetized animals, where the higher
autonomic structures and behavioural patterns are involved, a full-
fledged "defence reaction" usually results from stimulation of such nociceptive fibres.

The "depressor type" of nociceptive fibre, on the other hand, reflexly induces, via ventral parts of the medullary depressor area, an over-all sympathetic inhibition combined with a vagal bradycardia, which, when intense, simulate the cardiovascular changes seen in the fainting reaction.

Temperature Fibres

Sudden cooling of the skin produces reflex piloerection and cutaneous vasoconstriction. Some reflex vasoconstriction is seen even in anaesthetized or decerebrated animals, so some of the reflex connections required exist at medullary and even spinal levels. In the intact animal, however, by far the most important reflex connections for this group of thin afferent fibres (mainly $A\gamma$ and δ) are established in the hypothalamic thermoregulatory centres. Information from the skin thus reflexly helps to produce adjustments of cutaneous blood flow appropriate for the stabilization of body temperature (see Chapters 19 and 25).

"Touch" and "Pressure" Fibres

These afferent fibres, mainly the thick myelinated type, probably exert no reflex effects on the medullary cardiovascular centre itself. In the intact individual, however, the afferent message from such fibres may create an emotionally charged situation and a behavioural response that triggers vivid cardiovascular changes, which in extreme cases may even cause either a defence reaction or emotional fainting. Just consider the violent changes of heart rate that a light but unexpected touch by a lover's hand may sometimes produce. In decorticate animals in which the hypothalamic integration centres are released from cortical inhibition, even light touch may trigger an intense defence reaction (see Chapter 19).

Other Types of Afferent Fibres

It is not known whether "pressor" and "depressor" groups of somatic afferents contain, besides nociceptive fibres, fibres which influence cardiovascular performance. It is possible that such fibres might signal local chemical changes in the tissues and that others, which provide information about muscle tension and limb and joint movements, may reflexly influence cardiovascular regulation.

Such possibilities have been considered in interpreting the cardiovascular changes of exercise. The mere movement of a limb, or the contraction of a muscle group, causes little or no reflex circulatory effect in experimental animals. Nevertheless, the widespread and intense activation of such afferent fibres during heavy exercise in the intact individual may provide a pattern of afferent input which reflexly excites the cardiovascular sympathetic neurones.

Peripheral chemoreceptors have been suggested from time to time on the basis of the results of injections of drugs and acids. Usually the doses employed have excited nociceptive fibres. Nevertheless, recent reports suggest that more specific fibres of true chemoreceptor nature may be concealed among the "somatic pressor" and "somatic depressor" afferents. Thus, it is known that muscle exercise moderately increases both the local concentration of potassium ions and the tissue osmolarity; these local chemical changes are important in contributing to the production of exercise hyperemia (Chapter 22). Khayutin (1964), Baraz *et al.* (1968), and Wildenthal *et al.* (1968) have found that changes of local potassium concentration, quantitatively compatible with those which occur in exercise, cause reflex stimulation on the cardiovascular sympathetic discharge. The importance of such effects in the intact animal cannot be fully assessed at present, but the existence of such afferents can no longer be denied.

References

Baraz, L. A., V. M. Khayutin, and J. Molnár (1968). "Analysis of the stimulatory action of capsaicin on receptors and sensory fibres of the small intestine in the cat," *Acta Physiol. Acad. Scient. Hung.* **33,** 225–35.

Biscoe, T. J., and M. J. Purves (1967). "Observations on chemoreceptor activity," *J. Physiol.* **190,** 413–24.

Coleridge, J. C. G., and C. Kidd (1960). "Electrophysiological evidence of baroreceptors in the pulmonary artery of the dog," *J. Physiol.* **150,** 319–31.

Coleridge, J. C. G., A. Hemingway, R. L. Holmes, and R. J. Linden (1957). "The location of atrial receptors in the dog," *J. Physiol.* **136,** 174–97.

Daly, M. de Burgh, and B. H. Robinson (1968). "An analysis of the reflex systemic vasodilator response elicited by lung inflation in the dog," *J. Physiol.* **195,** 387–406.

Daly, M. de Burgh, and M. J. Scott (1963). "The cardiovascular responses to stimulation of the carotid body chemoreceptors in the dog," *J. Physiol.* **165,** 179–97.

Daly, M. de Burgh, C. J. Lambertsen, and A. Schweitzer (1954). "Observations on the volume of blood flow and oxygen utilization of the carotid body in the cat," *J. Physiol.* **125,** 67–89.

Ead, H. W., J. H. Green, and E. Neil (1952). "A comparison of the effects of pulsatile and non-pulsatile blood flow through the carotid sinus on the reflexogenic activity of the sinus baroreceptors in the cat," *J. Physiol.* **118,** 509–19.

Green, J. H. (1954). *Baroreceptor and chemoreceptor control of the circulation.* Ph.D. Thesis, University of London.

Green, J. H., and E. Neil (1953). From Keele, C. A., and E. Neil (1965). Sampson Wright's *Applied Physiology,* 11th ed., p. 142. London: Oxford University Press.

Heymans, C., and E. Neil (1958). *Reflexogenic areas of the cardiovascular system.* London: Churchill.

Johansson, B. (1962). "Circulatory responses to stimulation of somatic afferents," *Acta Physiol. Scand.* **57,** Suppl., 198.

Kenney, R. A., and E. Neil (1951). "The contribution of aortic chemoreceptor mechanisms to the maintenance of arterial blood pressure of cats and dogs after haemorrage," *J. Physiol.* **112,** 223–28.

Kezdi, P. (1967). "Baroreceptors and hypertension," *Proc. Int. Symp.,* p. 460, Dayton, Ohio, 1965. New York: Pergamon.

Khayutin, V. (1964). *Vasomotor reflexes,* p. 376. Moscow.

Korner, P. I., J. P. Chalmers, and S. W. White (1967). "Some mechanisms of reflex control of the circulation by the sympatho-adrenal system," *Circ. Res.* **XX–XXI,** Suppl., 3, 157–72.

Landgren, S. (1952). "The baroreceptor activity in the carotid sinus nerve and the distensibility of the sinus wall," *Acta Physiol. Scand.* **26,** 35–56.

Ledsome, J. R., and R. J. Linden (1967). "The effect of distending a pouch of the left atrium on the heart rate," *J. Physiol.* **193,** 121–29.

Neil, E., and N. Joels (1961). "The impulse activity in cardiac afferent vagal fibres," *Arch. für exp. Path. und Pharmak.* **240,** 453–60.

Paintal, A. S. (1953). "A study of right and left artrial receptors," *J. Physiol.* **120,** 596–610.

Paintal, A. S. (1963). "Vagal afferent fibres," *Ergebn. Physiol.* **52,** 75–156.

Pearce, J. W., and J. P. Henry (1955). "Changes in cardiac afferent nerve-fibre discharges induced by hemorrhage and adrenaline," *Am. J. Physiol.* **183,** 650.

Reis, D. J., and K. Fuxe (1968). "Adrenergic innervation of the carotid sinus," *Am. J. Physiol.* **215,** 1054–57.

Torrance, R. W. (1968). *Arterial chemoreceptors.* Oxford: Blackwell.

Wildenthal, K., D. S. Mierzwiak, N. S. Skinner, Jr., and J. H. Mitchell (1968). "Potassium-induced cardiovascular and ventilatory reflexes from the dog hindlimb," *Am. J. Physiol.* **215,** 542–48.

19

Nervous Control of the Circulation:
III   Cortico-hypothalamic Influences

General Considerations

Medullary servocontrol of the cardiovascular system was recognized in 1866. The concept of higher "autonomic" control of the circulatory system was introduced in 1910, when Karplus and Kreidl showed cardiovascular effects caused by hypothalamic stimulation (see Uvnäs, 1960a; Peiss, 1965).

Hess began his classical exploration of diencephalic mechanisms using topical stimulations in conscious animals in the 1920's (see Hess, 1948). In 1928 Philip Bard presented his important studies of the hypothalamic involvement in the rage response ("defence reaction") and showed how decortication "releases" the hypothalamic structures (see Bard, 1960). Even trifling stimuli can then cause vigorous expressions of rage, involving tachycardia and hypertension accompanied by spitting, clawing, tail lashing, piloerection, etc. Bilateral selective removal of the "neocortex" rendered the experimental animals unduly docile, providing that the "paleocortex" (largely the limbic system) remained intact, which suggested that some neocortical structures lower the threshold of the rage reaction.

However, bilateral removal of the limbic cortex or of the amygdaloid nucleus converted the placid creature into one betraying undue savagery. Evidently these structures contain neurones which tonically inhibit the

hypothalamic mechanisms responsible for aggressive or defensive behaviour. Bronk *et al.* (1940) provided an important landmark in the
physiology of autonomic nervous control (Fig. 19-1) with their analyses
of the effects of hypothalamic stimulation on sympathetic discharge.

It is now known that the hypothalamus contains a number of important
"centres" from which—as if they were "push-button" systems—specific
and well integrated response patterns may be provoked. Those which

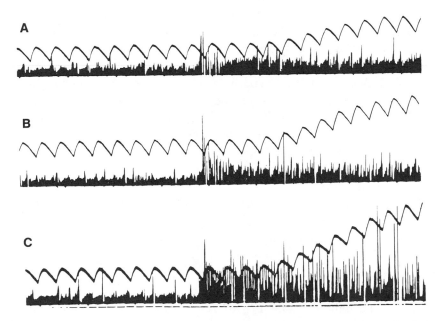

Fig. 19-1. The effects on arterial blood pressure and on sympathetic discharge
to the heart of hypothalamic stimulation at increasing intensities. (From
Bronk *et al.*, 1940. By permission.)

particularly involve the cardiovascular system will be briefly outlined
below, after a survey of some general principles.

These hypothalamic response patterns, some of which have relay stations
of considerable complexity at mesencephalic and lower brain stem levels
as well, usually involve somatomotor and hormonal components as well
as autonomic pathways so linked together that they adjust the organism
as a whole to face particular situations in an appropriate manner. This

necessitates an integrated influence, not only of interoreceptors and extero-
receptors, but telereceptors as well, in turn calling for intimate interaction
between cortical, hypothalamic, lower bulbar and spinal structures via
excitatory and inhibitory connections and feedback loops; the entire
system of autonomic "centres" works as a well co-ordinated unit.

Feedback mechanisms seem to exist at all levels: some of them will be
outlined here. Although the cardiovascular proprioceptors exert their
dominant influence at medullary level, Koch (1931) showed that a pronounced rise in carotid sinus pressure provoked a sleep-like state in the
unanaesthetized dog. Dell *et al.* (1954) found that carotid sinus hypertension reflexly depressed the ascending reticular system of the brain stem.
Zanchetti (1961) and his group showed that the baroreceptors exert a
damping influence on the hypothalamic structures responsible for the
defence reaction. Apparently even the cerebellum is involved in this complex feedback control of the bulbar-suprabulbar structures governing the
cardiovascular control (Moruzzi, 1940; Zanchetti and Zoccolini, 1954;
Reis and Cuenod, 1965). It seems that many of the principles of bulbar-
suprabulbar control of the somatomotor system apply to the autonomic
nervous system as well.

The hypothalamic neurone pools (which seem to show considerable
morphological overlaps, making their discriminate topical excitation or
destruction by means of electrodes difficult) additionally govern such
important mechanisms as water intake and loss, food intake, temperature
regulation, sexual control and behaviour, and the responses to imminent
danger.

These hypothalamic responses represent efferent expressions with no
truly emotional correlates of diencephalic location, for this requires cortical
involvement, but all the *external* signs of, for example, fear or rage are
present. Thus, after a topical stimulation of the defence area in a conscious
cat—which itself transforms a gentle creature into an apparently ferocious
beast attacking blindly—the animal seems merely puzzled by what happened, is immediately gentle again, and is easily stroked. The stimulation
provokes a typical "sham rage" response by artificially exciting the efferent
hypothalamic "push-button" system, bypassing the cortical structures
which alone allow the appreciation of the true emotions and which are the
normal source of excitation of the hypothalamus via their descending
connections.

Thus, superimposed on the hypothalamic integration stations—with their "push-button" systems for eliciting particular response patterns—the cortical autonomic areas exert their influence via excitatory and inhibitory pathways, some of which may exert a tonic influence judging from the release phenomena seen after decortication.

The cortical autonomic areas are particularly situated in the *limbic system*—the phylogenetically old "paleocortex", which surrounds the diencephalon like a ring (Fig. 19-2). The limbic system appears to be the main progenitor of the complex inherited behavioural patterns ("instincts")—critically important for the survival of the individual and the species—and of emotions and emotional behaviour, which are closely associated with the instincts.

The most important parts of the limbic system, with respect to cardio-vascular control, are found in (1) anterior parts of the cingulate gyrus, (2) posterior parts of the orbital cortex, (3) the insula, and (4) anteromedial

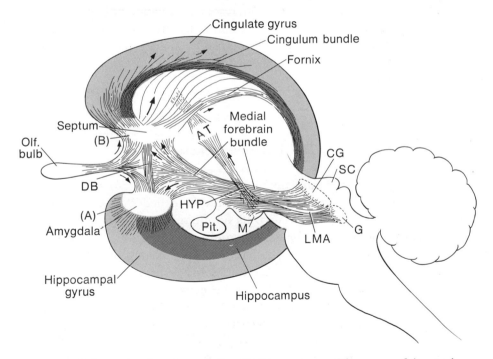

Fig. 19-2. Schematic drawing of the limbic system with some of its major connections via the medial forebrain bundle (MFB) to the hypothalamus and midbrain. (From MacLean, 1958. By permission.)

parts of the temporal lobes with the amygdala and the surrounding pyriform cortex. Parts of the motor-premotor cortex also contribute (see Delgado, 1960). These cortical structures influence the cardiovascular system via their hypothalamic connections, and they may also establish more direct pathways running in the internal capsule and the pyramids. But little is known so far.

The fact that different cortical autonomic response patterns may be provoked from a variety of cortical areas (see below) strongly suggests a high degree of functional differentiation, directing the efferent systems of the organism into more or less "emotionally charged" behavioural patterns, where the cardiovascular adjustments often form an important link. As Sherrington wrote in "The Integrative Action of the Nervous System": "Yet heightened beating of the heart, blanching or flushing of the blood vessels, the pallor of fear, the blush of shame . . . all these are prominent characters in the pantomime of natural emotion." Social life may have taught us to suppress most of the somatomotor expressions of our emotions ("poker face"), but we can do little about either the autonomic or the hormonal components of the phylogenetically ancient paleocortical-hypothalamic response patterns: further, they seem much the same in ducks, cats, rats, and in man.

The Defence Reaction

Few of the cortico-hypothalamic response patterns are so spectacular as that provoked by imminent danger—the so-called "defence reaction" (see Abrahams *et al.*, 1964)—with its fulminant mobilization of the total resources of the organism for flight or fight.

Though integrated at the hypothalamic level, stimulation of the amygdala can induce the reaction also, and some results suggest that closely similar cardiovascular responses may be evoked from the motor cortex (Fig. 19-3). Topical stimulation of the hypothalamic integration area, or its projections, excites the sympathetic cholinergic vasodilator fibres to the skeletal muscles, while the adrenergic fibres to virtually all other cardiovascular sections are excited (Eliasson *et al.*, 1951) with profound inotropic and chronotropic effects on the heart (Smith *et al.*, 1960). Some features of this response are shown in Figs. 19-4 and 19-5. The ensuing

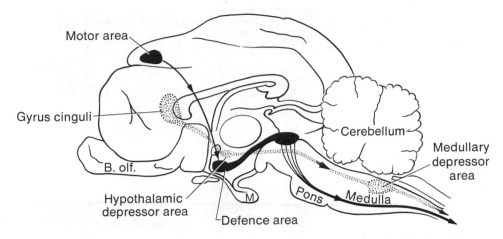

Fig. 19-3. Schematic illustration of the corticospinal connections for the "defence reaction" (black) (modified from Uvnäs 1960b), and the inhibitory responses (dotted) (modified from Löfving, 1961), the latter connections being presumably responsible for "playing dead" reactions and possibly for emotional fainting in man.

pressure rise excites the baroreceptors, though their reflex inhibitory effect on the heart is strongly suppressed by the defence response at the bulbar level, presumably a consequence of synaptic "occlusion" (Hilton, 1963). Baroreceptor modulation of the vascular bed seems to be only little affected, with the interesting result of further increasing cardiac output for a given neurogenic drive on the heart (Kylstra and Lisander, 1970); thus, if anything, this differentiated interaction appears to potentiate the hypothalamically induced cardiovascular performance.

While the autonomic-hormonal component is largely the same for the hunters and the hunted, the somatomotor component admittedly varies, depending on whether one is a lion, mouse, ostrich, or man. Imagine a gazelle grazing, which hears a twig crackle under the foot of a predator. The immediate somatomotor response is perhaps only an alerting reaction, but at the same time the full-fledged cardiovascular-hormonal changes are put into action—being probably already prominent in the predator, lurking in the grass. Another cautious move from his side and the gazelle explodes into an all-out flight response, his cardiovascular system being already prepared to give the nutritional supply needed.

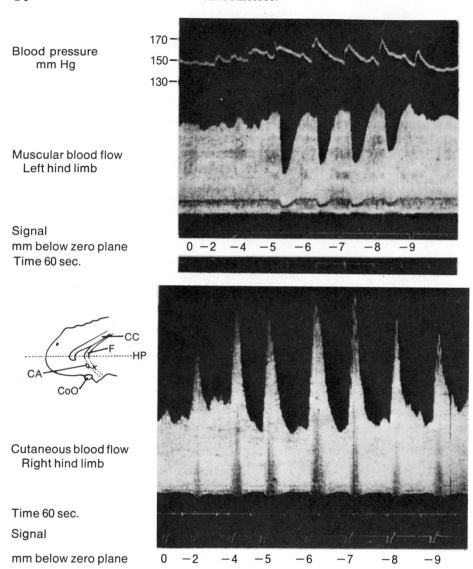

Blood pressure
mm Hg

170 —
150 —
130 —

Muscular blood flow
Left hind limb

Signal
mm below zero plane
Time 60 sec.

0 −2   −4   −5   −6   −7   −8   −9

CC
F
HP
CA
CoO

Cutaneous blood flow
Right hind limb

Time 60 sec.

Signal

mm below zero plane   0   −2   −4   −5   −6   −7   −8   −9

Fig. 19-4. Dorsoventral extension of points in and around the hypothalamic defense area, yielding vasodilator responses in muscles and vasoconstrictor responses in skin. (From Eliasson *et al.*, 1951. By permission.)

Fig. 19-5. Cardiac responses to hypothalamic stimulation, involving the nervous structures integrating the defence reaction, as compared with the cardiac response to exercise. (From Rushmer and Smith, 1959. By permission.)

It has sometimes been argued that not much could be gained by such anticipatory cardiovascular adjustments: the muscular effort would—so goes the argument—be virtually as good without it. This overlooks the fact that a split-second gain, though of little use in comfortable civilized life, may determine whether the gazelle escapes the killer; quite an

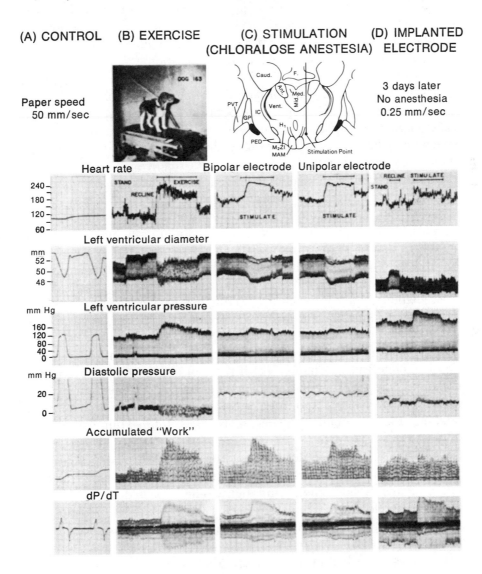

important "marginal" gain for the gazelle. Beyond doubt, this cardio-vascular-hormonal anticipatory adjustment is of utmost importance for survival in the animal kingdom, and not infrequently for man as well. Not for nothing does the Bible teach us to differentiate between the quick and the dead.

Civilized man, admittedly less exposed to the law of the jungle, nevertheless shows much the same response when under strain. The average candidate for an oral examination manifests tachycardia, cutaneous vasoconstriction, often associated with perspiration ("cold sweat"), dry mouth with viscid salivary secretion and an over-all jumpiness which reveals excessive cortico-hypothalamic discharge; urinary or blood analyses will reveal the full spectrum of hormonal changes. Experimental studies of emotional stress in man (when forced to do mental arithmetic, for example) have shown that exactly the same cardiovascular changes occur as in experimental animals (Brod *et al.*, 1959).

The cardiovascular changes of the defence reaction by no means call for extreme distress or danger to be fully displayed. They are already evident even with the trifling stimuli required to produce an alerting response (Abrahams *et al.*, 1964). They occur repeatedly in daily life—except presumably in that of Trappist monks—such as in moments of tense expectation and those of a pleasant nature. "Like greyhounds straining in the slips" (Shakespeare, *Henry V*), the command "ready" to an athlete puts his circulation going—if he has any feeling for the excitement of competition. Everyone must have heard of the pretty, if conceited, nurse who always deducted ten from the pulse rate of her male patients.

As the load on the heart may increase manyfold within a few seconds (Tension Time Index, Chapter 12) if responses of this nature are intense (Folkow *et al.*, 1968), it is not surprising that elderly gentlemen—with choleric temperaments and furred coronaries—may drop dead while watching their football favorites score (see John Hunter's remark, Chapter 23).

A civilized man, whose defence reaction is aroused by repeated arguments with his boss, reluctantly suppresses the somatomotor component and avoids both flight and fight. The repeated autonomic-hormonal-metabolic mobilization thus occurs largely "in vain", as no rapid burn-off occurs, much against nature's intentions. It is possible that such dissociated patterns, often repeated over years, may lead to pathophysiological states (see Charvat *et al.*, 1964). Abrahams *et al.* (1964) noted that the cardiovascular response of cats can easily be conditioned, and will then remain stable; this finding might be of considerable interest and relevance in man as well. It has also been shown that weak but oft-repeated stimulation of the hypothalamic defence area may lead gradually to a hypertensive state, which exists even when no stimulations are performed (Folkow and Rubinstein, 1966). A sensible reaction to emotional stress might be to exchange some harmless physical mayhem, such as kicking in a cupboard door, for the justifiable homicide of a pestering anatagonist, thus maintaining some of the proprieties but letting nature have its course. It must be remembered also that "Furor fit laesa saepius patientia".

The "Playing Dead" Reaction

Some species confronted by imminent danger display the "playing dead" reaction. In the opossum it is so common as to be sometimes called "playing possum", but a great variety of species—particularly the young (such as deer kids)—manifest this response in some danger situations, especially when "cornered". The animal drops suddenly as if dead: flaccid, almost apnoeic, with arterial hypotension and bradycardia. This behavioural response, the opposite of the "defence reaction", serves, nevertheless, to protect the individual. A predator may not even find its prey or is misled by the apparently dead animal and, if not of the scavenging type, will turn away after sniffing the "carcase". However, the "carcase" may suddenly jump up and display a most vivid and efficient flight reaction.

The cat does not normally manifest the "playing dead" reaction. Nevertheless, stimulation of certain parts of the anterior cingulate gyrus (Fig. 19-6) causes an over-all sympathetic inhibition together with vagal bradycardia, resulting in striking hypotension (Löfving, 1961). The loss of vasoconstrictor tone is most striking in the muscle vessels, causing such a fall in resistance that, despite the lowered pressure, the muscle blood flow *increases* phasically (Fig. 19-6). Exactly this haemodynamic change occurs in fainting man (see below).

The corticofugal pathway responsible passes via the anterior hypothalamus immediately dorsorostral to the "defence reaction area" and thence to the medial bulbar reticular formation to reach the "medullary depressor area" (see Fig. 17-1, p. 311). The pattern of inhibition induced by anterior cingular gyrus stimulation can be closely mimicked by stimulation of the medullary depressor area or the sino-aortic afferents. A lesion in the medullary depressor area abolishes the responses provoked by either

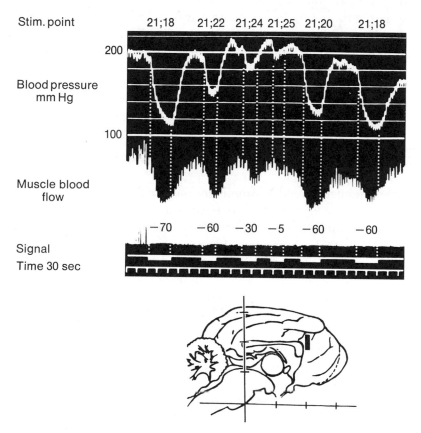

Fig. 19-6. Effects on arterial blood pressure and skeletal muscle blood flow of topical stimulation at different points within the depressor area of the cingulate gyrus (see map). The experiment is performed on a curarized and lightly anaesthetized cat, deprived of the vagal nerves and the baroreceptor modulation and with the cholinergic vasodilator fibres blocked. Ordinates for blood flow record *inversely* proportional to flow. Note the considerable increase of muscle blood flow despite the profound fall in blood pressure. Numbers on the blood flow recording indicate the percentage decreases in flow resistance. (From Löfving, 1961. By permission.)

cingulate or sino-aortic stimulation, although the reflex sympathetic excitatory responses induced by chemoreceptor stimulation remain unaffected. This medially placed medullary structure seemingly provides a final common path for canalizing sympatho-inhibitory discharges, whether these stem from cortical, hypothalamic, or sino-aortic baroreceptor sources, or even from the discharge of "somatic depressor" afferents (see Chapter 18).

Stimulation of the "cingulate depressor region" causes a striking reduction of somatomotor activity, in addition to autonomic effects (such as sympathetic inhibition and cardiac parasympathetic excitation). Not only is there a reduction of skeletal muscle tone, but the conscious animal subjected to such topical stimuli displays a depression of breathing and shows less somatomotor behavioural responses to provocation.

The cingulate inhibitory area thus seems responsible for the "playing dead" reaction. This reaction, though intense in some species, is probably a pattern present in all species, even, for instance, in the cat, although the carnivores rarely "play dead". Man too appears to exhibit this response pattern. Thus, some emotional shocks, rather than provoking defence reactions, provoke a feeling of weakness, dizziness, a need for slumping down motionless in a chair, which may even lead to an emotional faint. The haemodynamic response in fainting is very similar to that produced by topical stimulation of the cingulate gyrus. Some individuals, when confronted with certain types of stressful situations, are especially prone to respond by slumping into a faint, thereby gaining respite from the "slings and arrows of outrageous fortune"—at least temporarily.

Other Emotional Responses in Man

Emotional responses in man have many features, and of these the full-blown defence reaction and emotional fainting are only the most dramatic ones. Thus, hostility and resentment may cause marked vasodilatation of vessels in the gastrointestinal mucosa, evidently mediated via the vagal and pelvic nerves (Chapter 26). Wolf and Wolff (1943) described the striking colour changes in the exposed gastric mucosa of their gastrostomized patient Tom, when he had been upset by the clinic secretary.

Blushing—responsible for the first adumbration of the idea that vessel calibre was influenced by nerves—has received the attention of biologists (including Charles Darwin) for years, but is still not satisfactorily explained. It can certainly be vivid and sudden enough to suggest specific vasodilator fibres, but it is not entirely impossible that it is an effect of kallidin-bradykinin, released from sweat glands which are suddenly activated by cortico-hypothalamic excitation via their cholinergic sympathetic nerves. Blushing, however, is not confined to the skin of the face and neck. Thus, a male medical student who had volunteered to have a sigmoidoscope passed, on hearing that a woman medical student was peering through the instrument, developed a marked erythema of his colonic mucosa (Davenport, 1961).

The Feeding Response

The hypothalamus contains centres governing food intake, constituted by a medially placed "satiety centre" in reciprocal balance with a lateral "hunger centre" (see Brobeck, 1960; Anand, 1961; see also Fig. 19-7). Topical stimulation of the "hunger centre" initiates searching for food and food intake, accompanied by an increase in gastrointestinal motility and secretion due to the vagal discharge. Stimulation of this region in the lightly anaesthetized animal causes a moderate rise of blood pressure, tachycardia, and vasoconstriction of the muscles, together with an increased blood flow to the gastrointestinal tract (Folkow and Rubinstein,

---

Fig. 19-7. Effects on cardiovascular and gastrointestinal functions of topical stimulations in the hypothalamic area (upper hatched area of the schematic drawing of the cat's hypothalamus) from which feeding responses were obtained in the awake animal. Note the increased intestinal motility, the raised blood pressure, the moderate muscle vasoconstriction, and the obvious increase of intestinal blood flow (upper recording). The lower recording, by comparison, illustrates the effects of stimulating pathways involved in the defence reaction (lower hatched section in the diagram). Note the inhibited gastrointestinal motility, the rise in blood pressure, the decrease in intestinal blood flow and increase of muscle blood flow. (From Folkow and Rubinstein, 1965. By permission.)

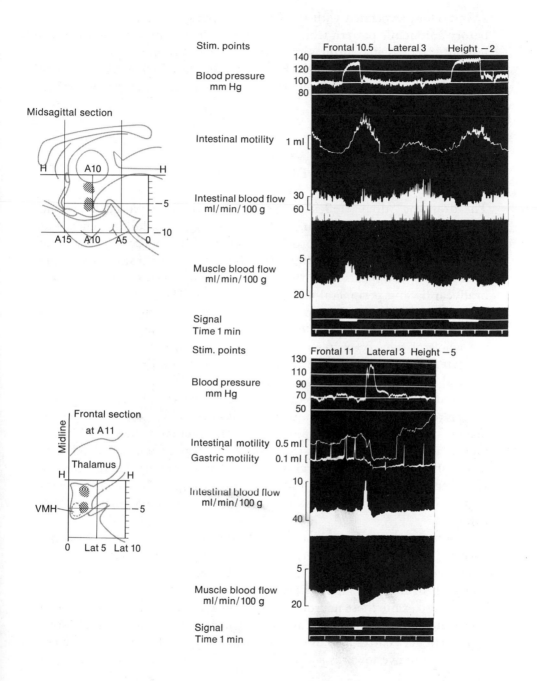

1965). Thus, associated with the feeding response there occurs an anticipatory autonomic pattern which favours the blood supply to the gastrointestinal tract, elicited at the same time as the gastrointestinal function is
increased via the vagal nerves (Fig. 19-7). Similarly, when dogs eat they
display tachycardia and some rise of blood pressure (Rushmer *et al.*,
1960).

The Diving Response

The dramatic "diving reflex" response—beautifully explored by Irving
and Scholander (see Andersen, 1966)—is *basically* a medullary reflex, but
in expert divers it is often so profoundly affected by cortico-hypothalamic
influences that it is best described in this context. The framework of the
diving response appears to be the "primary chemoreceptor" reflex: vagal
bradycardia and peripheral vasoconstriction (see Chapter 18).

In principle, the diving response implies that the cardiovascular system
becomes transformed into a "heart-brain circuit", which delivers almost
the whole of the oxygen reserves in the blood and lungs to these vitally
important tissues. In order to do so, something more than the gradually
evolved chemoreceptor reflex is needed.

Three important prerequisites must be satisfied: (1) the *onset* of the
diving reflex must be so prompt that initial oxygen losses to peripheral
tissues are minimized. (2) Vasoconstriction in other tissues must be so
intense as virtually to abolish their usage of oxygen from the blood, and
this is imperative in the exercising skeletal muscles. (3) There must be
some mechanism which can gradually provide the brain and heart with
all the oxygen-carrying venous blood from the restricted peripheral circulation.

Expert divers display an *immediate* bradycardia and vasoconstriction,
once their nostrils are submerged. In fact, any "active" suppression of
spontaneous respiration appears to trigger this response, and it might be so
that such neurogenic suppressions of the respiratory centre by axon collaterals also excite those neurone pools of the cardiovascular centres which
constitute the efferent links for the chemoreceptor reflex (see Folkow,
1968). Higher centres may also trigger this response; for example, a mere
threatening move towards a seal will do so. This shows the cortico-hypo-

thalamic influences. Further, upper brain stem stimulation in ducks may simulate the cardiovascular response of diving, although stimulation of nearby areas may elicit a defence reaction.*

In diving, twentyfold (or more) decreases in cardiac output, at maintained arterial and raised venous pressures, can be seen (Fig. 19-8) and blood flow to the peripheral tissues virtually stops, even in the exercising muscles. The vasoconstrictor fibre impact is extremely powerful, and muscle performance relies on myoglobin oxygen stores for short dives and on anaerobic metabolism for more prolonged dives. Cardiac function is thus greatly reduced, involving both vagal bradycardia and a powerful negative inotropic effect of vagal origin, which affects the ventricular myocardium so that stroke volume may be reduced, despite the raised filling pressure(Folkow and Yonce, 1967).

The greatly reduced cardiac output, and hence the oxygen stores of blood and lungs, are preferentially delivered to the brain and the myocardium, but the needs of the myocardium are by now greatly reduced. In the periphery, only the cutaneous A-V shunts (usually implicated in thermal regulation) are patent. They allow a small peripheral blood flow, which, losing no oxygen to the peripheral tissues, helps to maintain a slow flow of venous blood back to the heart for subsequent distribution to the brain.

When the diver surfaces, these changes are reversed within seconds (Fig. 19-8). A sudden sympathetic drive on the heart, coupled with an elimination of cardiac vagal tone and an inhibition of peripheral vasoconstrictor fibre discharge, provides a *huge* cardiac output to all the tissues, repaying the oxygen debt and flooding the blood with the acid metabolites earlier trapped.

* This led to the following critical verse by Professor S. M. Hilton:

> The duck he could't care less
> About Feigl's and Folkow's distress
> He doesn't know why
> He should dive or just fly
>   His brain is a terrible mess.

The criticism was found justified, but the experiments had their bright side, so the answer was:

> To scratch a duck in his brain
> Is a cry in the desert in vain
> But when he is dead
> And the cook goes ahead
>   The effort appears much more sane.

The efficiency of this remarkable response is perhaps best illustrated by some simple figures. With an intact diving response the domestic duck may stay submerged for 15 minutes; if the response is disrupted it drowns in 2 to 3 minutes. A seal may survive 20 to 30 minutes of submersion and some

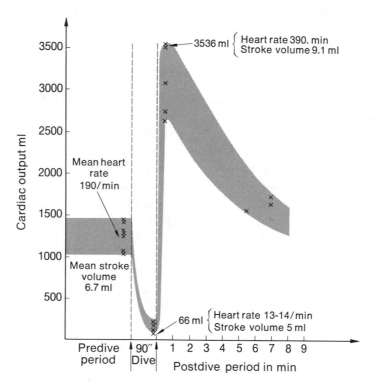

Fig. 19-8. Diagram illustrating the changes in cardiac output, heart rate, and stroke volume before, during, and after 90-second submersion of the head of a duck. (From Folkow *et al.*, 1967. By permission.)

whale species 1 to 2 hours. Yet, their brains are not much more tolerant of hypoxia than is that of man. It is all a matter of so adjusting the cardiovascular system as to provide the oxygen reserves virtually only to the central nervous system and a few other sensitive tissues.

The Thermo-regulatory Centres

The "thermo-regulatory" hypothalamic neurones provide graded and
selective adjustments of the sympathetic constrictor discharge to the skin
vessels (see Ström, 1960), as described in Chapter 25. The selectivity of their
responses is yet another example of differentiated adjustments of sympathetic discharge. Fig. 19-9 illustrates how well graded to the local
temperature of the heat loss centre such cutaneous vascular adjustments

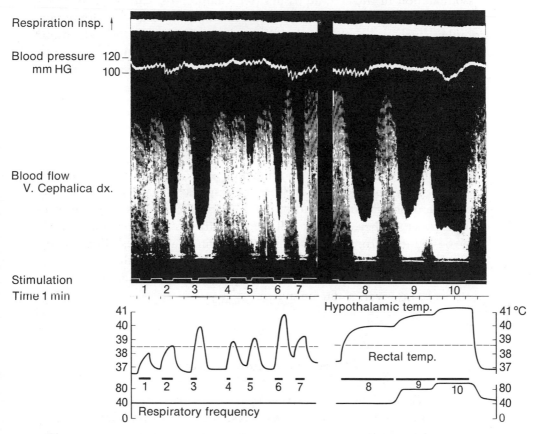

Fig. 19-9. The effect of graded diathermic heating of the hypothalamic heat
loss centre upon cutaneous blood flow in the forelimb. (From Ström, 1950.
By permission.)

can be, although the animal is under anaesthesia, which itself depresses the sensitivity of the hypothalamic neurones involved. In a conscious animal similar quantitative responses of the peripheral sympathetic nerves would probably be provoked by much smaller increments of central thermal stress.

Sexual Responses

Vasodilatation in the erectile tissues (see Chapter 16) can be induced by topical stimulation of particular areas in the limbic system - hypothalamus complex, such as in the medial preoptic region of the hypothalamus (MacLean *et al.*, 1960). Stimulation of these brain structures appear to integrate the complete behavioural pattern necessary for copulation.

Other Cortico-hypothalamic Patterns

Topical stimulations in the hypothalamus and cingulate gyrus can produce over-all vasoconstrictor and pressor responses, characterized also by muscle vasoconstriction instead of the dilatation seen in the defence reaction. Further, rather complex differential patterns of a "pressor" nature may be induced from various parts of the cingulate gyrus (Fig. 19-10), again illustrating the potentiality for specific adjustments that the cardio-vascular nervous control is capable of. The functional significance of these patterns is, however, so far unknown.

The Motor-premotor Cortex

Hoff and Green (1936) found that stimulation of the motor cortex may evoke pressor and cardioacceleratory responses. Wall and Davis (1951) concluded that stimulation of the sensorimotor cortex causes autonomic excitation and, as stated earlier, circulatory changes, simulating those seen in the defence reaction, may be provoked by stimulation of the motor cortex in dogs (Unväs, 1960). There is much evidence to indicate that the initial phases of exercise, particularly when they are accompanied by alarm or alertness, are characterized by a considerable sympathetic "drive". This sympathetic drive, which emanates partly from the highest

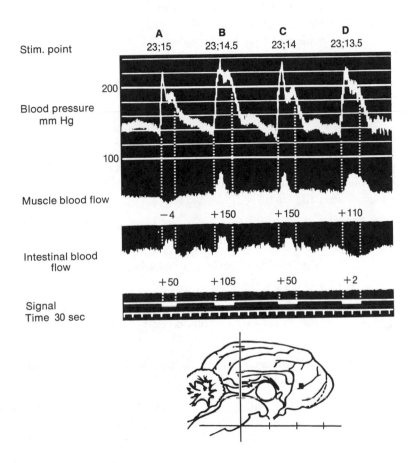

Fig. 19-10. Effects on arterial blood pressure, skeletal muscle, and intestinal blood flows of topical stimulations at different points within the pressor area of the cingulate gyrus. Note that the patterns of response can vary considerably (compare A and D) with small shifts of the electrode position. The numbers on the blood flow recordings indicate the percentage changes in blood flow resistance. The animal was prepared in the same way as that in Fig. 19-6. (From Löfving, 1961. By permission.)

brain centres, is "parallel-coupled" with the cortical excitation of the skeletal musculature. This "centrogenic" sympathetic drive seems to be mainly relayed in the hypothalamus, for Smith *et al.* (1960) observed that the tachycardia and hypertension of exercise were greatly reduced after elective hypothalamic lesions.

The details of cardiovascular control exercised by the higher neuraxis are not yet clear, but their study is likely to prove rewarding, not the least in interpreting problems of pathophysiology.

References

Abrahams, V. C., S. M. Hilton, and A. W. Zbrozyna (1964). "The role of active muscle vasodilatation in the alerting stage of the defence reaction," *J. Physiol.* **171,** 189–202.

Anand, B. K. (1961). "Nervous regulation of food intake," *Physiol. Rev.* **41,** 677–708.

Andersen, H. T. (1966). "Physiological adaptations in diving vertebrates," *Physiol. Rev.* **46,** 212–43.

Bard, P. (1960). "Anatomical organization of the central nervous system in relation to control of the heart and blood vessels," *Physiol. Rev.* **40,** Suppl. 4, 3–26.

Brobeck, J. R. (1960). "Regulation of feeding and drinking," *Handbook of Physiology*, 1, Neurophysiology **II,** 1197–1206.

Brod, J., V. Fencl, Z. Hejl, and J. Jirka (1959). "Circulatory changes underlying blood pressure elevation during acute emotional stress (mental arithmetic) in normotensive and hypertensive subjects," *Clin. Sci.* **18,** 269–79.

Bronk, D. W., R. F. Pitts, and M. G. Larrabee (1940). "Role of hypothalamus in cardiovascular regulation," *A. Res. Nerv. & Ment. Dis. Proc.* **20,** 323–41.

Charvat, J., P. Dell, and B. Folkow (1964). "Mental factors and cardiovascular diseases," *Cardiologia*, **44,** 124–41.

Davenport, H. W. (1961). *Physiology of the digestive tract.* Chicago: Year Book Med. Publ.

Delgado, J. M. R. (1960). "Circulatory effects of cortical stimulation," *Physiol. Rev.* **40,** Suppl. 4, 146–71.

Dell, P., M. Bonvallet, and A. Hugelin (1954). "Tonus sympathique, adrénaline et contrôle reticulaire de la motricité spinal," *Electroencephalog. clin. Neurophysiol.* **6,** 599–618.

Eliasson, S., B. Folkow, P. Lindgren, and B. Uvnäs (1951). "Activation of sympathetic vasodilator nerves to the skeletal muscles in the cat by hypothalamic stimulation," *Acta Physiol. Scand.* **23,** 333–51.

Folkow, B. (1968). "Circulatory adaptations to diving in ducks," *Proc. Intern. Union of Physiol. Sci.* **6,** XXIV Intern. Congress., Washington, 23–24.

Folkow, B., and E. H. Rubinstein (1965). "Behavioural and autonomic patterns evoked by stimulation of the lateral hypothalamic area in the cat," *Acta Physiol. Scand.* **65,** 292–99.

Folkow, B., and E. H. Rubinstein (1966). "Cardiovascular effects of acute and chronic stimulations of the hypothalamic defence area in the rat," *Acta Physiol. Scand.* **68,** 48–57.

Folkow, B., and L. R. Yonce (1967). "The negative inotropic effect of vagal stimulation on the heart ventricles of the duck," *Acta Physiol. Scand.* **71,** 77–84.

Folkow, B., N. J. Nilsson, and L. R. Yonce (1967). "Effects of 'diving' on cardiac output in ducks," *Acta Physiol. Scand.* **70,** 347–61.

Folkow, B., B. Lisander, R. S. Tuttle, and S. C. Wang (1968). "Changes in cardiac output upon stimulation of the hypothalamic defence area and the medullary depressor area in the cat," *Acta Physiol. Scand.* **72,** 220–33.

Hess, W. R. (1948). *Die funktionelle Organisation des vegetativen Nervensystems.* Basle: Benno Schwabe & Co. Verlag.

Hilton, S. M. (1963). "Inhibition of baroreceptor reflexes on hypothalamic stimulation," *J. Physiol.* **165,** 56–57 P.

Hoff, E. C., and H. D. Green (1936). "Cardiovascular reactions induced by electrical stimulation of the cerebral cortex," *Am. J. Physiol.* **117,** 411–22.

Koch, E. (1931). *Die reflektorische Selbsteuerung des Kreislaufes.* Berlin: Springer.

Kylstra, P., and B. Lisander (1970). "Differentiated interaction between the hypothalamic defence area and baroreceptor reflexes," *Acta Physiol. Scand.,* **78,** 386–92.

Löfving, B. (1961). "Cardiovascular adjustments induced from the rostral cingulate gyrus," *Acta Physiol. Scand.* **53,** Suppl., 184.

MacLean, D. P. (1951). "Contrasting functions of limbic and neocortical systems of the brain and their relevance to psychophysiological aspects of medicine," *Am. J. Med.* **25,** 611–23.

MacLean, D. P., D. W. Ploog, and B. W. Robinson (1960). "Circulatory effects of limbic stimulation, with special reference to the male genital organ," *Physiol. Rev.* **40,** Suppl. 4, 105–12.

Moruzzi, G. (1940). "Paleocerebellar inhibition of vasomotor and respiratory carotid sinus reflexes," *J. Neurophysiol.* **3,** 20–32.

Peiss, C. N. (1965). "Concepts of cardiovascular regulation," in *Nervous control of the heart.* Baltimore: Williams & Wilkins.

Reis, D., and M. Cuenod (1965). "Central neural regulation of carotid baroreceptor reflexes in the cat," *Am. J. Physiol.* **209,** 1267–77.

Rushmer, R. F., A. O. Smith, Jr., and E. P. Lasher (1960). "Neural mechanisms of cardiac control during exertion," *Physiol. Rev.* **40,** Suppl. 4, 27–34.

Smith, O. A., Jr., S. J. Jabbur, R. F. Rushmer, and E. P. Lasher (1960). "Role of hypothalamic structures in cardiac control," *Physiol. Rev.* **40,** Suppl. 4, 136–41.

Ström, G. (1950). "Influence of local thermal stimulation of the hypothalamus of the cat on cutaneous blood flow and respiration rate," *Acta Physiol. Scand.* **20,** Suppl., 70, 47–76.

Ström, G. (1960). "Central nervous regulation of body temperature," *Handbook of Physiology,* 1, Neurophysiology **II,** 1173–96.

Uvnäs, B. (1960a). "Central cardiovascular control," *Handbook of Physiology,* 1, Neurophysiology **II,** 1131–62.

Uvnäs, B. (1960b). "Sympathetic vasodilator system and blood flow," *Physiol. Rev.* **40,** Suppl. 4, 68–76.

Wall, P. D., and G. D. Davis (1951). "Three cerebral cortical systems affecting autonomic function," *J. Neurophysiol.* **14,** 507–17.

Wolf, S., and H. G. Wolff (1943). *Human gastric function.* New York: Oxford University Press.

Zanchetti, A. (1961). "Reflex mechanisms regulating hypothalamic autonomic activity and emotional behaviour, their importance in circulatory homeostasis," *Proc. Intern. Symp. on the Pathogenesis of Essential Hypertension*, pp. 191–98. Prague, Czechoslovakia: State Medical Publ. House.

Zanchetti, A., and A. Zoccolini (1954). "Autonomic hypothalamic outburst elicited by cerebellar stimulation," *J. Neurophysiol.* **17,** 475–83.

20

Regulation of Blood Volume

General Considerations

The blood volume of a 70 kg man is 5.5 litres (75 to 80 ml/kg body weight), and in an adult woman it is slightly lower (some 70 ml/kg body weight). These volumes stay remarkably constant. Of the 5.5 litres in adult man 55 to 60% of the blood—3 to 3.5 litres—is in the plasma and the remainder in the red cells. The problem of the regulation of these plasma and red cell volumes cannot be considered without referring to the situation of the control of body water as a whole, for the body compartments are closely interrelated in many respects. Several recent reviews covering different aspects of blood volume regulation are available (Gregersen and Rawson, 1959; Sjöstrand, 1962; Gauer and Henry, 1963; Chien, 1967; Gauer *et al.*, 1970).

External Fluid Exchange

The average daily intake of water is of the order of 2 to 2.5 l. Further, every day 6 to 8 litres of fluid enter the G.I. tract in the form of digestive secretions, but these are reabsorbed, with the exception of 100 to 200 ml, which are excreted in the faeces. Similarly, the kidneys filter say 170 litres daily but reabsorb all but some 1.5 litres. By insensitive evaporation from the skin and the lungs about 0.5 to 0.7 litres are lost. These figures give the rough daily balance of external water exchange (Fig. 20-1). They hold for temperate climate conditions. Those for tropical conditions are discussed below.

The kidneys constitute the main regulator on the output side. Of the 170 litres filtered, the proximal tubules absorb about 85%. The final adjustment of the sodium uptake occurs in the distal tubules and

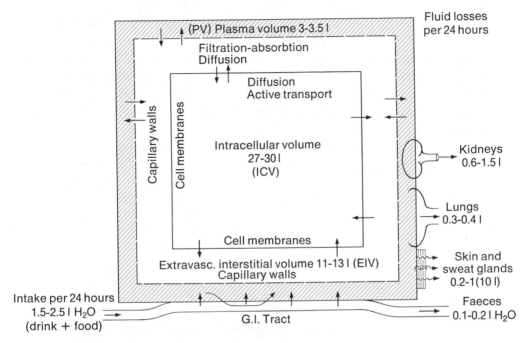

Fig. 20-1. Schematic drawing illustrating the different fluid spaces and their interrelationships, together with the daily fluid intake and losses by means of the varying routes.

is governed by aldosterone. This hormone therefore secures the maintenance of sodium chloride, the *"osmotic skeleton" of the extracellular space.*

Some 20 litres reach the distal and collecting tubules. Largely due to the antidiuretic hormone (ADH)—secreted by the hypothalamic osmoreceptors and extruded via the axoplasma of the hypothalamo-hypophyseal tract—18.5 litres are reabsorbed, leaving 1.5 litres of urine to be excreted. Without ADH life would be socially impossible.

In hot climates the sweat output may reach 1 to 2 litres per hour, entailing the active secretion of a hypotonic sodium chloride solution. Clearly such fluid losses must be sustained primarily from the extracellular fluid volume as a whole and secondarily from readjustments between intracellular and extracellular fluid compartments. This leads to hypertonicity. The hypothalamic osmoreceptors respond appropriately to the tonicity of the body fluids. Hypertonicity thus evokes thirst, to which low-pressure "volume" receptors (see below) contribute, and therefore leads to water intake. Hypertonicity induces also an outpouring of ADH and maximal water reabsorbtion from the fluid in the renal collecting tubules. This is not complete, however, for there is an obligatory volume of 500 to 600 ml required in man for the excretion of urea and other waste products. The remark that "the urinary output in Baghdad is a puff of dust", though memorable and though giving the sense of this problem, is not accurate.

Water retention does not normally occur over long periods, for osmolar factors and osmoreceptor regulation prevent it—the fluids of the body must be isotonic over a finite period, and for the extracellular space sodium chloride provides the "osmotic skeleton" referred to above. If a subject in water balance drinks one litre of water, it is absorbed within 20 to 30 min. If it remained in the bloodstream it would cause a 33% dilution of the plasma, but of course it permeates the entire body water space, suppresses the secretion of ADH by the osmoreceptors, and is voided in the urine within 90 minutes or so.

Exchange between Different Fluid Compartments

During a 24 hour period the heart pumps perhaps 8000 to 9000 litres of blood round the circulation, and of this some 20 litres of fluid escape from the capillaries by transudation, to be returned via the capillaries (16 to 18 litres) and the lymph (2 to 4 litres). The diffusion exchange is many times that of the total blood flow (see Chapter 8).

Still, the fluid component of the blood, the plasma volume (PV, 3 to 3.5 l), is kept in equilibrium with the much greater bulk of fluid in the extravascular interstitial volume (EIV, 9 to 12 l) and the intracellular volume of fluid (ICV, 27 to 30 l). Water can pass freely throughout the body—indeed this is the basis of measurement of *total body water* (TBW) by the use of D_2O (see Fig. 20-1).

ICV cannot be measured directly but is obtained by subtraction of the extracellular volume ECV, determined by dilution techniques, from the TBW.

The substances used to determine ECV are obviously those which purport to remain extracellular. Sodium thiosulphate is one—its use in dilution techniques yields a figure of 13 to 14 litres for ECV. Sodium thiocyanate, on the other hand, gives a value of 16 to 17 litres. The important fact is that there are some 13 to 16 litres of ECV of which PV constitutes 3 to 3.5 litres (or 40 to 50 ml/kg/body weight).

PV can be measured directly by estimating the degree of dilution observed following the intravenous injection of the dye T 1834 (Evans blue), or some other tracer, which largely remains in the plasma compartment (e.g. Risa = radioactive iodinated serum albumin). Red cell mass can similarly be estimated directly by determining the degree of dilution of radioactively labelled red cells (^{51}Cr-labelling).

The relative constancy of the blood volume presupposes a constancy of red cell mass and, more important in the present context, a constancy of the plasma volume. Certain pathological conditions are attended by plethora—e.g. cardiac failure, cirrhosis, and nephrosis. Conversely, due to sweating thermal stress causes general dehydration, as does insufficient secretion of corticoids (Addison's disease). This lowers the blood volume by diminishing the stocks of body water, with the terminal result that the viscosity of the polycythaemic blood adds considerably to the work done by the heart, while, at the same time, its filling seriously deteriorates.

Mechanisms Involved in Regulation

The important factors which determine blood volume are (1) the control of the fluid exchange between plasma and interstitial fluid, (2) the control of the fluid exchange between plasma and external environment (mainly via the kidneys), and (3) the control of the red cell volume.

Fluid Exchange between Plasma and Interstitial Fluid

Hydrostatic and colloid osmotic pressures normally balance each other in the capillaries (Chapter 8). A gross disturbance of this balance is, of course, induced in dependent body regions due to the rise in hydrostatic pressure, but several mechanisms tend to offset this disturbance (Chapter 16).

Apart from such shifts in the hydrostatic capillary pressure, it is governed by the pre/postcapillary resistance ratio. A preponderant vasodilatation of the precapillary vessels (or constriction of the postcapillary ones) raises this pressure and fluid filters from the vascular compartment. Functional hyperaemia, such as in exercise, leads to such an increase in capillary pressure. The precapillary resistance vessels are more susceptible to the action of local metabolites than are the postcapillary ones. Further, the higher w/r ratio of the precapillary vessels implies bigger luminal changes for a given smooth muscle relaxation (Chapter 5). The result is a *fall* in the pre/postcapillary resistance ratio and a *rise* in the capillary pressure. In exercise this occurs to such an extent that haemoconcentration ensues, to which the hyperosmolarity within the active muscles contributes (Chapter 22). Within 15 to 20 minutes of heavy exercise up to 15% of the plasma volume can be transiently "lost" in this way—likewise, venous back pressure, as in heart failure, increases fluid transudation.

Conversely, an *increase* in the pre/postcapillary resistance ratio, such as occurs upon reflex increases in vasoconstrictor fibre discharge in some tissues, results in an uptake of fluid from the tissue spaces. Such reflex increases of the pre/postcapillary resistance ratio are especially marked in skeletal muscle (Öberg, 1964), and this tissue has the largest interstitial fluid depot of them all, rendering it especially suited for delivering such "autotransfusions" from the extravascular space. This appears to constitute a steadily operating mechanism for the reflex control of the blood volume (see **Fig. 20-2**).

Fig. 20-2. A. Stepwise increases in reflex muscle vasoconstriction with consequent increases in fluid absorption (volume curve) as a response to stepwise reductions in blood volume (2 ml/kg) at A, B, and C. Reflex adjustments occur even in A where the blood loss has not lowered the arterial mean pressure. Retransfusion at D and E. (The muscle region studied is cross-circulated to keep its regional arterial and venous pressures constant.)
B. Same procedure as in 20-2A but no crossperfusion. At the signal, bleeding (10 ml/kg) with intact vasoconstrictor fibre supply in A but with the sympathetics cut in B. Note that fluid absorption occurs only as long as the reflex increase in pre/postcapillary resistance ratio can occur. (From Öberg, 1964. By permission.)

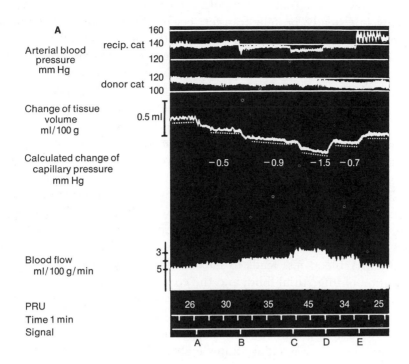

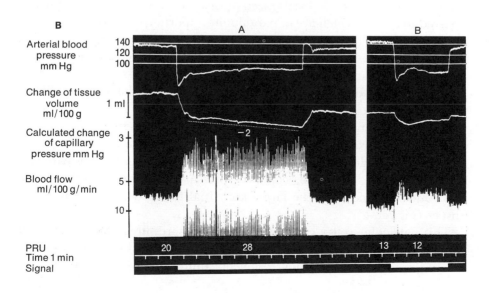

Protein does escape from the capillaries—up to 200 g/day (Chapter 8). This slow but steady protein transfer, essentially via the *large* capillary pores, cannot regain access to the blood via the capillaries but is returned to the blood via the lymphatics. If this were not the case the osmotic pressure difference across the capillary walls would gradually vanish, in which case it would be impossible to maintain a proper plasma volume. This occurs upon obstruction, or major leakage, in the main lymphatic trunks. Thus, the plasma proteins constitute the *"colloid osmotic skeleton" of the plasma compartment*, just as sodium chloride constitutes the "osmotic skeleton" of the entire extracellular fluid compartment. No doubt there must exist a strict control of the total amount of plasma proteins, since blood loss is known to be followed by an increased production of such proteins. Exactly how this very important regulation is effected is not known. Presumably one of the mechanisms might be related to the plasma protein concentration itself, acting perhaps as a feedback on albumin production. A blood loss leads to haemodilution by means of the reflex mobilization of interstitial fluid, and the consequent reduction of albumin concentration may constitute one of the means by which the liver release of albumin is stimulated.

Local vascular adjustments are also of importance, as exemplified by the autoregulatory precapillary adjustments which occur in the legs and which counteract regional fluid losses across the capillaries (Chapter 16). Superimposed on such local mechanisms are the reflex adjustments, referred to above, which are of paramount importance for over-all plasma volume control. Thus, a fall in blood pressure, or even a slight reduction in pulse pressure, reduces the impulse activity of the mechanoreceptors of the aortic and carotid sinus. This in turn increases the sympathetic vasoconstrictor fibre discharge and a series of important changes take place. As mentioned, it appears that the muscle vascular circuit is most sensitively affected, and this not only helps to increase the systemic resistance, but, more importantly, the vasoconstrictor fibre discharge to this circuit produces a considerable and well sustained increase of the pre/postcapillary resistance ratio. Therefore, capillary pressure falls and a well graded absorbtion of fluid from the large interstitial fluid "depot" of this tissue ensues (Fig. 20-2).

This particular reflex effect from the "high-pressure" receptors in fact precedes those affecting other circuits and the venous capacitance side, where the reflex discharge increase is not quite so marked except at very strong reflex excitation (Browse *et al.*, 1966; Hadjiminas and Öberg, 1968). Thus, reflex mobilization of tissue fluid appears to have some "priority" over increases of over-all flow resistance and even over the adjustments of the capacitance vessels, with respect to the arterial receptors, at least. Considering the fact that restitution of blood volume is *the* adequate way to maintain cardiovascular homeostasis after fluid loss, such a high degree of sensitivity of the reflex adjustments of the pre/postcapillary resistance ratio in skeletal muscle appears appropriate.

Not only *arterial* mechanoreceptors but also those situated in the veno-atrial junctions in the "low-pressure side" of the system are involved in the control of the blood volume. These latter receptors are well suited to "sense" the *filling* of the system, situated as they are in distensible walls just at the entrance for the filling of the heart. However, the filling of the system is indirectly sensed also on the high-pressure side, for a reduced venous filling means a reduced stroke volume in the steady state, hence a more narrow arterial pulse pressure and even a reduced mean pressure.

The suggestion that a nervous control of the blood volume is exercised from the central veins was advanced by Peters as early as 1935, at a time when no such receptors were known. Since 1943, however, there has been increasingly detailed evidence of such receptors from histological, electrophysiological, and cardiovascular investigations. As stated in Chapter 18, these nerve endings of vagal origin are found in the subintima and subendocardial regions of the junctions of the venae cavae and right atrium and of the junctions of the pulmonary veins with the left atrium.

Electrophysiological methods show that the impulse activity of these nerve endings is *decreased* by diminishing the venous return and *increased* by circulatory plethora. Such changes of their afferent activity are accompanied by reflex sympathetic discharge changes, similar to those evokable from the systemic arterial receptors; increased impulse discharge of most of the atrial receptors causes an inhibition of sympathetic activity, etc. (Heymans and Neil, 1958). Recent experiments (Öberg and White, 1970) suggest that these low-pressure cardiac receptors affect the pre/postcapillary adjustments of the muscle circuit less markedly than do the arterial receptors. On the other hand, the low-pressure receptors appear to exert a relatively more powerful reflex influence on the *renal* vascular circuit (and on the heart), which presumably aids in their control of renal fluid losses (see below). Both the "low-pressure" receptors and the "high-pressure" receptors appear to influence the systemic capacitance vessels to about the same extent. This type of quantitatively differentiated reflex effect is schematized in Fig. 20-3.

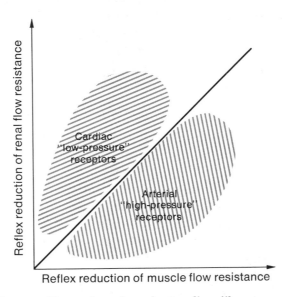

Fig. 20-3. Diagram illustrating that the cardiac "low-pressure" receptors— for a given extent of reflex muscle vasodilatation which is used as a "reference" —produce a stronger reflex vasodilatation in the kidney than the arterial "high-pressure" receptors. These, in turn, adjust with particular sensitivity the filtration-absorption equilibrium in the large muscle tissue mass (Fig. 20-2A). Both sets of receptors exert about equal reflex effects on the veins. (From Öberg and White, 1970. By permission.)

Control of the Exchange between Plasma and External Environment

Cardiovascular Receptors

There is evidence that the arterial receptors, besides their reflex effect on the renal vascular circuit referred to above, play a more direct role with respect to the renal influence on the blood volume. Gauer *et al.* (1954) showed that negative pressure ventilation induced diuresis and attributed this effect to the increased left atrial filling which attended such artificial ventilation. They proved that the effect was reflex in origin by abolishing it by cutting the left cardiac vagi. Furthermore, they showed that artificial stretching of the left atrio-pulmonary venous junction induces either an increased impulse discharge from the left atrial receptors (Henry and Pearce, 1956) or the diuretic effect.

There arose the proposition that these vagal afferents—besides relaying in the medullary centres and causing the cardiovascular reflexes mentioned above and in Chapter 18—also relay to ascending fibres which reach hypothalamic levels and influence the osmoreceptive centres responsible for the control of ADH secretion. Thus, an increase in the circulating blood volume would inhibit ADH secretion with the result that a greater fluid loss would ensue. The reverse would occur in anhydraemia. More recent studies have further substantiated this concept of low-pressure receptor control of the blood volume (Gupta *et al.*, 1966).

It would seem likely that aldosterone secretion is reflexly affected in a similar manner by a "neuro-hormonal" reflex arch, but such a possibility is still being debated. No doubt some mechanism of this general effect does exist, since shifts in fluid alone are of little relevance if the "osmotic skeleton" of the fluid, sodium chloride, is not shifted as well. However, changes in aldosterone secretion might be mainly a consequence of reflex effects—from "low-pressure" as well as "high-pressure" receptors—on the renal vasoconstrictor fibre discharge, with consequent shifts in renin release and angiotensin production (see below).

In any case, the "neuro-hormonal" reflex effects on the ADH secretion is certainly not the only mechanism involved. This is clear from the fact that the effect of negative pressure in producing diuresis is in part present even when the ADH concentration in the blood is kept maximal by ADH infusion (Ledsome *et al.*, 1961). The effect is undoubtedly dependent upon vagal afferents, as vagotomy abolishes it. It would seem likely that the above mentioned reflex adjustments of the renal circuit from the cardiac "volume" receptors may in part explain this phenomenon. A preferential reflex vasoconstrictor fibre inhibition in this circuit would increase not only renal blood flow but also the glomerular filtration rate. This, in itself, would increase the urinary output, other things being equal. Moreover, since even very slight changes in renal vasoconstrictor fibre discharge appear to be instrumental in changing renin release (Bunag *et al.*, 1966) there might be secondary effects on sodium chloride absorption as well.

Renal Factors

The kidney itself elaborates two hormones which influence blood volume. One is *erythropoietin*, responsible for the stimulation of the stem cells of the bone marrow which elaborate the erythrocytes. The other is *renin*, which is synthetized in the cells of the "Polkissen", situated in the wall of the afferent arteriole to the glomerulus.

Renin is a proteolytic enzyme with no direct pressor effect of its own. It acts on α_2-globulin substrate in the plasma to produce angiotensin I—a decapeptide which is converted to angiotensin II by a chloride-activated enzyme in the plasma (see Page and McCubbin, 1968). Angiotensin II, again, is an octapeptide and a very powerful vasoconstrictor agent. It acts preferentially on the systemic precapillary resistance vessels. Probably of even greater significance, it powerfully stimulates the liberation of aldo-sterone from the zona glomerulosa of the adrenal cortex (see below).

Renin granules in the juxtaglomerular apparatus (JGA) increase in number and more renin is released when the blood pressure falls, when the pulse pressure is reduced, or when the renal vessels are even slightly constricted by their sympathetic fibres (Bunag *et al.*, 1966). Thus, an in-creased production and liberation of the enzyme appears to occur in circumstances in which it would act appropriately. Some regard the JGA as a built-in baroreceptor of non-nervous type which, like the neural receptors, acts in response to the distortion of the wall produced by the pulse pressure. Tobian (1960) has suggested that chronic changes in the sodium and water content of the wall may render the wall less susceptible to such phasic stretches and may lead to inappropriate features of renin release. Be that as it may, the renin system contributes to the regulation of blood volume, perhaps less by influencing the precapillary vessels and hence capillary hydrostatic pressure appreciably—except perhaps in blood loss, etc.—but especially by altering the *secretion of aldosterone*.

As mentioned, no retention or loss of water of any considerable degree can be achieved over a long period without there being an accompanying change of the skeleton of sodium. Indeed, there is evidence that sodium conservation, as ultimately controlled by aldosterone, is the primary factor

---

Fig. 20-4. Schematic illustration of blood volume control (time sequence):
1st line of defence: reflex adjustments of cardiovascular effectors "around" the available blood volume.
2nd line of defence: mobilization of interstitial fluid depots by reflex vascular adjustments (compare Fig. 20-2A).
3rd line of defence: reflex neuro-hormonal adjustments of renal losses; of water-salt intake; of blood cell and plasma protein prod-uction.

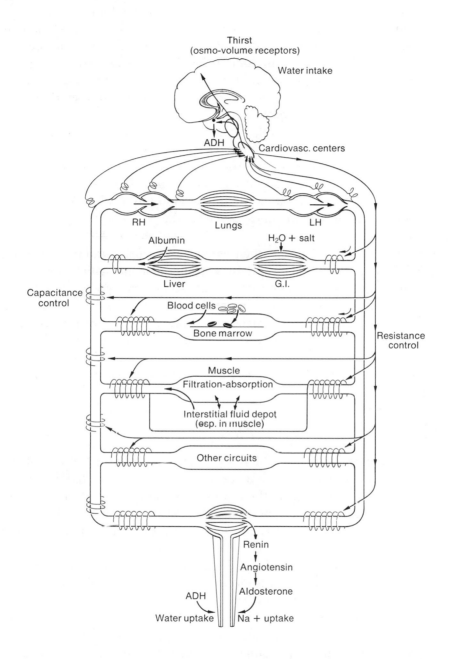

and that water is largely retained passively. The sodium which is not absorbed in the proximal tubule gains access to the distal tubule where its absorption, again active, is adjusted by aldosterone. A deficiency of aldosterone is characterized by sodium loss in the urine with consequent depletion of the extracellular fluid, including the plasma volume. Conversely, an excessive secretion of aldosterone induces sodium retention and as a consequence water retention.

It can readily be understood, then, that a vascular monitoring system (the JGA)—as influenced by the renal vasoconstrictor fibre effects on the vessels, in turn controlled by the various cardiovascular receptors—signals either plethora or a deficiency of plasma volume. This JGA mechanism controls via angiotensin the secretion of aldosterone, being of utmost value in adjusting sodium and therefore water excretion and plasma volume.

Certain clinical conditions, such as congestive heart failure, cirrhosis, and nephrosis, are characterized by chronic oedema, which may be of enormous degree. Each is associated with a secondary hyperaldosteronism and hypoproteinaemia. Only if mercurial diuretics (which reduce renal sodium reabsorption) or spirolactones (which act competitively with aldosterone for the "receptor" sites of the distal tubule responsible for the reabsorption of sodium) are used can this oedema be satisfactorily reduced by the natural process of renal excretion of sodium accompanied passively by that of water.

Control of Red Cell Volume

Erythropoietin is the hormone which is primarily responsible for the red cell mass. It has long been known that chronic hypoxia is associated with polycythaemia, but until recently the mechanism was attributed to the direct effect of oxygen lack on the bone marrow. However, tissue culture preparations of marrow stem cells show no response to the pO_2 of the nutrient medium. Evidence is plentiful now that the hypoxic proliferation of the red cell series is *hormonally* induced (see Linman and Bethell, 1960). Erythropoietin is a glycoprotein with the electrophoretic mobility of an α-globulin, produced mainly by the kidney but possibly elsewhere as well. Its exact site of production is not known.

Chronic renal disease is frequently accompanied by severe anaemia, due presumably to the destruction of the sites of erythropoietin production.

Conversely, anaemias of non-renal origin, such as hypoplastic anaemia, leukaemia, and Cooley's anaemia, are associated with high plasma concentrations of erythropoietin. Use has been made of this by inducing anaemia in animals by ionizing radiation or by administering the haemolytic substance phenylhydrazine. This calls forth an increased secretion of erythropoietin which can then be isolated from the plasma. Erythropoietin probably exerts its action on the transformation of the bone marrow primitive stem cell to the proerythroblast.

Normally, then, a feedback system exists in the adjustment of the red cell mass. A reduction in the red cell concentration of the blood induces an increased output of erythropoietin and vice versa. Patients with congenital heart disease who are cyanosed have polycythaemia. It is probable that the erythropoietin production sites are sensitive to the local pO_2. Polycythaemia is a feature of hypoxia when the situation is chronic.

It is appropriate that the blood which supplies the requirements of the body is regulated both in *volume* and *composition* by the combined activity of many parts of the central nervous system and the endocrine system (Fig. 20-4). For, as Goethe wrote, "Das Blut is ein ganz besonderer Saft".

References

Browse, N. L., J. T. Shepherd, and D. E. Donald (1966). "Differences in response of veins and resistance vessels in limbs to same stimulus," *Am. J. Physiol.* **211**, 1241–47.

Bunag, R. D., I. H. Page, and J. W. McCubbin (1966). "Neural stimulation of release of renin," *Circ. Res.* **19**, 851–58.

Chien, Shu (1967). "Role of the sympathetic nervous system in hemorrhage," *Physiol. Rev.* **47**, 214–88.

Gauer, O. H., and J. P. Henry (1963). "Circulatory basis of fluid volume control," *Physiol. Rev.* **43**, 423–81.

Gauer, O. H., J. P. Henry, H. O. Sieker, and W. E. Wendt (1954). "The effect of negative pressure breathing on urine flow," *J. Clin. Invest.* **33**, 287–96.

Gauer, O. H., J. P. Henry, and C. Behn (1970). "The regulation of extracellular fluid volume," *Ann. Rev. Physiol.* **32**, 572–94.

Gregersen, M. I., and R. A. Rawson (1959). "Blood volume," *Physiol. Rev.* **39,** 307–42.

Gupta, P. D., J. P. Henry, R. Sinclair, and R. von Baumgarten (1966). "Responses of atrial and aortic baroreceptors to nonhypotensive hemorrhage and transfusion," *Am. J. Physiol.* **211,** 1429–37.

Hadjiminas, J., and B. Öberg (1968). "Effects of carotid baroreceptor reflexes on venous tone in skeletal muscle and intestine of the cat," *Acta Physiol. Scand.* **72,** 518–32.

Henry, J. P., and J. W. Pearce (1956). "The possible role of cardiac atrial stretch receptors in the induction of changes in urine flow," *J. Physiol.* **131,** 572–85.

Heymans, C., and E. Neil (1958). "The reflexogenic areas of the cardiovascular system," London: Churchill.

Ledsome, J. R., R. Linden, and W. J. O'Connor (1961). "The mechanisms by which distension of the left atrium produces diuresis in anaesthetized dogs," *J. Physiol.* **159,** 87–100.

Linman, J. W., and F. H. Bethell (1960). *Factors controlling erythropoiesis*, pp. 3–208. Springfield, Ill.: Charles C. Thomas.

Öberg, B. (1964). "Effects of cardiovascular reflexes on net capillary fluid transfer," *Acta Physiol. Scand.* **62,** Suppl., 229.

Öberg, B., and S. White (1970). "Circulatory effects of interruption and stimulation of cardial vagal afferents," *Acta Physiol. Scand.*, in press.

Page, I. H., and J. W. McCubbin (1968). *Renal hypertension*. Chicago: Year Book Med. Publ.

Peters, J. P. (1935). *Body Water*. London: Baillière, Tindall and Cox.

Sjöstrand, T. (1962). "Blood volume," *Handbook of Physiology*, 2, Circulation **I,** 51–62.

Tobian, L. (1960). "Interrelationships of electrolytes, juxtaglomerular cells and hypertension," *Physiol. Rev.* **40,** 280–91.

21

Pulmonary Circulation

The Arab scholar Ibnul-Nafiess (1208–1288 A.D.) provided the first adequate description of the pulmonary circulation (see Fig. 21-1).

The entire cardiac output is pumped through the low-pressure pulmonary circuit; the mixed venous blood is oxygenated and its excess of
CO_2 is removed by exchange between the capillaries and the alveoli.
This is the sole function of the pulmonary circuit; the nutrition of the lung
tissues is satisfied by the systemic bronchial circuit. Though such a function is seemingly simple it requires the provision of a circuit whose structural characteristics are unique (for references see Fishman, 1963; Daly
and Hebb, 1967).

Physical Characteristics

Some of these have been detailed in Chapters 5 and 6; additional structural and physical features are given here.

General Design

The pulmonary vascular bed offers only a small resistance to flow. Although the cardiac output may increase fivefold from its resting value, the
pressure head, which secures pulmonary flow, rises only slightly from its

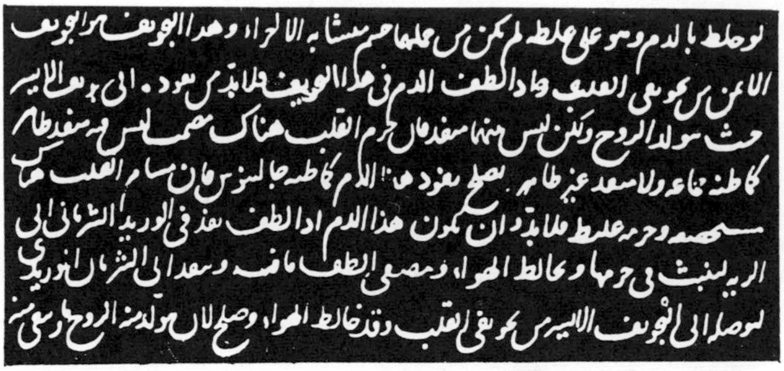

Fig. 21-1. A photographic reproduction of the original manuscript of the Arab scholar Ibnul-Nafiess (1208–1288 A.D.) who discovered the pulmonary circulation of the blood. A translation (kindly furnished by Dr. F. S. Nashat) is added for those readers who might have troubles with their Arabic.

". . . And this is the right one of the two cavities of the heart. If blood were to be purified here it must pass to the left cavity where the soul is generated. But there is no passage between these two cavities. The mass of the heart there is dull and has no visible apertures, as some people thought, nor invisible openings suitable for the passage of blood, as Galen thought. The pores of the heart in this region are scaled and its mass is heavy. Then it is necessary that blood, to be purified, has to pass through the arterial vein to the lungs where it penetrates into its mass, mixes with air, and the better part of it is purified. It then passes into the venous artery to reach the left cavity of the heart."

value of 10 to 15 mm Hg in the resting circulation. Transmural pressures are correspondingly low and are relatively little modified by hydrostatic factors. The wall-lumen ratio is small compared with that in the systemic precapillary resistance vessels.

The pulmonary arterial compartment is thin-walled and wide and contains almost as much blood as does the pulmonary venous compartment; its resistance is not much higher either. This arterial compartment is characterized mainly by the elastic content of its wall, and in the larger branches the smooth muscles of the wall seem to be disposed in such a manner as to limit the wall distensibility (see Chapter 6) rather than to produce extensive changes of calibre. The smallest pulmonary arterioles, quite unlike those of the systemic circuit, contain little or no contractile elements; those that are found are most abundant in the precapillary vessels of 50 to 500 μ radius, and these vessels abut the respiratory bronchioles. The close proximity of this adjustable "resistance" section to the alveoli themselves is important: it has a great deal to do with the adjustment of the regional blood flow to the local gaseous exchange (see below). The smooth muscles of these resistance vessels are reasonably well supplied by adrenergic constrictor fibres.

The venules and veins also contain little smooth muscle. Both the arteries and the veins are "end-vessels", with few if any collaterals. This explains why the wedging of a fine-bore catheter (passed via the right heart) into the smallest arterial branch reflects the pulmonary venous pressure fairly well ("pulmonary wedge pressure"). Were there abundant collaterals, the pressure recorded would simply reflect that at the closest ramification level of the arterial tree.

Although the pulmonary venous contractile elements are sparse and in some species relatively insignificant, venous "capacitance" responses may nevertheless be achieved indirectly by a primary constriction of the pre-capillary vessels. The fall of pressure downstream causes a passive elastic recoil of the veins and may even lead to a partial collapse of the vessel wall, which serves to expel pulmonary venous blood into the left atrium. To this comes the blood that may be expelled by active contraction of the arterial compartment, which by its mere size may substantially add to the capacitance function in this particular circuit (see below). Though relatively small, the mobilizable fraction of the pulmonary blood volume, whether displaced by active or passive means, serves as a reservoir for the left heart. When the left heart increases its force of beat, some of its increase of stroke volume is secured by reducing its systolic reserve and some by ladling more blood from the pulmonary circuit. Such mechanisms "take up the slack" until systemic venous return is boosted by the muscle pump and by sympathetic venoconstriction.

Vascular Distensibility

The high distensibility of the circuit allows a facile accommodation of large changes in flow and volume but invites unusually large disturbances whenever significant hydrostatic factors interfere. In resting man in the recumbent position the pulmonary blood volume is 600 ml; forced expiration against a resistance lowers this to perhaps 200 ml and forced inspiration raises it to 1000 ml.

Pressure-flow resistance curves show that the pulmonary "resistance" vessels are very distensible (Fig. 21-2). Resistance to flow, here as elsewhere,

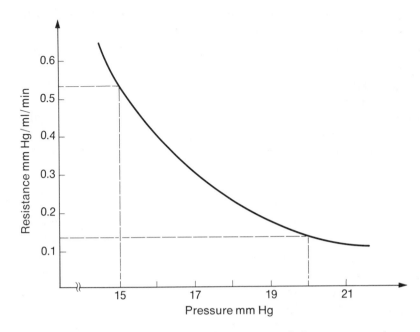

Fig. 21-2. Approximate relationship between perfusion pressure (or trans-mural pressure) and flow resistance in an isolated, blood-perfused lung lobe of the dog. Note the marked reduction of resistance for such moderate rises in pressure (15–20 mm Hg) as may occur during exercise. (From Edwards, 1951. By permission.) It may partly be due to rounding of semicollapsed lumina (compare Fig. 5-10B).

is governed by two factors in the Poiseuille formula, L and r. Inspiration lowers the flow resistance so long as the lung expansion does not exceed 50% of the maximum. The mean luminal widening, especially that which occurs in the larger vessels, is sufficient to overcome the increase in L by increasing the average "effective" r^4. Still deeper inspiration, which continues to increase the pulmonary blood volume, is accompanied by an *increase* in pulmonary flow resistance, which is offered particularly by the small "alveolar" vessels. The average radius for the pulmonary vascular bed appears now to be almost maximally stretched by the expanding lung parenchyma while the average vascular length is still increasing. However, in ordinary breathing, or even during exercise hyperventilation, inspiration *increases* the regional blood content (see Chapter 10; Fig. 10-5) but *decreases* the regional flow resistance. The forces involved and the *r-L* interrelations are complex, however, and the experimental results are not in entire agreement (Fishman, 1963).

During positive pressure ventilation, as during surgery, the rise of alveolar pressure hinders systemic venous return. Both cardiac and pulmonary blood volumes fall. However, as the pulmonary circuit is normally entirely enclosed in the thorax, neither its pressure head nor the transmural pressure is primarily affected by the raised alveolar pressure. The effects of the raised intrathoracic pressure on the *pulmonary* circuit are secondary to the pooling of more blood in the extrathoracic systemic veins.

Coughing is associated with a simultaneous rise in pressure in the thorax, abdomen, and cerebrospinal canal. Although the intrathoracic pressure may briefly reach 150 mm Hg, the pressure gradient responsible for pushing blood along the pulmonary vessels is again not affected. This intrathoracic pressure rise *is* transmitted, however, to the systemic peripheral vessels, and this causes here a brief but marked increase in the transmural distending pressure.

Uneven Perfusion-ventilation

Although the hydrostatic pressure differences are fairly small in the lungs —the apex and the base are placed, respectively, only some 15 cm above and below the atrioventricular heart level in erect man—even these small differences in transmural pressure are of profound importance for pulmonary blood flow and volume distribution, because of the high distensibility of these vessels. About the same differences in transmural pressure occur between the uppermost and lowermost lungs in man lying on his side. The small pulmonary vessels are exposed to the alveolar air ("alveolar vessels"), which provides no tissue fluid which can offset part of the hydrostatic factors. The full impact of the changed intravascular pressure therefore influences their radius and/or luminal configuration.

This explains why pulmonary blood flow in standing man is normally greater in the bases than in the apices (West and Dollery, 1960). An experiment using radioactively labelled CO_2 ($^{15}CO_2$) and scanning techniques shows such regional differences in pulmonary blood flow. The subject takes a deep breath and holds it for 15 sec; the slope of the tracing recorded by a pair of scintillation counters placed antero-posteriorly at different levels of the lung shows the regional blood flow (Fig. 21-3). Alternatively, ^{133}Xe in saline solution can be injected into the right atrium, and the xenon, owing to its low solubility, is evolved from the lung capillaries.

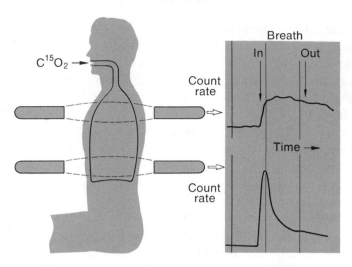

Fig. 21-3. Measurement of regional pulmonary blood flow and ventilation using radioactive CO_2. Pairs of scintillation counters examine the anterior-posterior cores of the lung. The counting rate at the end of inspiration is proportional to the ventilation of the lung in the counting field, and its volume; the slope of the tracing during breath-holding (clearance rate) measures the regional blood flow. (From West, 1963. By permission.)

An *ideal* O_2-CO_2 exchange calls for *a perfusion-ventilation ratio of unity throughout the lung*. The effect of these hydrostatic factors on the vessel calibre complicates gas exchange and particularly influences the oxygenation of the blood. There may be lung regions which are ventilated but not perfused ("*parallel-coupled dead space*")—the lung apex is in fact often very close to this situation in standing man—and those which are perfused but not ventilated ("*blood shunts*"). Such extremes are pathophysiological variants, but considerable distortions of the "ideal" perfusion-ventilation ratio occur even in normal circumstances, although local physiological adjustments (see below) achieve some measure of compensation.

Uneven perfusion-ventilation is of little consequence in the elimination of CO_2, for the underventilation of one blood fraction is largely offset by the overventilation of another, and the mixed arterial blood ejected by the left ventricle may still display a normal CO_2 content. The situation is more complex with oxygen. *Moderate* degrees of uneven perfusion-ventilation do not matter much, for the characteristic S-shape of the Hb-O_2 dissociation curve allows nearly complete saturation of haemoglobin even in the underventilated parts of the lungs. With more extreme underventilation, however, the haemoglobin in such regions is only partly saturated with O_2, and in the overventilated regions nothing can be gained beyond full oxygenation: the mixed arterial blood thus shows a reduced O_2 content, as if some of the blood had traversed a right-left shunt.

Fortunately, physiological mechanisms exist which help to offset these physical consequences of the pronounced vascular distensibility in the lungs. Thus, whenever a lung region is underventilated (and/or over-perfused)—leading to a lowered alveolar pO_2 and raised pCO_2—the local bronchiolar smooth muscles relax, while those of the local precapillary vessels constrict (see also Chapter 16). The converse occurs in lung sections exposed to a relative overventilation. Such local responses (see below) of the contractile elements adjust both the ventilation and the circulation so that the "ideal" perfusion-ventilation ratio is approached. The assignation which blood and air enjoy in the lungs can only be satisfactorily consummated because of these complex physiological adjustments.

Capillary Function in the Lungs

The pulmonary capillaries—which have a maximal combined surface area of some 90 m^2 in man—are relatively wide in bore, and short, and they form dense networks around the aveoli (Chapter 5). Their endothelium is of the "continuous" type (Chapter 8) with a combined alveolar-capillary interface which is only 0.25 to 0.5 micron thick. Their total blood content is some 70 to 100 ml (12 to 15% of the average blood volume in the lungs). Despite the shortness and wide bore of the individual tubes, this pulmonary capillary section seems to furnish most of the (admittedly low) pulmonary flow resistance (Fig. 21-4). The remaining resistance is about equally shared by vessels placed upstream and downstream, respectively (e.g. Agostini and Piiper, 1962), except when a precapillary constriction occurs.

The order of magnitude of the pulmonary capillary flow was first established by the use of a nitrous oxide inhalation.

$$\text{Flow} = \frac{\text{Volume of nitrous oxide absorbed per min}}{\text{Solubility coefficient of } N_2O/\text{Mean alveolar content of } N_2O}$$

However, the method suffered severe practical limitations, and the N_2O method fell into disuse until Lee and Du Bois (1955) introduced the body plethysmograph. This technique pictures the pulmonary capillary flow as vigorously pulsatile (Fig. 21-5), as is the case in the whole circuit, mainly because of the very low resistance to flow. The method depends on the extreme solubility of N_2O in blood. When a nitrous oxide mixture is inhaled it is immediately taken up by the blood entering the pulmonary capillaries. The subject sits in an air-tight chamber and rebreathes from a

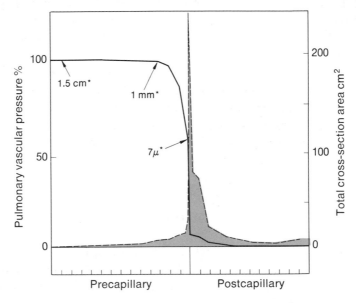

Fig. 21-4. Hypothetical relationship between blood pressure in per cent of initial level (solid line) and cross-sectional area (shaded) in pulmonary vascular bed of the dog. Vascular diameters at key points are indicated by asterisks. The major drop in blood pressure seems to occur in the region of the pulmonary capillaries. (From Fishman, 1963. By permission.)

bag (containing the nitrous oxide mixture) which is also within the chamber. The pressure in the chamber falls owing to the absorption of N_2O (Fig. 21-5A). He stops breathing for a few seconds and the pressure record shows a pulsatile tracing (Fig. 21-5B). By recording the ECG simultaneously it can be seen that gas absorption, and hence the capillary blood flow, is higher during systole than diastole. As the concentration of the gas and its solubility in blood are known, the instantaneous blood flow can be calculated.

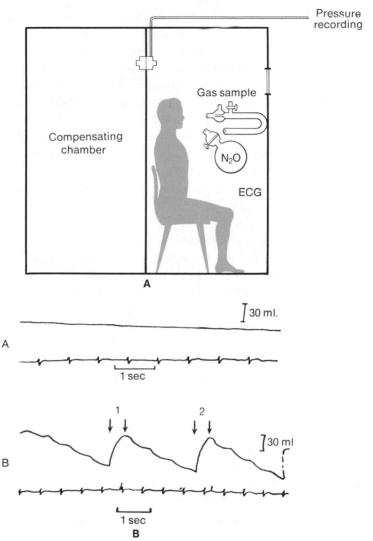

Fig. 21-5A. Diagram of a body plethysmograph.

Fig. 21-5B. Plethysmograph volume changes and electrocardiogram while subject held his breath on room air (A) and on nitrous oxide (B). Note in B that the uptake of nitrous oxide is pulsatile with heart rate. The plethysmograph was opened to the atmosphere between arrows at (1) and (2). The record, although obtained as the change in pressure in the plethysmograph, was converted to volume change by calibrating with a syringe attached to the plethysmograph (records retouched). (From Lee and DuBois, 1955. By permission.)

Blood spends 0.75 to 1 sec in the pulmonary capillaries in resting man, but in exercise the transit time is reduced to about 0.33 sec (Chapter 5). These values can also be calculated from measurements of alveolar capillary gas exchange and the kinetic data of CO-Hb combination (Roughton, 1945). During heavy exercise the pO_2 difference across the alveolar walls increases somewhat due to the shortened capillary transit time. However, efficient blood oxygenation still occurs thanks to the S-shape of the Hb-O_2 dissociation curve. The situation is different for a man climbing Mount Everest. Suppose that the partial oxygen pressure is so low that he is close to the steep part of his Hb-O_2 dissociation curve even during rest. The reduced capillary transit time during climbing may now lead to a considerable drop in his Hb saturation, with cyanosis, dizziness, and weakness as a result.

While the entire capillary surface is available for the passage of the lipid-soluble O_2 and CO_2, the pulmonary capillary endothelium is unusually "tight" with respect to intercellular porosity. This is evident both from diffusion studies (Chinard *et al.*, 1962) and from recent measurements of the filtration-absorption events in isolated perfused lungs (Fig. 21-6; see also Hauge *et al.*, 1966). An approximate computation of the filtration transfer across comparable capillary surface area in lung tissue and skeletal muscle suggests a decidedly *lower* pore density in the lung, while the slow but definite passage of protein indicates that the pore radius may be about the same.

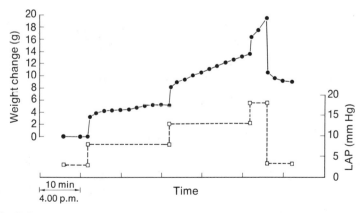

Fig. 21-6. Effect upon vascular capacity and transcapillary fluid exchange of elevations in left atrial pressure (LAp) in the isolated rabbit lung. ●—● weight change; □ – – – □ LAp. (From Hauge *et al.*, 1966. By permission.)

These results suggest that a typical Starling equilibrium is displayed by the pulmonary capillaries. This equilibrium occurs at a capillary pressure which is lower than that in the systemic capillaries, with a minute filtration to, and absorption from, narrow, but protein-rich, tissue spaces. Presumably these "slits" gradually expand towards the edges between alveoli and bronchioli, to become slowly drained via the more substantial interstitia around the bronchial capillary network. Thus, the alveoli themselves receive no lymphatics, for the pulmonary lymph vessels— which drain a fairly protein-rich lymph—stop short at the level of the atria of the respiratory bronchiole, from which the alveoli debouch.

It was earlier assumed that the tiny tissue spaces around the pulmonary capillaries were safely "dry", because plasma colloid-osmotic pressure (π_{pl}) so greatly exceeds pulmonary capillary pressure (Pc); the possible presence of a tissue fluid compartment was largely neglected. If this were so, however, filtration would not occur until Pc exceeded π_{pl}; but Fig. 21-6 shows that *any* rise of Pc causes some filtration, even though this may be transient. In most situations a new equilibrium is soon reached, presumably when the high colloid-osmotic pressure in the narrow interstitial space is sufficiently lowered by this transuded fluid.

A gross increase of capillary pressure—and/or capillary damage— overcomes this efficient equilibrium and causes manifest engorgement of the interstitial space and even gross pulmonary oedema. Thus, when pulmonary venous and capillary pressures are raised, as occurs with an attack of left heart failure, pulmonary oedema develops rapidly. Such an attack typically begins while the patient is asleep. In the recumbent position, the volume of blood—and the transmural pressure—in the heart and lungs are greater than they are in the erect posture, and these factors predipose to the attack. As stated before, the effects of hydrostatic pressure are transmitted to the lung vascular bed largely unopposed by any concomitant changes in tissue pressure. For example, in the recumbent side position, parts of the lower lung are about 15 cm below the level of the heart and the pressure in these pulmonary capillaries may be nearly as high as 20 mm Hg. Any additional rise caused by the early stage of left heart failure tends to cause pulmonary oedema, which is thus first seen in dependent parts of the lungs.

The maintenance of a filtration-absorption equilibrium across intact capillaries in the lung requires the presence of erythrocytes in artificial perfusing fluids. Otherwise the perfused lung quickly develops oedema, and electron microphotographs show damage of the capillary endothelial cells and widened intercellular gaps (Lunde, 1967). There might be some important, but unknown, metabolic connection between red cells and the capillary endothelium which is required for the integrity of the capillary walls.

Local Control of Pulmonary Vessels

Lung vessels show little of "basal tone" (see Chapter 16) in the resting equilibrium; consequently, adaptation to an increased flow (such as in exercise) appears to be a matter mainly of *passive* effects; i.e. the effect of an increased transmural pressure on the highly distensible vessels (Fig. 21-2). Thus, the cardiac output may increase three to four times without there being much rise in the mean pulmonary arterial pressure. As the pulmonary flow increases, the initial slight rise in pressure appears to expand and/or "round up" the vessels. The pulmonary arterial pressure then shows a plateau somewhat lower than its initial peak value.

Clearly the pulmonary vascular resistance has decreased, but there is no certainty as to how this is brought about. As mentioned above, "active" vasodilatation is probably of minor importance in the normal lung. Intravascular pressure no doubt increases somewhat and there may be some decrease in mean intrapleural pressure as a result of the increased respiratory movements. Both these factors will raise the transmural pressure in the pulmonary circuit. It is therefore likely that a passive widening of patent vessels is the most important factor, but some opening of vessels that are closed during resting conditions may also contribute.

The situation is very complex, however, as the kinetic energy imparted to the system may exceed the potential energy in the flow situation present during exercise. Moreover, interconversions of kinetic and potential energy along the course of the vascular circuit undoubtedly occur. These are difficult problems to explore, partly because calculations of the pulmonary vascular resistance and the transmural pressure are only valid if we have *simultaneous* records of pulmonary arterial, left atrial, and pleural pressures, and of pulmonary flow, and we do not have such records.

The pulmonary vascular smooth muscles are unique with respect to their reactions to a series of local chemical and blood-borne humoral factors. The most important of these is perhaps the response to hypoxia, first described by Euler and Liljestrand (1946) and analysed in great detail by Duke (1957). The local effect of hypoxia on the precapillary smooth muscle is one of *constriction*, the very opposite of that in systemic vessels (see Chapter 16).

In unanaesthetized man and animals, acute hypercapnia has no effect on the pulmonary flow and resistance, but in anaesthetized animals, passively ventilated at constant ventilation volume, CO_2 added to the mixture evokes pulmonary vasoconstriction. In the latter case the degree of acidaemia induced by the CO_2 is greater than that in the spontaneously breathing animal, which can of course increase its ventilation under the CO_2 stimulus. Like hypoxia, acidosis of any type causes pulmonary vasoconstriction.

The small precapillary vessels—those that are supplied with smooth muscle and are responsible for the adjustments to hypoxia—are juxtaposed to the respiratory bronchioles and can therefore respond to a lowered pO_2 in these air passages. Perfusion of the pulmonary vessels with hypoxic blood also produces such vasoconstriction, but *not* if the pO_2 in the alveoli is kept high, which leads to oxygenation of the bloodstream (Duke, 1957). Thus, the precapillary smooth muscles primarily "sense" the situation in the adjacent *air passages*, and this situation, in turn, determines the extent to which the hypoxic blood arriving will be oxygenated. This is important, for otherwise the severely reduced venous blood of heavy exercise would cause vasoconstriction as it traversed these pulmonary arterioles. Fortunately, however, such arteriolar tone is determined by the pO_2 of the adjacent air passages.

It has been much debated how this pulmonary vasoconstrictor response to hypoxia is elicited; especially whether it is mediated by a local release of some specific constrictor agent. A whole series of substances—many of which are vasodilators in the systemic circulation—produce pulmonary vasoconstriction, such as noradrenaline, serotonin (5-HT), ATP, histamine, plasmakinins (e.g. Hauge *et al.*, 1966). Interestingly enough, histamine and plasmakinins do *not* increase capillary permeability in the lungs (Waaler 1968), in contrast to their effects on most systemic capillaries. Only prostaglandin (PGE_1) and, at least in some species, adrenaline *decrease* pulmonary flow resistance. However, both the catecholamines tend to *decrease* pulmonary blood volume (Hauge *et al.*, 1967), a capacitance response which is of advantage for left heart filling.

Now, the responses to nearly all of the constrictor substances mentioned can be blocked, in one way or the other, *without* affecting the constrictor response to hypoxia. However, according to Hauge (1968), antihistaminic agents block the pulmonary constrictor response to hypoxia in the rat without affecting the response to other pulmonary constrictor agents. On the other hand, Duke (1969) could not confirm this in experiments in the cat. Hauge also found that histamine liberators, which greatly reduce the pulmonary histamine content, eliminate selectively the constrictor response to hypoxia in both rats and cats, while histaminase inhibitors tend to potentiate selectively the hypoxic vasoconstriction. He has drawn attention to the possibility that endogenous histamine may mediate the pulmonary vascular response to low oxygen tensions; further experiments are needed to settle this interesting question.

Chronic hypoxia is associated with a marked increase in pulmonary arterial pressure and with a later development of right ventricular hypertrophy. Cattle living at high altitudes (8000 feet or more) develop brisket disease, in which pulmonary hypertension, severe right ventricular failure, and oedema of the brisket are the outstanding features. Thick pulmonary precapillary vessels develop in high-altitude dwellers, and even children born and raised at high altitudes show pulmonary hypertension (compare Chapter 31).

Pulmonary Vasomotor Fibre Control

Innervation

The pulmonary vessels are fairly richly supplied with adrenergic vasoconstrictor fibres wherever smooth muscles are present. This involves large and small arteries, large arterioles, and the venous compartment, though the smooth muscle cover here is scant and, in some species, almost absent. It is further known (see above) that the adrenergic transmitter, noradrenaline, via α-receptors, can considerably enhance the flow resistance and decrease the blood volume of the lungs.

It has proved difficult, however, to demonstrate pulmonary vasoconstrictor fibre effects. This stems from the fact that the bronchial circulation has not been separately perfused in the "isolated lung" preparation, artificially perfused by a pump. The viability of the sympathetic nerves to the pulmonary vessels depends on their getting a blood supply from the bronchial vessels. Daly and co-workers (see Daly and Hebb, 1967) perfused the bronchial circulation separately and, if necessary, interrupted this

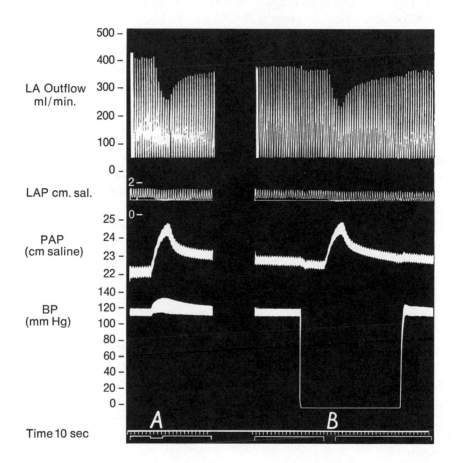

Fig. 21-7. The effect of electrical stimulation of the stellate ganglion on pulmonary vascular resistance. The innervated isolated left lung of a dog was perfused with blood through the pulmonary artery at a constant head of pressure and through the bronchial arteries. No ventilation of the lung. Two stimulations (A and B) of the left stellate ganglion caused a fall in blood flow through the lungs (top record). Note that the second response (B) was obtained while there was no blood flowing through the bronchial circulation, i.e. at zero bronchial arterial blood pressure (BP). LA, left atrial; PA, pulmonary artery; P, pressure. (From Daly, 1958. By permission.)

perfusion only for the brief period required to obtain control values of pulmonary blood flow before and after a short burst of stimuli delivered to the stellate ganglion, from which course the pulmonary sympathetic fibres (Fig. 21-7). In such preparations it was possible to explore the vaso-constrictor fibre effect in great detail.

It then appears that the neurogenic effects on pulmonary flow *resistance* are usually quite weak; even maximal discharge rates seldom increase the resistance more than some 30% or so (Fig. 21-8; see also Daly and Hebb, 1967). This may, however, be in keeping with the fact that the main pulmonary flow resistance resides in the capillaries and vessels closely adjacent, which lack contractile elements. Hence, neurogenic constrictions confined to *larger arteries and veins*—which are almost equal in volume and together contain the major part of the pulmonary blood content but do not add much to resistance—may after all be substantial. Such considerations direct the interest to a nervous control primarily of pulmonary *capacitance* function. Thus it appears likely that the vasoconstrictor nerves, without much affecting pulmonary flow resistance, may actively expel considerable fractions of the pulmonary blood reservoir to the left heart; haemodynamically, this may well be the really important function of this vascular innervation. Furthermore, the fact that the capacitance of the arterial side matches that of the venous side has another great advantage. Capacitance constrictor responses unavoidably increase flow resistance somewhat—if the resistance is not predominantly effectuated by means of *longitudinal* smooth muscles, as might be the case in some of the veins of the G.I. tract. Now, as these unavoidable resistance increases in connection with the expulsion of blood might be placed about equally on the pre-capillary and postcapillary sides in the lungs, there would be no secondary decrease in pre/postcapillary resistance ratio and hence no increase of pulmonary *capillary* pressure as a result of such a capacitance response (see Chapter 16).

Reflex Control

Reflexes affecting the pulmonary vascular resistance have been demonstrated. Baroreceptor stimulation (aortic or carotid sinus) induces reflex dilatation of the pulmonary vessels, whereas chemoreceptor stimulation provokes reflex pulmonary vasoconstriction. There is evidence that the sympathetic nerves provide a slight tonic vasoconstriction of the pulmonary vessels except, perhaps, during complete rest. The reflex effects described

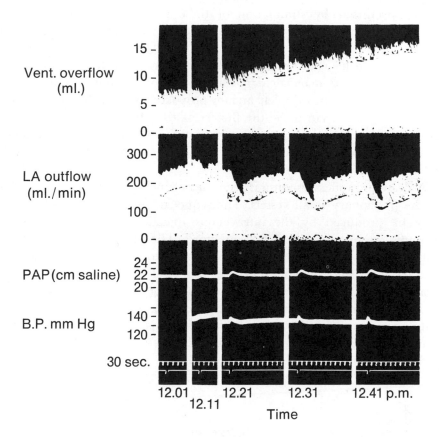

Fig. 21-8. Effects of high-frequency sympathetic stimulation on the pulmonary blood flow resistance, as evidenced by a reduced pulmonary blood flow (LA outflow) and raised pulmonary arterial pressure (PAP). At top and bottom recordings of ventilation and systemic blood pressure. (From Allison *et al.*, 1961. By permission.)

above are abolished by stellatectomy and are therefore mediated by the sympathetic nerves (Daly and Hebb, 1967).

As described in Chapter 18, the pulmonary trunk and the right and left pulmonary arteries are the site of adventitially placed vagal mechanoreceptors, which are similar in appearance to those in the carotid sinus and aortic arch. An increase in pressure in the pulmonary artery provokes bradycardia and hypotension, and, in general, the cardiovascular reflex effects produced by stimulation of these pulmonary baroreceptors is qualitatively similar to those that may be provoked from the sino-aortic areas.

Linden and his colleagues (Chapter 18) have provided clear evidence that the stimulation of vagal mechanoreceptors at the junction of the pulmonary veins with the left atrium provokes tachycardia. These vagal receptors would seem to be the fingers of the afferent arm of the Bainbridge reflex. Vagal receptors in a similar site—perhaps the same ones—when stimulated induce diuresis and would seem to be concerned in the regulation of blood volume.

A dramatic reflex response is seen on producing multiple microemboli in the pulmonary small vessels. The sequel to such microemboli (which may be produced by the intravenous injection of starch grains, for example) is an extraordinary tachypnoea. The afferent fibres are vagal, and they must be small for they resist cooling to 3°C. Phenyl diguanidine injected intravenously will excite these fibres, as will 5-hydroxytryptamine (Paintal, 1955). It has been suggested, but not proved, that these nerve endings are situated immediately adjacent to, but not in, the smallest pulmonary arterioles (in which the starch grains lodge). It is possible that platelet disintegration liberates 5-HT and causes excitation of these nerve endings.

References

Agostini, E., and J. Piiper (1962). "Capillary pressure and distribution of vascular resistance in isolated lung," *Am. J. Physiol.* **202,** 1033–36.

Allison, P. R., I. de Burgh Daly, and B. Waaler (1961). "Bronchial circulation and pulmonary vasomotor nerve responses in isolated perfused lungs," *J. Physiol.* **157,** 462–74.

Chinard, F. P., T. Enns, and M. F. Nolan (1962). "The permeability characteristics of the alveolar capillary barrier," *Trans. Ass. Am. Physns.* **72,** 253–61.

Daly, I. de B. (1958). "Intrinsic mechanisms of the lung," *Quart. J. Exp. Physiol.* **43,** 2–26.

Daly, I. de B., and C. O. Hebb (1967). *Pulmonary and bronchial vascular systems.* Baltimore: Williams and Wilkins.

Duke, H. N. (1957). "Observations on the effects of hypoxia on the pulmonary vascular bed," *J. Physiol.* **135,** 45–51. (London.)

Duke, H. N. (1969). "The pulmonary pressor response to hypoxia in isolated perfused lungs of cats; the influence of mepyramine maleate and semicarbazide," *J. Physiol.* **200,** 133–35P.

Edwards, W. S. (1951). "The effects of lung inflation and epinephrine on pulmonary vascular resistance," *Am. J. Physiol.* **167,** 756–62.

Euler, U. S. von, and G. Liljestrand (1946). "Observations on the pulmonary arterial blood pressure in the cat," *Acta Physiol. Scand.* **12,** 301–20.

Fishman, A. P. (1963). "Dynamics of the pulmonary circulation," *Handbook of Physiology,* 1, Circulation **II,** 1667–1743.

Hauge, A. (1968). "Studies on the effect of acute hypoxia on pulmonary vascular resistance," *Norw. Monographs Med. Sci.* Oslo: Universitetsforlaget.

Hauge, A., P. K. M. Lunde, and B. A. Waaler (1966a). "Transvascular fluid balance in the lung," *J. Physiol.* **186,** 94–95P.

Hauge, A., P. K. M. Lunde, and B. A. Waaler (1966b). "The effect of bradykinin, kallidin, and eledoisin upon the pulmonary vascular bed of an isolated blood-perfused rabbit lung preparation," *Acta Physiol. Scand.* **66,** 269–77.

Hauge, A., P. K. M. Lunde, and B. A. Waaler (1967). "Effects of catecholamines on pulmonary blood volume," *Acta Physiol. Scand.* **70,** 323–33.

Lee, G. de J., and A. B. Dubois (1955). "Pulmonary capillary blood flow in man," *J. Clin. Invest.* **34,** 1380–90.

Lunde, P. K. M. (1967). "Edema development in perfused rabbit lungs," *Norw. Monographs Med. Sci.* Oslo: Universitetsforlaget.

Paintal, A. S. (1955). "Impulses in vagal afferent fibres from specific pulmonary deflation receptors," *Quart. J. Exp. Physiol.* **40,** 89–111.

Roughton, F. J. W. (1945). "The average time spent by the blood in the human lung capillary and its relation to the rates of CO uptake and elimination in man," *Am. J. Physiol.* **143,** 621–33.

Waaler, B. A. (1968). Personal communication.

West, J. B. (1963–64). "Distribution of gas and blood in the normal lungs," *Brit. Med. Bull.* **19–20,** 53–58.

West, J. B., and C. T. Dollery (1960). "Distribution of blood flow and ventilation-perfusion ratio in the lung, measured with radioactive CO_2," *J. Appl. Physiol.* **15,** 405–10.

22

Muscle Circulation

General Considerations

No vascular circuit has been subjected to more intense study than that of skeletal muscle. For example, by skilful use of the plethysmograph many of the basic principles of vascular control have been elucidated in studies on man's limbs by Lewis, Barcroft, Greenfield, and their groups (see reviews below).

The muscle vascular bed is extensive and shows a tremendous range of blood flow, from that seen in circumstances of powerful vasoconstriction, as in haemorrhage, to that evinced in intense muscular exercise, where maximal vasodilatation occurs. When the entire muscle mass is involved in intense exercise, it imposes the greatest single load on cardiovascular performance met with in the intact organism. Excellent reviews covering studies of muscle circulation are available and should be consulted for details (e.g. see Barcroft, 1963; Hudlická, 1967).

Dimensions

Muscles constitute 40 to 50% of the tissue mass in an average man. Their oxygen usage at rest, 50 to 60 ml/min, or 20% of total oxygen

399

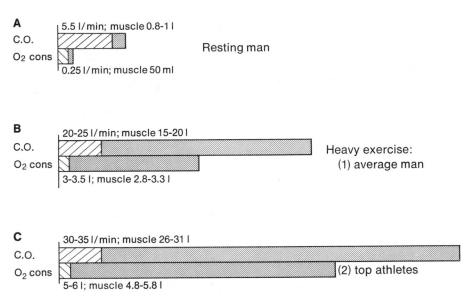

Fig. 22-1. Schematic illustration of the distribution of blood flow and oxygen to skeletal muscles during rest (A), heavy exercise in average man (B), and in top athletes (C).

consumption, is supplied by a blood flow of 800 to 1000 ml, implying some 25 to 30% extraction of the arterial O_2 content.

In average subjects performing maximal steady-state exercise, the oxygen usage is 3 to 3.5 l/min, of which 90% or more is consumed by the muscles. In such circumstances the muscle blood flow is of the order of 15 to 20 l/min, with a cardiac output about 20 to 25 l/min. Corresponding figures for athletes in top training—runners, cyclists, etc.—can be as high as 5 to 6 l/min for oxygen usage, 25 to 30 l/min for muscle blood flow, and 30 to 35 l/min for cardiac output (Fig. 22-1). In such situations each 100 ml of blood traversing the muscles gives up at least 80 to 90% of its arterial oxygen of 20 ml, implying that muscle metabolism operates at quite low oxygen tensions in these circumstances, despite the Bohr shift.

Fulminant maximal exercise, such as that undertaken by the 100 metre sprinter, the finishing cyclist, or an animal startled by a predator, entails metabolic requirements of the muscle which may exceed the powers of blood and oxygen supply by a factor of 3 to 5. For such activities to be covered by aerobic metabolism, a cardiac output of at least 100 to 150 l/min would be required, and this is an impossible demand on a 300 g pump. Such fulminant exercise is therefore mainly anaerobic and its duration necessarily shortlived. Muscle glycogen is broken down to lactic acid, and even the local stores of energy-rich phosphate compounds become reduced. These local chemical changes effectively terminate the exercise. Restoration of the status quo is effected during recovery as some of the lactic acid produced is oxidized while the major part of it is resynthetized to glycogen, mainly in the liver. The *"oxygen debt"* incurred during exercise can be measured by determining the oxygen used in excess of the resting value during the recovery phase; such an oxygen debt may be of the order of 18 to 20 litres. Most aspects of cardiovascular dynamics and muscle blood flow during exercise in man have recently been reviewed (Bevegård and Shepherd, 1967; Åstrand and Rodahl, 1970).

Phasic and Tonic Skeletal Muscles

Two types of muscle fibre, rapid *phasic* ("white") and slow *tonic* ("red"), are present in varying proportions in most muscles. About 80 to 85% of the total muscle mass seems to be composed of the phasic type of fibre; exact figures are difficult to give, particularly since there may be no strict borderline between the two types of muscle.

Phasic units constitute the bulk of the forearm and calf muscles in man; similarly, the gastrocnemius muscle in the cat is primarily composed of phasic fibres. Studies of such muscles in man and in experimental animals reveal that their maximal flow capacity is 40 to 60 ml/100 g/min at a pressure head of 100 mm Hg: their maximal capillary surface area seems to be almost 7000 cm²/100 g, with 300 to 400 capillaries per cubic millimetre. During heavy exercise, when mean arterial pressure is raised 10 to 20%, the maximal blood flow through all the phasic muscles in average man is perhaps 12 to 16 litres per min; it is some 30% higher in athletes, mainly because they have a proportionally greater muscle mass. A further gain in pressure head, and flow, is obtained in the legs during running, skiing, etc., due to the action of the muscle pump on the veins (see below). This increases total muscle flow even more.

Tonic units are mainly used during prolonged periods of steady activity, as is required in the maintenance of posture. Such activity needs relatively less oxygen than heavy rhythmic activity of phasic units, being achieved by a low frequency of asynchronous contraction of the rather "slow" muscle units. Tonic muscles may comprise only some 15 to 20% of the total muscle mass, but they are characterized by a larger vascular bed and capillary surface area than those of the phasic muscles. Results obtained in animals by Hilton (1966) and others indicate that the vascular bed of tonic muscle is perhaps 2 to 3 times larger than that of phasic muscles and the maximal flow through tonic muscles may be 100 to 150 ml/100 g/min with a correspondingly larger capillary surface area. If we assume that these figures also hold true for man, the results suggest that a flow of 5 to 8 l/min would occur through the total vascular bed of all the tonic muscles if maximal vasodilatation were achieved and if the muscle contractions did not mechanically interfere with the flow. However, normally the muscle contractions *do* interfere, and this reduces the figure by perhaps 30 to 50% (see below). Tonic muscles, mainly engaged as they are in sustained postural contractions, can nevertheless perform their work aerobically thanks to their larger vascular bed and lower oxygen demands, and they do not usually incur notable oxygen debts.

Skeletal muscle vascular beds have a relatively low regional blood volume—3 to 4 ml/100 g even when maximally dilated, and, in the average situation, only about 2.5 to 3 ml/100 g. Nevertheless, the sheer bulk of the muscle mass means that potentially about a litre of blood may be present in the muscles during maximal vasodilatation. In exercise, however, the massaging action of the muscle pump is of great importance in squeezing the blood back to the heart (see Chapters 6 and 10); the sudden interruption of such activity may therefore imply considerable venous pooling of blood in dependent muscle (and skin) regions, to such an extent that fainting occurs.

Resting Vascular Tone

In resting (predominantly phasic) muscle the average flow in man is 2 to 5 ml/100 g/min, according to the current level of vasoconstrictor fibre discharge. Elimination of vasoconstrictor discharge increases the flow to 6 to 9 ml/min in phasic muscles; basal myogenic tone in these phasic muscles is high. Tonic muscles usually show a far higher resting flow, in some as high as 30 to 50 ml/100 g/min (Hilton, 1966). The reason for this is not known; the oxygen uptake of tonic muscles during rest is not much higher than that of phasic muscles.

Vasoconstrictor discharge to resting muscle seems to be of the order of 0.5 to 1 impulse/sec in the recumbent position, but it rises to perhaps 2 to 3/sec in the upright position. Maximal discharge, which is approximately 6 to 10/sec, lowers muscle flow to some 15% of its normal value in resting phasic muscles (Folkow, 1955). Tonic muscles possess a vascular bed far less subject to the quantitative effects of vasoconstrictor discharge, for maximal discharge only reduces blood flow to perhaps 40 to 50% of its value in normal conditions.

The vasoconstrictor fibres further increase the pre/postcapillary ratio in skeletal muscle vessels and lower the mean capillary pressure considerably. This increases the absorption of fluid from the interstitium—and the interstitial fluid "depot" of skeletal muscle is larger than in any other tissue. Blood volume can therefore be efficiently varied by this type of indirect neurogenic control of the exchange between blood and extravascular fluid (see Chapters 16 and 20). On the postcapillary capacitance side the constrictor fibres can mobilize about 40% of the blood content; all these neurogenic effects are illustrated in Fig. 22-2 (Mellander, 1960).

Autoregulation of myogenic tone, particularly that of the precapillary vessels, is usually well established in skeletal muscles, and it is, as mentioned in Chapter 16, partly responsible for the surprisingly good compensation of gravity effects manifested by both the muscle and the cutaneous microcirculation in standing man. The increase of transmural pressure in the leg muscle vessels and capillaries is largely offset by a local increase of precapillary myogenic tone, reducing the fraction of the capillary bed which is patent, and thus minimizing the tendency to oedema (see Chapter 8).

Exercise Hyperaemia

Maximal exercise may increase the muscle blood flow from a resting value of 2 to 5 ml/100 g/min, to an average value of 50 to 75 ml/100 g/min, if the increase in pressure head is also taken into account. Such hyperaemia is much the same in normal and sympathectomized limbs and is therefore not of neural origin; local chemical changes act in concert to secure this

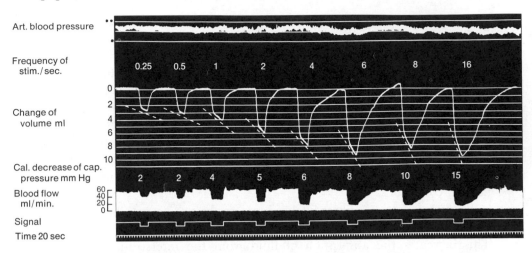

Art. blood pressure

Frequency of stim./sec.

Change of volume ml

Cal. decrease of cap. pressure mm Hg

Blood flow ml/min.

Signal

Time 20 sec

Fig. 22-2. Effects on resistance and capacitance vessels and on net transcapillary fluid shift in skeletal muscle during vasoconstrictor fibre stimulation at increasing rates. The dashed lines, parallel to the second phase of volume change, indicate the corresponding rates of transcapillary influx of extravascular fluid, due to the neurogenic increase of the pre/postcapillary resistance ratio. The maximal capacitance response reached at 6 imp/sec; the maximal resistance response first between 8-16 imp/sec. (From Mellander, 1960. By permission.)

increase in flow. This by no means denies that, in some situations of "arousal" or alarm, central nervous influences may contribute to the initiation of the hyperaemia (see Chapter 19).

Exercise hyperaemia is associated with a dilatation of the precapillary resistance vessels and an increase in the capillary bed due to the relaxation of the "sphincters". Hence there is an increase in the capillary surface area, even though capillary permeability remains the same. The postcapillary vessels show little if any relaxation and must be considered as relatively impervious to the metabolites liberated locally (see Kjellmer, 1965). This pattern of vasodilatation leads to a capillary pressure rise, producing filtration, to which is added an osmotic fluid transfer from the blood to the interstitial space of the muscles (see below). Such factors explain why the plasma volume decreases as much as 10 to 15% even after a brief period of intense exercise.

Any chemical factor to be considered as a candidate for eliciting exercise hyperaemia must be able to mimic its various features when infused intra-arterially into a muscle vascular bed. Further, it must be shown to be released into the interstitium during exercise in such concentrations as to be of real relevance. So far, only two locally produced factors have fulfilled these two important criteria—local hyperosmolality and locally released potassium ions—and hyperosmolality seems the more powerful.

Exercise causes an intracellular breakdown of larger molecules into an increased number of smaller molecules, increasing osmolality within the skeletal muscle fibres, which draws fluid from the interstitium. This is reflected as an increased osmolality of the venous effluent, in turn reflecting the change in the muscles and their interstitial fluid (Mellander *et al.*, 1967). It was also shown in this study that such a change causes shrinkage of the vascular smooth muscles and that this shrinkage inhibits myogenic activity and its propagation (see also Chapters 15 and 16). In this way, vasodilatation, most prominently manifest in the precapillary vessels, is established in proportion to the level of exercise and the hyperosmolality produced. When the degree of vasodilatation is plotted against the osmolality increase, exercise and intra-arterial infusions of non-specific

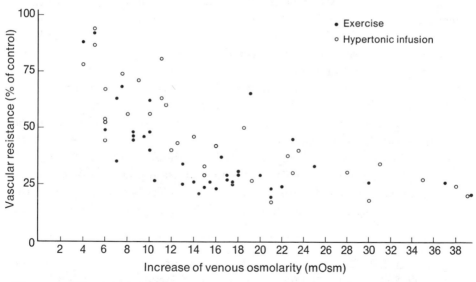

Fig. 22-3. The relationship between increase of venous osmolality and fall in muscle flow resistance in graded exercise, as compared with graded intra-arterial infusion of unspecific hypertonic solutions. Note the close similarity in degree of vasodilatation for a given increase of osmolality, whether produced by exercise or hypertonic infusions. (From Mellander *et al.*, 1967. By permission.)

hyperosmolar solutions produce almost identical effects, and intense exercise can increase local osmolality some 15% above the normal value of about 300 mOsm (Fig. 22-3).

The potency of hyperosmolality is therefore so great that it suggests the factor may be of predominant importance in the *establishment* of hyper-aemia at the onset of exercise, at least; however, as the hyperaemia *develops*, transfer of fluid from the increased blood stream will tend to again lower the osmotic pressure somewhat, and, apart from this, it seems likely that other factors are involved as well. For example, the release of K^+ from the exercising muscle cells is often so pronounced that it may contribute considerably to the hyperaemia (Kjellmer, 1965). Skinner and Powell (1967) have shown, too, that local hypoxia considerably potentiates the vasodilator effect of potassium, and oxygen tension is doubtless greatly reduced in skeletal muscles during intense exercise. Other influences, such as local increase in H^+, may contribute. Further, adenosine compounds are fairly powerful vasodilators, but it is debatable whether such agents normally cross the cell membranes in concentrations high enough to produce significant vasodilator effects in skeletal muscle; the situation seems to be a different one in the myocardium (see Chapter 23). Moreover, such agents relax the postcapillary vessels in skeletal muscle, and since postcapillary vessels are little affected in exercise hyperaemia, that fact speaks against adenosine involvement. Lastly, there is no evidence of either kinin or histamine release, and these agents increase capillary permeability, which remains unchanged in exercise (Fig. 22-4).

Tonic muscle vessels show much lower basal vascular tone in resting conditions than do phasic muscle vessels, and therefore the *relative* flow increase in exercise is usually less (Hilton, 1966), although the *absolute* flow figures may greatly surpass those in exercising phasic muscles thanks to the larger vascular dimensions of tonic muscles. It is possible that the relative importance of the "metabolic" factors involved in producing

---

Fig. 22-4 A & B. Relationship between (A) reduction in flow resistance and in-crease of volume (i.e. dilatation of capacitance vessels): and (B) increase of capillary filtration coefficient (CFC, reflecting opening of more capillaries and/or increased permeability) for exercise, K^+, histamine, acetylcholine, ATP and bradykinin. Note that of these, only K^+ (and hyperosmolality) mimic the pattern of response produced by exercise. (From Kjellmer, 1965. By permission.)

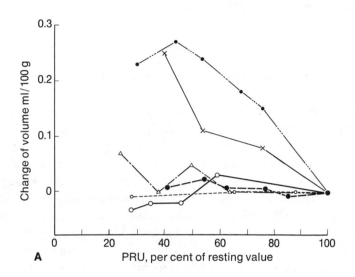

A

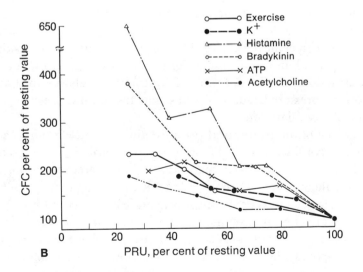

B

exercise hyperaemia in phasic muscle is not the same as that in tonic
muscle; the metabolism of tonic muscle is in several critical respects different from that of phasic muscle.

Mechanical Interference with Exercise Hyperaemia

Obviously, contractions raise the tissue pressure within the muscle fascia
and temporarily impede arterial inflow while squeezing out blood from
the veins (see also Chapter 6). Indeed, blood flow may stop entirely during
intense contractions of phasic muscles, but the very intermittency of such
contractions in most situations ensures that flow passes through the dilated
vessels during the relaxation periods. However, muscle blood flow is no
doubt markedly reduced during the very phase when oxygen usage is
highest. On the other hand, the intracellular myoglobin, recharged during
the "relaxation hyperaemic phase", delivers its oxygen during the contraction phase. Only when phasic muscle is involved in strong contractions
sustained beyond a period of 5 to 10 sec does the local myoglobin "accumulator" action fail to cover the aerobic requirements of the muscle. Then
anaerobic metabolites accumulate, leading to fatigue and ischaemic pain.
Hence, the forearm muscles, which are mainly of phasic type, rapidly
tire when one carries a heavy suitcase, even though, with intermittent
contractions, they can achieve far larger performances without exhaustion.
The flow rate per minute and unit weight will thus depend on the in-
tensity of contractions, on the duration of contractions relative to that of
relaxation, on the pressure head, on the vascular transmural pressure, and
on the extent of vasodilatation.

The importance of the transmural pressure and the muscle pump calls
for some further considerations. (These are also discussed in Chapters 6
and 10.) When an average sized man stands in the erect position, the
transmural vascular pressure at the calf level is raised some 70 to 80 mm
Hg in both the arterial and venous compartments. Since maximally dilated
resistance vessels are only slightly distended by transmural pressures above
normal because their "rigid jackets" are then stretched, such passive
reductions of regional flow resistance increase flow at most some 10%
above that seen when the vasodilated leg is placed at heart level.

However, besides this slight gain in flow by vascular distension in the dependent limbs, there is a considerable gain in effective *pressure head* as well. The muscular contractions empty the well-filled veins towards the heart, thereby markedly but phasically lowering the raised venous pressure. Providing the venous valves are competent, blood surges into the emptied veins from the arterial side during muscular relaxation, until they are again filled at the original transmural pressure level. Thus, intermittent phases of markedly reduced venous pressure are created in the dependent leg during rhythmic exercise, which lowers the *average* venous pressure considerably and hence raises the effective perfusion pressure and flow correspondingly, as the arterial pressure at the calf level is also raised by some 70 to 80 mm Hg. This "venous milking" factor itself has been

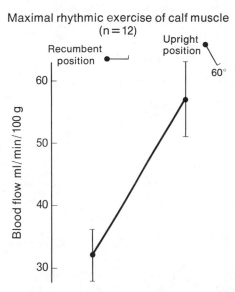

Fig. 22-5. The difference in blood flow in the calf muscles of man when heavy rhythmic exercise (once per sec, each contraction lasting 0.25–0.3 sec to mimic the situation during running) is performed in the recumbent position and in the upright position. Note the marked increase in flow ([133]Xenon clearance method) in the upright position, evidently due to the gain in effective perfusion pressure when mean venous pressure is lowered by the "muscle pump." In the *absence* of rhythmic exercise, there was no significant difference in maximal blood flow in the two positions, as measured during muscle rest immediately after heavy exercise performed during a period of ischaemia. (From Folkow *et al.*, 1971. By permission. Compare Fig. 10-3.)

shown to increase flow through the exercising calf muscles of man some 50 to 60% beyond the flow produced by the same heavy rhythmic exercise performed in the recumbent position (Fig. 22-5). It is likely that such factors explain why heavier loads of rhythmic leg work can be tolerated in the erect position than when the subject is recumbent and also why somewhat higher figures for cardiac output are reached during heavy exercise in the erect position.

The situation for tonic muscles during exercise is different. No doubt their activity is usually more prolonged, with sustained periods of mechanical interference with their blood supply. On the other hand, tonic muscles rarely show a discharge rate above 15 to 20 sec, even at maximal

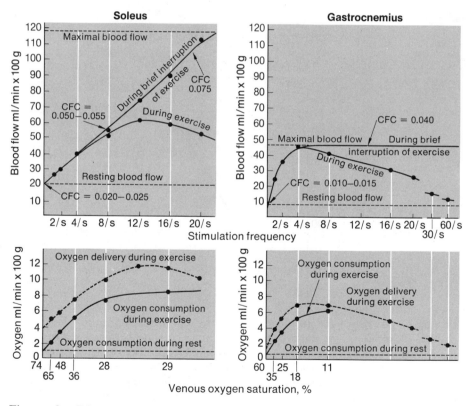

Fig. 22-6. Diagram illustrating average values for CFC, "free" and "mechanically interfered" blood flow, oxygen delivery and consumption in the "tonic" soleus, and "phasic" gastrocnemius muscles of the cat during rest and graded exercise. (From Folkow and Halicka, 1968. By permission.)

activation, and have, correspondingly, a relatively low oxygen require-
ment. In addition, their maximal flow capacity is far higher than that of
phasic muscles and their flow suffers less mechanical interference by the
contraction. Even their maximal energy requirements can therefore
almost always be covered by aerobic metabolism. Some of the differences
between phasic and tonic muscles are schematically illustrated in Fig.
22-6.

Interaction between Neurogenic Vasoconstriction and Local Factors in Exercise Hyperaemia

In most mammals, and in man, during heavy steady-state exercise it
makes little difference to their muscle blood supply whether the sympathetic vasoconstrictor fibre discharge is present or not. This is an important
point. It has been fully realized in man by measuring the "blood debt"

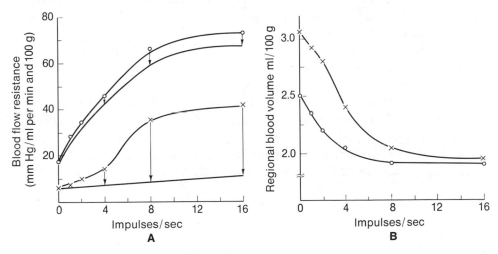

Fig. 22-7. The effects of graded sympathetic stimulation on muscle flow
resistance (A) and on blood volume in the muscles (B).
Circles = values during rest; crosses = values during exercise. The transformation from the initial peak responses to the steady state responses is indicated by
the arrows. It is clear that the vasoconstrictor fibres have very little effect on
muscle flow resistance during *steady state* exercise, even at intense fibre discharge,
while the effects on the capacitance side of the constrictor fibres are only little
affected by exercise. (From Kjellmer, 1965. By permission.)

(i.e. the total blood flow in excess of resting flow) that can be measured in the post-exercise period. That measured in, say, the left arm, normally innervated, following a given quantitative work performance was little different from that measured in the sympathectomized right arm doing the same work. Further, as shown in Fig. 22-7, the muscle blood flow during moderate or heavy steady-state exercise of an animal's leg is almost unaffected by even intense vasoconstrictor discharge. The tone of the precapillary resistance vessels then becomes almost wholly subservient to the influence of local factors, which thereby dictate the flow changes. However, the postcapillary vessels are far less affected by their local environment and remain dominated by neurogenic influences (Kjellmer, 1965).

Diving species exhibit a striking contrast (see Chapter 19). In such creatures muscle blood flow must be kept minimal during prolonged swimming under water, despite the tremendous increase in the concentration of local metabolites which such ischaemia entails (Scholander, 1942). This ischaemic state, calling for a high capacity for anaerobic metabolism, is partly achieved by a strong and effective neurogenic constriction of the major arteries that supply the muscle vascular beds. These vessels are geographically remote from the muscles and are not subjected to the chemical changes which occur in the interstitium surrounding the muscle vascular bed. In addition, the precapillary resistance vessels within the muscle receive an unusually dense innervation by vasoconstrictor fibres which presumably release overwhelmingly high amounts of noradrenaline. The catecholamine release not only keeps the muscle bed constricted, it also may exert a positive inotropic effect (the Orbeli effect) on the contracting muscles in such species (Folkow et al., 1966).

Reactive Hyperaemia

Following the release of a temporary arrest of muscle blood flow, the flow increases to a point above control resting level. The effect is quickly manifested, and, on reaching a peak, it declines exponentially. It is caused by the accumulation of "metabolites" and by the oxygen lack itself, and, further, by the reduction in the mechanical facilitation of precapillary myogenic tone consequent upon the lowering of the transmural pressure. This last factor probably accounts for a considerable part of the often pronounced but evanescent dilatation which ensues upon an arterial occlusion of even a few seconds' duration. Longer lasting circulatory arrest is followed, appropriately, by a more sustained hyperaemia which is predominantly of chemical origin since the accumulation of metabolites is then larger. These events thus involve the same local mechanisms as those responsible for the autoregulation of blood flow (see Chapter 16).

Neurogenic and Hormonal Vasodilatation

Vasodilatation of neurogenic origin may be caused by reflex inhibition of resting vasoconstrictor discharge or by excitation of cholinergic sympathetic vasodilator fibres.

Of these perhaps the first is the more common. Usually the sudden reflex inhibition of vasoconstrictor activity will cause only a moderate increase in flow because the basal myogenic tone of the precapillary vessels is itself so high in resting conditions. However, if vasoconstrictor discharge has been high, as in the circumstances of haemorrhage or of venous pooling resulting from prolonged immobile standing, then the local metabolite concentration is more considerable. A sudden loss or inhibition of vasoconstrictor discharge then allows the blood to surge through vessels whose myogenic tone is lowered. The sudden inhibition of sympathetic tone which, together with vagal bradycardia, seems to constitute the fainting reaction (see Chapter 19) may for such reasons lead to a transient muscle flow "overshoot", often observed in this situation.

Cholinergic sympathetic vasodilator fibres, of considerable importance in some animal species (e.g. cat and dog), are excited in the defence reaction (see Chapter 19; see also Uvnäs, 1960; Abrahams et al., 1964). This reaction is accompanied by an inhibition of the vasoconstrictor discharge to the resistance vessels in skeletal muscles only, produced reflexly via the baroreceptors once mean arterial and pulse pressures rise as a consequence of the central nervous drive on the other vascular circuits and on the heart. This potentiates the impact of the vasodilator fibres, and muscle blood flow may increase to as much as 75% of that found in maximal vasodilatation in animals (Fig. 22-8). It is not known with any certainty to what an

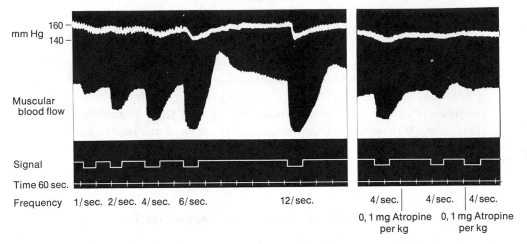

Fig. 22-8. The effect of the cholinergic vasodilator fibres in the sympathetic nerve supply to the cat's muscle blood vessels. The fibres are stimulated at increasing rates, the constrictor fibres being blocked by α-receptor blocking drugs. Note the blocking effect of atropine on the dilator response. Drop recorder—ordinate writer, the height of the ordinates being *inversely* proportional to the blood flow. (From Folkow, 1952. By permission.)

extent such vasodilator fibres reach the muscle vessels in man; it appears, however, that alarm situations may induce substantial muscle vasodilation also in this species (Blair *et al.*, 1959).

These vasodilator fibres inhibit the tone of the precapillary resistance vessels in the defence reaction, hence forming part of an "anticipatory", over-all cardiovascular adjustment, so designed as to deliver an increased cardiac output mainly to the muscles, facilitating an all-out muscle exertion. Once the skeletal muscles become active, this neurogenic vasodilation is reinforced by the exercise hyperaemia, which also opens the precapillary "sphincters" and secures an increased capillary surface area. If the stimulus which starts the defence reaction is not followed by exercise, the neurogenic vasodilation tends to become nullified by a locally induced "autoregulatory escape" of the resistance vessels (Djojosugito *et al.*, 1968). On the other hand, the defence reaction also involves a secretion of adrenaline from the suprarenal medulla, and this adrenaline dilates the muscle resistance vessels by coupling with their β-receptors; the neurogenic vasodilatation, although it is of itself of short duration, may sometimes be considerably prolonged by the influence of the adrenaline liberated.

References

Abrahams, V. C., S. M. Hilton, and A. W. Zbrozyna (1964). "The role of active muscle vasodilatation in the alerting stage of the defence reaction," *J. Physiol.* **171,** 189–202.

Åstrand, P. O., and K. Rodahl (1970). *Textbook of work physiology.* New York: McGraw-Hill.

Barcroft, H. (1963). "Circulation in skeletal muscle," *Handbook of Physiology*, 2, Circulation **II,** 1353–85.

Bevegård, B. S., and J. T. Shepherd (1967). "Regulation of the circulation during exercise in man," *Physiol. Rev.* **47,** 178–213.

Blair, D. A., E. W. Glover, A. D. M. Greenfield, and I. C. Roddie (1959). "Excitation of cholinergic vasodilator nerves to human skeletal muscles during emotional stress," *J. Physiol.* **148,** 633–47. (London.)

Djojosugito, A. M., B. Folkow, B. Lisander, and H. Sparks (1968). "Mechanism of escape of skeletal muscle resistance vessels from the influence of sympathetic cholinergic vasodilator fibre activity," *Acta Physiol. Scand.* **72,** 148–56.

Folkow, B. (1952). "Impulse frequency in sympathetic vasomotor fibres correlated to the release and elimination of the transmitter," *Acta Physiol. Scand.* **25,** 49–76.

Folkow, B. (1955). "Nervous control of the blood vessels," *Physiol. Rev.* **35,** 629–63.

Folkow, B., and H. D. Halicka (1968). "A comparison between 'red' and 'white' muscle with respect to blood supply, capillary surface area and oxygen uptake during rest and exercise," *Microvascular Res.* **1,** 1–14.

Folkow, B., K. Fuxe, and R. R. Sonnenschein (1966). "Responses of skeletal musculature and its vasculature during 'diving' in the duck: peculiarities of the adrenergic vasoconstrictor innervation," *Acta Physiol. Scand.* **67,** 327–42.

Folkow, B., U. Haglund, M. Jodal, and O. Lundgren (1971). "Blood flow in the calf muscles of man during heavy rhythmic exercise," *Acta Physiol. Scand.* In press.

Hilton, S. M. (1966). "The search for the cause of functional hyperaemia in skeletal muscle," in *Circulation in Skeletal Muscle* (ed. O. Hudlická), pp. 137–

44. Institute of Physiology, Czechoslovak Academy of Sciences. Prague: Pergamon.

Hudlická, O., ed. (1966). *Circulation in Skeletal Muscle*. Institute of Physiology, Czechoslovak Academy of Sciences. Prague: Pergamon.

Kjellmer, I. (1965). "Studies on exercise hyperaemia," *Acta Physiol. Scand.* **64,** Suppl., 244.

Mellander, S. (1960). "Comparative studies on the adrenergic neurohormonal control of resistance and capacitance blood vessels in the cat," *Acta Physiol. Scand.* **50,** Suppl., 176.

Mellander, S., B. Johansson, S. Gray, O. Jonsson, J. Lundvall, and B. Ljung (1967). "The effects of hyperosmolarity on intact and isolated vascular smooth muscle. Possible role in exercise hyperaemia," *Angiologica*, **4,** 310–22.

Scholander, P. F. (1942). "Scientific results of marine biological research," *Hvalrådets Skrifter*, **22.** Oslo.

Skinner, N. S., and W. J. Powell (1966). "Action of oxygen and potassium on vascular resistance of dog skeletal muscle," *Am. J. Physiol.* **212,** 533–40.

Uvnäs, B. (1960). "Central cardiovascular control," *Handbook of Physiology*, 1, Neurophysiology **II,** 1131–62.

23

Coronary Circulation

General Considerations

The coronary circuit supplies a tissue that is continuously active, cannot sustain an oxygen debt, and is vitally more important than any other. The metabolic requirements of the myocardium in heavy exercise increase fourfold or fivefold; in top-class athletes such demands may briefly reach a sevenfold level. The mechanical squeezing of the coronary vessels during systole greatly impedes the blood supply to the left ventricle, whereas the diastolic period is inevitably reduced by tachycardia. Clearly, satisfactory nutrition of the left ventricle poses serious problems.

Two recent reviews, (Gregg and Fisher, 1963; Berne, 1964) and a symposium on the coronary circulation (Marchetti and Taccardi, 1967) should be consulted for details.

Vascular Organization and Dimensions

The myocardium of average man, some 300 g of tissue, is dominated by the thick-walled left ventricle. Blood flow is delivered by means of the two coronary arteries. In dogs there is a striking preponderance of left coronary arterial supply—some 85% of the *total* myocardium—but this is not the case in man. Only 20% of men studied have a left coronary artery pre-ponderance, while 50% show right preponderance, and 30% show a balance between the two arteries.

The left coronary artery in man divides into a left circumflex branch and an anterior descending branch. The circumflex branch ends in a posterior descending branch, while the anterior descending branch courses the intraventricular groove to reach the apex, yielding septal branches in transit. Thus the left coronary artery mainly supplies the left ventricle in man. The right coronary artery passes along the right atrioventricular sulcus towards the back of the heart, where it gives off descending branches to both ventricles. At the apex, terminal divisions of the various arteries pass inward to supply the inner layers of the myocardium and the papillary muscles.

The coronary arteries can deliver enormous blood flows to the myo-cardium. Direct measurements in exercising dogs show that the left ventricular blood flow in maximal dilatation is at least 300 to 400 ml/min/ 100 g. Similar figures are probably reached in athletes during intense exercise (see below). Myocardial O_2 delivery is in such situations some 80 ml/min/100 g and the O_2 uptake is perhaps 60 to 65 ml/min/100 g. These high flow values are reached despite the fact that left ventricular flow is greatly reduced during systole, and systole may occupy almost two-thirds of the heart cycle during intense tachycardia. "True" coronary flow resistance (i.e. when no mechanical obstruction is present) in this situation is probably below 0.2 PRU_{100} (see below). This should be compared with the maximal flow figures in phasic skeletal muscle, corresponding to PRU_{100} values in skeletal muscle, which are some 8 to 12 times higher (Chapter 22).

The density of the capillary network and the combined capillary surface area are correspondingly larger. Thanks to the thin myocardial fibrils and the density of the capillary network, there are at maximal vasodilatation 2500 to 4000 capillaries/mm³ (the higher figure applies to the deeper wall layers of the left ventricle) compared with 300 to 400 in phasic skeletal muscle (Fig. 23-1A). The maximal *diffusion* distances are thus nowhere greater than 10 μ. Recent PS measurements (Winbury et al., 1965) fully confirm these figures (see Renkin, 1967) and the total capillary surface area of the human heart seems to be some 20 m² (Fig. 23-1B).

Despite this richness of the myocardial blood supply, it is a striking fact that coronary arterial interconnections at the different levels of arborisa-

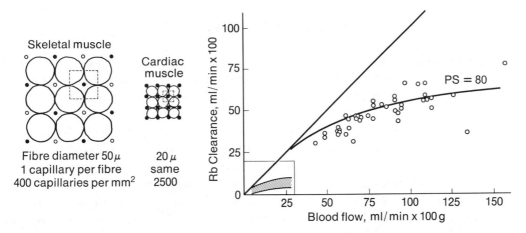

Fig. 23-1. A. Diagram illustrating relative capillary densities in skeletal and cardiac muscle.

B. Capillary clearance-flow relation for ^{86}Rb in cardiac muscle (Winbury et al., 1965; by permission) compared with the range for skeletal muscle shown in insert. (From Renkin, 1967. By permission.)

tion are so poor that in an acute coronary obstruction such collaterals can supply less than 10% of normal flow even when fully dilated (see Linder, 1966). This is usually too little, and infarction may therefore ensue, especially if the affected segment is large, when flow to central parts is very poor.

As the myocardium is so richly vascularized, it is not surprising that the average myocardial blood content is as high as some 8%. There are twice as many venous as arterial channels and they interconnect far more than the arterial ones. The major venous drainage—particularly that of the left ventricle—occurs via the coronary sinus, but considerable parts of the right ventricle are drained via the anterior cardiac veins which empty individually into the right atrium. Some deeper myocardial veins have minor communications directly with the heart cavities (Thebesian and sinusoidal channels), but their functional importance is obscure.

This short, wide-bore circuit has a mean transit time of only 6 to 8 sec in resting man, and this is reduced by at least 50% during intense exercise. This rapid coronary "recirculation" complicates the situation in measurements of cardiac output by the dye dilution technique.

Coronary Blood Flow During "Rest"

In resting man, where each ventricle expels about 5.5 l/min at a frequency about 70/min and a stroke volume around 80 ml, the coronary blood flow is 60 to 80 ml/min/100 g, with a myocardial O_2 consumption of some 7 to 9 ml/min/100 g.

The high ratio between the coronary flow during "rest", 60 to 80 ml/min/100 g, and that during maximal dilatation, 300 to 400 ml/min/100 g, indicates that there is a pronounced basal tone of the precapillary resistance vessels (and probably also of the precapillary "sphincters"), despite the considerable and steady production of vasodilator metabolites. If myocardial arrest is induced by potassium (itself a vasodilator in most circuits), while the coronary vessels are perfused from another animal, myocardial blood flow is as low as some 15 ml/min/100 g ($7PRU_{100}$), despite the fact that mechanical flow interference is now absent. Then the oxygen consumption is 1.5 to 2 ml/min/100 g—about twice the value for resting tonic skeletal muscle and three times that for phasic muscle. This resting O_2 usage is, of course, partly a function of fibre length.

Thus the inherent resistance vessel tone of the coronary circuit is high indeed during myocardial arrest, and is still fairly pronounced in the heart beating during resting conditions. Maximal heart activity, with flows up to 400 ml/min/100 g, implies up to thirtyfold decreases of flow resistance compared with the situation during myocardial arrest.

Mechanical Interference with Coronary Blood Flow

Blood flow in skeletal muscle (Chapter 22) suffers a mechanical interference from the muscle contractions, and this is the case in the heart as well. The stronger the contractions and the higher the tissue pressure, the more the flow will be impeded. As the coronary vessels are perfused at aortic pressure —and as the left ventricular contractions furnish this pressure—it follows that the left ventricular blood flow is far more affected by systole than is that of the "low-pressure" right ventricle and the atria. This is especially so in the deeper part of the left ventricular wall, where tissue pressure is highest during systole (Kirk and Honig, 1964). Here flow actually ceases during systole. Consequently, as peak systolic tissue pressure is higher than peak systolic blood pressure, oxygen tension is usually the lowest in subendocardial parts of the left ventricular wall; the *average* O_2 tension in the wall is some 30 mm Hg with a transmural gradient of 10 to 15 mm Hg. As a compensatory measure the capillary network is as mentioned, somewhat denser in the deeper part of the wall and the myoglobin content is larger (see also Myers and Honig, 1964).

The principal difference between left and right ventricular blood supply during resting conditions is illustrated in Fig. 23-2. Thus systolic flow to the right ventricle may be as large as, or even larger than that during diastole, simply because the rise in aortic pressure head during systole may completely overcome the relatively moderate rise in intramural tension of the right ventricle.

Clearly, this can never be the case for the left ventricle, as the aortic systolic pressure head is the result of the left ventricular wall tension during

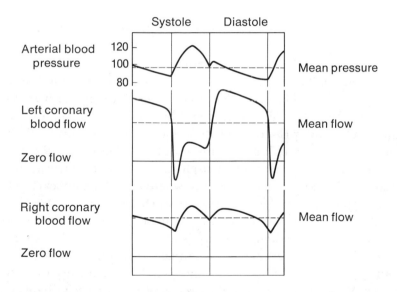

Fig. 23-2. Approximate relationship between arterial blood pressure and phasic blood supply to the left and right ventricles throughout the cardiac cycle. Note the far stronger mechanical interference with the blood supply of the left ventricle during systole, an interference which is especially marked in the subendocardial portions.

systole; this must therefore always impede flow markedly, especially in the deeper parts of the wall. As a rough average, systolic coronary supply to the left ventricle is only some 20 to 30% of the diastolic supply, and this percentage often tends to *decrease* when heart activity is increased (compare first and fourth panel in Fig. 23-3). A left ventricular segment—supplied by a partially obstructed coronary branch which creates a dilated "low-pressure circuit" beyond the pathological hindrance—may easily have its vessels completely obstructed during systole and is thus even more dependent on diastolic flow than is the normally perfused myocardium.

In each case the presence of myoglobin-bound oxygen implies an "accumulator action", which furnishes sufficient oxygen for the high demands during systole and which is rapidly recharged with oxygen during the abundant flow of diastole (compare skeletal muscle; Chapter 22).

Coronary Flow Adjustments to Myocardial Activity Level

In the coronary circuit, as in most vascular beds, the basal tone of the resistance and sphincter sections is exposed to the powerful "negative feedback" inherent in the steady local addition of vasodilator metabolites (Chapter 16). Here should be considered both the fundamental variables of PO_2, pCO_2, and pH—dependent not only on the current balance between flow and metabolism but also on the composition of the arterial blood—and the steady production from the contracting myocardium of more "specific" vasodilator metabolites, where adenosine appears to be of particular importance in the coronary circuit (Berne, 1964).

In one sense the coronary vessels are in a lifelong state of exercise hyperaemia, moderate when the body is at rest but marked in strenuous exercise or in emotional excitement. Coronary resistance tone is usually so balanced to the metabolic rate that some 50 to 60% of the arterial oxygen is extracted. When myocardial activity is increased the vessels dilate almost proportionally so that the O_2 extraction is only slightly increased; in other words, the vessels dilate sufficiently to maintain a rather constant local oxygen tension until the limit set by maximal dilatation is reached. Then a further increase of activity inevitably increases the O_2 extraction and reduces the myocardial O_2 tension. This has led to the assumption that the coronary smooth muscles may be especially sensitive to pO_2 and that this factor might be the most important regulator of coronary blood flow. It no doubt appears that the coronary vascular smooth muscles adjust more sensitively to pO_2 changes than those, for example, of skeletal muscle vessels.

On the other hand, the sensitive coronary adjustments to shifts in pO_2 are not necessarily a consequence of pO_2 alone. They might be due also, or even mainly, to some key vasodilator "metabolite" which increases in concentration whenever pO_2 falls and vice versa. It appears, as mentioned, as if adenosine may play such a role in the local control of the coronary circuit (Berne, 1964). It is further possible that most vasodilator factors that influence the skeletal muscle circuit (Chapter 22) are to some extent involved in the control of the coronary vessels. Here as elsewhere several dilator factors may co-operate to secure a vitally important regulation, and even the relative importance of these factors may vary in different situations.

As coronary vascular tone is so readily affected by the local chemical changes—induced by even small changes in myocardial metabolism—a primary reduction of coronary blood supply, at a *constant* myocardial metabolism, is followed by a vascular relaxation which serves a compensatory function. This is the important principle by which coronary artery stenosis is compensated: vasodilatation occurs downstream. However, this "uses up" part of the "blood flow reserve" even in resting conditions and correspondingly limits the vasodilator response to an increase of metabolism caused by exercise or emotional excitation.

The coronary vascular bed may thus be expected to display a pronounced "autoregulation of flow" if perfused at different pressures at *constant* myocardial metabolism, and for the same reasons as in other circuits (Chapter 16). Further, it displays, for these same reasons, a prompt and profound reactive hyperaemia even upon a brief arterial obstruction. However, the coronary vessels can, of course, hardly reveal their ability to autoregulate flow if the experimental exploration is so designed that the heart *itself* furnishes the varying pressure head for relating pressure to coronary flow. The reason is that myocardial metabolism then increases when pressure increases, and vice versa; in other words, pressure head and tissue metabolism change in parallel, which masks any ability of the vessels to autoregulate flow.

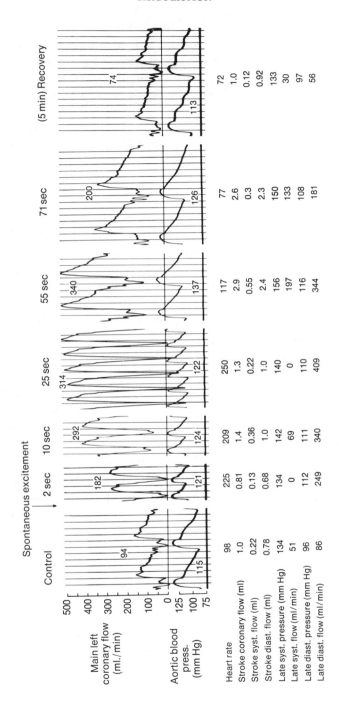

	Control	2 sec	10 sec	25 sec	55 sec	71 sec	(5 min) Recovery
Heart rate	98	225	209	250	117	77	72
Stroke coronary flow (ml)	1.0	0.81	1.4	1.3	2.9	2.6	1.0
Stroke syst. flow (ml)	0.22	0.13	0.36	0.22	0.55	0.3	0.12
Stroke diast. flow (ml)	0.78	0.68	1.0	1.0	2.4	2.3	0.92
Late syst. pressure (mm Hg)	134	134	142	140	156	150	133
Late syst. flow (ml/min)	51	0	69	0	197	133	30
Late diast. pressure (mm Hg)	96	112	111	110	116	108	97
Late diast. flow (ml/min)	86	249	340	409	344	181	56

Effect of Exercise and Emotional Excitement

The highest demands on coronary blood flow are met with in the left ventricle during intense exercise or during strong emotional excitement (Fig. 23-3). This may be illustrated by an arbitrary example in man. At rest mean arterial pressure is 100 mm Hg and cardiac output (C.O.) is 5.5 l, with a systolic period of perhaps 0.35 sec and a diastolic period of 0.5 sec at a heart rate about 70/min. Mean coronary flow is, say, 60 ml/min/100 g, where the mean diastolic flow level per unit time for the left ventricle is three times higher than that during systole. The diastolic perfusion period/min is $0.5 \times 70 = 35$ sec, and as much as 80 to 85% of left ventricular blood supply, about 50 ml of the 60 ml per min and 100 g, will thus take place during the diastolic period.

Suppose that the cardiac output increases fourfold, to 22 litres, during heavy exercise at a heart rate of 180/min and a mean arterial pressure of 115 mm Hg. At this high heart rate each cycle is only 0.33 sec and—despite a strong sympathetic discharge to the ventricles—systole is not reduced below 0.20 sec, leaving a diastolic period of only 0.13 sec. Thus, the systolic perfusion period/min is now $180 \times 0.2 = 36$ sec and the diastolic perfusion period/min is reduced to 24 sec. At the same time the work load on the left ventricle has increased perhaps fivefold (fourfold by the increased output alone, but arterial pressure was raised 15% and the metabolic cost for an increased pressure load on the heart rises out of proportion; see Chapter 12).

In order to avoid serious reduction in tissue pO_2 coronary flow has to increase about fourfold, i.e. to 240 ml/min/100 g. However, the mechanical obstructive effect of systole on coronary flow is prolonged, now occupying 60% instead of 40% of the cycle. Even if the relationship between mean diastolic and mean systolic flow levels were still 3:1, it would mean that the 24 sec of diastolic period per min must be allowed for the passage of 160 to

Fig. 23-3. Reproduction of sections from a continuous record in a conscious dog resting in left lateral position, 7 days postoperative, and showing the effect of spontaneous excitement on phasic main left coronary artery flow and phasic aortic blood pressure, using an electromagnetic flowmeter and Wetterer-Gauer manometer. Zero flow line = true zero. Vertical time lines 0.1 sec. Dog wt. 19.2 kg. (From Rayford, et al., 1965. By permission.)

170 ml of blood per 100 g of left ventricular myocardium, while only 70 to 80 ml will pass during the 36 sec of systolic period. Actually the difference between these figures may be even greater, as the ratio between mean diastolic and mean systolic flow levels usually *increases* during exercise.

This arbitrary example must be reasonably well in accord with what can be expected to occur in man. If one now assumes that the free flow during diastole reflects the "true" coronary flow resistance, one arrives at the following coronary resistance figures for this example:

$$\text{"True" flow resistance during rest} = \frac{100 \times 35}{50 \times 60} = 1.17 \ PRU_{100}$$

$$\text{"True" flow resistance during exercise} = \frac{115 \times 24}{170 \times 60} = 0.27 \ PRU_{100}$$

It is quite likely that coronary flow must increase still more in athletes, who may display some sixfold increases in cardiac output. It seems probable that the "true" coronary flow resistance in such subjects may be 0.2 PRU_{100} or even lower; i.e. allowing for a "free" coronary flow of 500 ml/min/100 g or more in the left ventricle and an "integrated" coronary flow (where the mechanical interference of the systole is taken into account) of at least some 350 ml/min/100 g. This, in turn, would imply a total arterial O_2 delivery to the heart (300 g) of some 200 ml/min (Fig. 23-4). This seems necessary, however, as a 300 g myocardium during rest consumes perhaps 20 to 25 ml O_2/min, and a sixfold increase in cardiac output associated with some rise in mean arterial pressure must inevitably imply *at least* a sevenfold increase in O_2 consumption, i.e. a total of 175 to 200 ml/min.

These considerations, based on actual cardiac output data in outstanding athletes, reveal that the figures discussed above for maximal coronary flow and oxygen delivery in man can hardly be exaggerated, because such highly trained subjects *do* cope with these enormous loads without signs of myocardial failure—and myocardial O_2 delivery is here imperative. In fact, as it is unlikely that *all* the O_2 is extracted from the blood at maximal performance, the myocardial blood supply of such top athletes is probably even beyond 400 ml/min/100 g in this situation.

High levels of heart rate are of potential disadvantage for the coronary blood supply, not only because of the shortening of the diastolic flow period, but also because the expulsion of a given cardiac output against

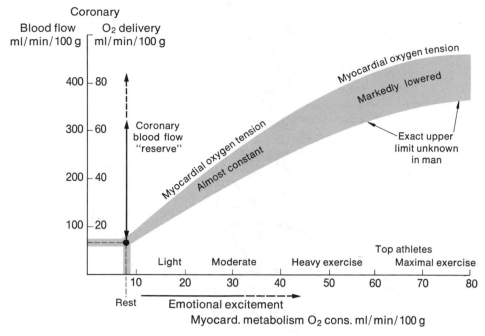

Fig. 23-4. Approximate relationship between myocardial metabolism (O_2 consumption/min/100 g myocardium) and myocardial blood supply and oxygen delivery. Due to the prompt coronary vasodilatation upon increased metabolism, tissue oxygen tension stays largely constant until the limit set by maximal dilatation is approached: then O_2 extraction increases and tissue oxygen tension falls.

a given aortic pressure is metabolically more "expensive" the higher the heart rate (Sarnoff *et al.*, 1958; see also Chapter 12). This is at least partly explained by the fact that the isometric contraction periods—not appearing as external work but certainly requiring a considerable O_2 consumption (Chapter 12)—increase in number/min with the heart rate and hence total myocardial O_2 consumption/min will increase as well. Such factors are usually not important in the healthy heart, because the situation is here easily met by a compensatory coronary dilatation. However, the above considerations may be relevant in coronary insufficiency, where the "flow reserves", inherent in compensatory coronary vasodilatation, may be already exhausted in covering the normal resting demands.

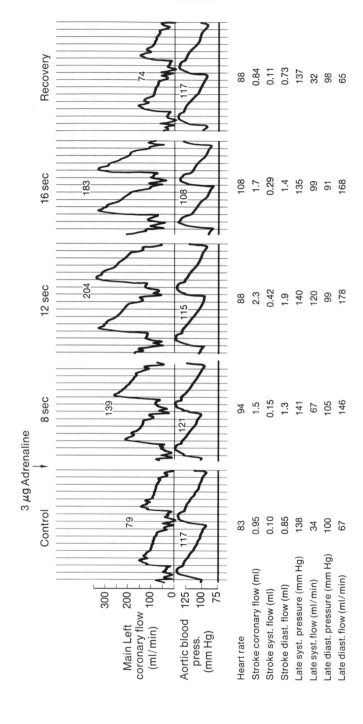

Neurogenic and Hormonal Control

Until recently, little was known about the *direct* nervous control of the coronary vessels, simply because direct sympathetic stimulation inevitably excites the myocardium as well; the increased metabolism causes vasodilatation (Fig. 23-3) which makes such constrictor effects as might be caused by a possible direct vascular innervation difficult to reveal.

Drugs blocking the adrenergic β-receptors, thus selectively eliminating the adrenergic effects on the myocardium, can be used to clarify the direct effects of sympathetic nerves on the coronary vessels (Feigl, 1967). After such a blockade, sympathetic fibres cause a fairly minor vasoconstriction of the coronary bed in the dog. Even at *maximal* stimulation rates the coronary flow resistance rises only by some 30%, and this effect is evanescent, being largely overcome by the local chemical vasodilator factors. These figures should be compared to those in resting skeletal muscle, where a maximal sympathetic discharge may increase the flow resistance sixfold or more. Even in skeletal muscle, however, intense metabolic activity will markedly overcome the influence of the vasoconstrictor fibres (Chapter 22).

Nevertheless, even though these slight neurogenic effects imply that the coronary vascular bed may be considered to be largely withdrawn from most centrally or reflexly induced restrictions of systemic blood flow, there might be pathophysiological situations where even such weak neurogenic restrictions of flow help to precipitate an anginal attack. It is, for example, possible that such a mechanism, perhaps combined with a reflex pressor response, explains the anginal effects which are provoked by cold winds in subjects who may tolerate moderate exercise fairly well, for such attacks of pain are usually indicative of relative myocardial ischaemia. Further studies are needed to explore the physiological and pathophysiological significance of the weak, but perhaps significant, vasoconstrictor fibre action on the coronary vascular bed. It is, moreover, not impossible that the coronary vasoconstrictor fibres exert a more powerful effect in man than in the dog.

Fig. 23-5. Effect of i.v. injection of about 0.2 μg adrenaline per kg bodyweight on blood pressure, heart rate, and on left coronary artery flow in a resting, conscious dog (electromagnetic flow meter). Note the marked increase of myocardial blood flow. (From Rayford *et al.*, 1965. By permission.)

Sympathetic cholinergic vasodilator fibres do not supply the coronary vessels, in contrast to the situation in the skeletal muscle bed (Feigl, 1967). Thus, even after α-receptor blockade as well as β-receptor blockade, sympathetic stimulation does not cause coronary vasodilatation. Neither does atropine administration enhance the weak vasoconstrictor effect obtained by sympathetic stimulation to the heart after complete β-receptor blockade. There is, however, recent evidence that the vagi supply vasodilator fibres to the coronary vessels (Feigl, 1969); their functional significance is unknown so far.

Blood-borne catecholamines—essentially adrenaline in man—affect, of course, both the myocardium and the coronary vessels. Even though the direct sympathetic innervation of the heart, for one and the same discharge rate, is several times more powerful than the effects induced by the blood-borne sympatho-adrenal component, the latter cannot be neglected. Like noradrenaline, adrenaline stimulates myocardial metabolism greatly and thus induces coronary vasodilatation indirectly (Fig. 23-5). Evidence indicates that adrenaline also exerts a *direct* dilator effect on the coronary vessels. However, adrenaline increases the O_2 demands of the heart so powerfully as to render its administration to subjects with coronary obstructions potentially lethal.

Aspects of Coronary Insufficiency

As subjects with coronary insufficiency display a compensatory dilatation below the hindrance, which covers their *resting* metabolic demands, they have already utilized part or all of their easily mobilized "blood flow reserve", inherent in the basal vascular tone which is normally pronounced. Sudden increases in heart metabolism—whether due to exercise or emotional excitement—then lead to serious *decreases* in the vital ratio of coronary flow to tissue metabolism. In the healthy subject this ratio is, as mentioned, kept largely constant over a wide range of cardiac activities by coronary vasodilatation (Fig. 23-6). A decrease of the ratio can precipitate an acute anginal attack or, in serious cases, such intense and widespread hypoxia that ventricular fibrillation and sudden death ensue. Animal experiments suggest that strong, sudden emotions may increase the work load on the heart perhaps threefold by means of the autonomic

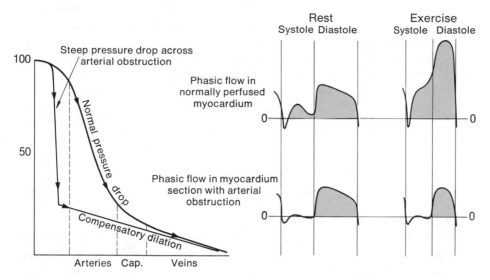

Fig. 23-6. Schematic illustration of the different haemodynamic situations for the normally perfused left ventricular myocardium and a myocardial section where an arterial obstruction has led to a virtually maximal vasodilatation distal to the hindrance even in the resting state. Virtually no systolic blood supply, the lack of ability to produce further vasodilatation, the shortened diastole, and the increased myocardial metabolism during exercise or emotional excitement cause prompt relative ischaemia, with nociceptive fibre stimulation when the ischaemia is intense.

discharge alone (e.g. Folkow *et al.* 1968). This puts strong emphasis on John Hunter's famous remark, based on his knowledge of his own temperament and his serious state of coronary obstruction: "My life is at the mercy of any rascal who chooses to annoy me" (see also Chapter 19).

It is well-known, however, that some vasodilator drugs, especially acute administration of nitrites, may effectively curb even intense anginal attacks. This is in all likelihood *not* primarily due to coronary vasodilatation, because all the vessels beyond a pathological stenotic region are probably already sufficiently relaxed thanks to the efficient action of the accumulated tissue metabolites, as are most of the collaterals. These metabolic factors are usually far more efficient coronary dilators by their presence in high concentrations at the proper point than are the amounts of vasodilator drugs which can be administered by the bloodstream.

The therapeutic value of the nitrites is rather a consequence mainly of reduced requirements for cardiac metabolism than due to an increased coronary flow. Nitrites may do this because their dilator action is especially powerful in the systemic venous compartment (Åblad and Mellander, 1963). This leads to a peripheral pooling of blood, reduced venous return and cardiac output and hypotension; myocardial oxygen demands are thus rapidly reduced, so that the poor coronary flow may again match the metabolic situation. In other words, such drugs help to re-establish balance in the vital ratio:

$$\frac{\text{coronary flow}}{\text{myocardial metabolism}}$$

mainly by decreasing the denominator.

From the physiological point of view it would further appear possible to "protect" the heart of coronary patients from unexpected emotional impacts in another way. Usually such individuals restrain themselves effectively from undue physical exercise, but the sudden load imposed on the heart by emotional explosions may be more difficult to avoid—which was John Hunter's personal experience. A certain amount of protection might be achieved here—if great caution is exercised—by a suitably balanced β-receptor blockade of the sympathetic effect on the myocardium, combined with an acute administration of nitrites to induce venous pooling when necessary.

References

Åblad, B., and S. Mellander (1963). "Comparative effects of hydralazine, sodium nitrite and acetylcholine on resistance blood vessels and capillary filtration in skeletal muscle in the cat," *Acta Physiol. Scand.* **58,** 319–29.

Berne, R. M. (1964). "Regulation of coronary blood flow," *Physiol. Rev.* **44,** 1–29.

Feigl, E. O. (1967). "Sympathetic control of coronary circulation," *Circ. Res.* **XX,** 262–71.

Feigl, E. O. (1969). "Parasympathetic control of coronary blood flow in dogs". *Circ. Rev.* **XXV,** 509–20.

Folkow, B., B. Lisander, R. S. Tuttle, and S. C. Wang (1968). "Changes in cardiac output upon stimulation of the hypothalamic defence area and the medullary depressor area in the cat," *Acta Physiol. Scand.* **72,** 220–33.

Gregg, D. E., and L. C. Fisher (1963). "Blood supply to the heart," *Handbook of Physiology*, 2, Circulation **II,** 1517–84.

Kirk, E. S., and C. R. Honig (1964). "Non-uniform distribution of blood-flow and gradients of oxygen tension within the heart," *Am. J. Physiol.* **207,** 661–68.

Linder, E. (1966). "Measurements of normal and collateral coronary blood flow by close-arterial and intramyocardial injection of krypton[85] and xenon[133]," *Acta Physiol. Scand.* **68,** Suppl., 272, 5–31.

Marchetti, G., and B. Taccardi, eds. (1967). *International symposium on the coronary circulation and energetics of the myocardium.* Basel/New York: Karger.

Myers, W. W., and C. R. Honig (1964). "Number and distribution of capillaries as determinants of myocardial oxygen tension," *Am. J. Physiol.* **207,** 653–60.

Rayford, C. R., E. M. Khouris, and D. E. Gregg (1965). "Effect of excitement on coronary and systemic energetics in unanesthetized dogs," *Am. J. Physiol.* **209,** 680–88.

Renkin, E. M. (1967). "Blood flow and transcapillary exchange in skeletal and cardiac muscle," in *International symposium on the coronary circulation and energetics of the myocardium* (ed. G. Marchetti and B. Taccardi). Basel/New York: Karger.

Sarnoff, S. J., E. Braunwald, G. H. Welch, Jr., R. B. Case, W. N. Stainsby, and R. Macruz (1958). "Haemodynamic determinants of oxygen consumption of the heart with special reference to the tension-time index," *Am. J. Physiol.* **192,** 148–56.

Winbury, M. M., D. Kissil, and M. Losada (1965). "Approaches to the study of nutritional blood flow extraction of Rb[86] by the heart and hind limb," in *Isotopes in experimental pharmacology* (ed. L. J. Roth), pp. 229–48. Chicago: University of Chicago Press.

24

Cerebral Circulation

General Considerations

The vascular circuit of the brain (for lit. see Sokoloff, 1959; Kety, 1960) may be considered as the most important of them all, at least in most people. Man's brain, which weighs about 1400 g in adults, receives some 50 to 60 ml/min/100 g of blood during "resting" equilibrium, or some 750 ml *in toto*. Thus, nearly 15% of resting cardiac output is delivered to an organ which constitutes only 2% of the body weight. The oxygen usage is 3 to 3.5 ml/min/100 g brain, or nearly 20% of the total oxygen usage during rest.

The internal carotid and vertebral arteries, forming the basilar artery, unite in the circle of Willis at the base of the brain and provide the entire blood supply in man. This arterial anastomosis is not fully efficient, for ligation of one of the internal carotids reduces the blood supply to the corresponding hemisphere so greatly that the impairment is sufficient to result in a stroke, except in young people. The circle of Willis provides six cerebral branches for distribution to the cortex, subcortex, and upper brain stem, while the basilar artery directly supplies the occipital lobes, cerebellum, pons, and medulla.

As the cranium is rigid (except in the young child), and as the brain is virtually incompressible, the combined volume of brain tissue, cerebrospinal fluid, and intracranial blood is nearly constant. The Monro-Kellie hypothesis states that the blood volume in the cranial cavity is approximately constant. This has occasionally made people doubt whether the cerebral blood flow can increase by vasodilatation. It is obvious, however, that the small volume increase occasioned even by substantial arteriolar dilatation which increases the flow is easily compensated for without causing any undue side effects simply by a minor compression of the far more voluminous veins.

Superficial and deep veins empty into the venous sinuses that lie between the dura mater and the bone. These veins have no valves and are kept open by the structure of the dura around their orifices. The blood drains from the brain mainly via the internal jugular vein, but also by channels which join the vertebral venous plexus and by anastomoses with the orbital and pterygoid plexuses. The discovery of these anastomoses invalidated the quantitative results claimed by Ferris (1941), who ingeniously employed the principle of occlusion plethysmography in attempting to measure cerebral blood flow. He measured the volume displacement of cerebrospinal fluid (through a lumbar puncture) which occurred on pumping up a pressure cuff fitted round the neck. The flow values deduced were too low, however, because of the impossibility of occluding the vertebral anastomoses or of preventing shifts of intracranial venous blood into the highly distensible veins of the face and scalp. (It is worth noting that vertebral anastomoses *can* deal with the entire venous return from the brain. Batson reported a case of complete obstruction of the upper part of the superior vena cava; the patient survived.)

Measurements of Cerebral Blood Flow in Man

The importance of cerebral tissue, the frequency of disturbances of its blood supply, and the particular technical difficulties inherent in measurements of the cerebral blood flow in man (see Sokoloff, 1959; Kety, 1960) justify a brief description of the methods employed (compare Chapter 7).

Schmidt pioneered in making important quantitative measurements of cerebral blood flow, using the bubble flow meter in monkeys, and these direct values were compared with those obtained with the nitrous oxide technique, showing the latter to be accurate and acceptable for use in man (Kety and Schmidt, 1948).

The subject breathes 15% N_2O in an oxygen-nitrogen mixture for 10 min, while at regular intervals six pairs of arterial (peripheral artery) and venous (internal jugular bulb) samples are withdrawn simultaneously and their N_2O concentrations analysed and plotted graphically (Fig. 24-1). The integrated A-V–nitrous oxide difference can be obtained

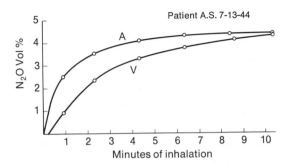

Fig. 24-1. Arterial and internal jugular blood concentrations of nitrous oxide in a human subject during the inhalation of 15 per cent nitrous oxide in oxygen. (From Kety and Schmidt, 1945. By permission.)

graphically or by calculation. When the brain is in equilibrium with the arterial blood with respect to N_2O, the arterial and venous N_2O concentrations become equal. As the partition coefficient of N_2O between blood and brain is unity, the N_2O amount per 100 g brain is known at this stage. As the cerebral uptake per unit tissue weight and the A-V difference for N_2O can thus be deduced, the Fick principle is applicable for measurement of the average cerebral blood flow (CBF).

$$CBF/min/100 \text{ g} = 100 \frac{\text{Amount of } N_2O \text{ uptake}}{(A\text{-}V) \ N_2O \text{ concentration}}$$

$$\therefore \quad CBF/min/100 \text{ g} = \frac{100 \ V_u \cdot S}{(A\text{-}V) \ dt}$$

where V_u is the venous N_2O concentration after equilibrium is reached in the brain tissue during time u and S is the partition coefficient for N_2O between blood and brain.

This method was the first to provide accurate quantitative data of the cerebral haemodynamics in man and it has been of the greatest importance.

Its disadvantages are that it can only be used in steady states and it does not reveal regional differences in flow. More recently the clearance of [85]Krypton or [133]Xenon (see Ingvar and Lassen, 1962)—administered either in the same way as N_2O or as a direct injection into the internal carotid artery—has proved to be most valuable, both because the recording process is less complex and because regional flow differences—and flow changes—may be recorded at least semiquantitatively if exact collimations of external scintillation monitoring systems are used (e.g. Ingvar and Risberg, 1967). Moreover, by multicomponent analysis, flows in grey and white matter may be separately assessed.

Capillary Permeability in the Brain

The capillary exchange vessels of the brain (and the retina, which is part of it) possess unique permeability characteristics, and this has led to the concept of the "blood brain barrier" (BBB; see Davson, 1963; Dobbing, 1963; Broman and Steinwall, 1967). This "barrier", together with that between the blood and cerebrospinal fluid, provides the brain with a specific "milieu interieur" of its own, based in part on facilitated and restricted diffusion conditions. These are combined with active transport mechanisms, almost as if the brain were supplied at strategical points with its own "renal tubular mechanisms" for active expulsion, helping to keep its particular chemical environment both constant yet different from that of the rest of the body. This is not the place to analyse all such complex mechanisms in detail (see the references quoted above and Fig. 24-2), but some aspects of the capillary transfer mechanisms may be considered briefly.

Lipid-soluble substances pass freely across the cerebral capillaries, as across capillaries elsewhere. The passage of many water-soluble substances, however, is restricted in a fashion not critically related to the relationship between their molecular size and that of capillary pores in general (see Chapter 8). Thus, glucose and amino acids pass readily, while, for example, mannitol or sucrose, and many ions, are almost completely barred. Crone (1965) has shown that the "nutritional" substances mentioned traverse a concentration gradient in a manner which deserves to be called "facilitated diffusion". It is interesting that the borders of the endothelial cells of the cerebral capillaries overlap markedly, with tight junctions showing no signs of pores, except in a few restricted parts of the brain (Brightman, 1970; see also Chapter 8). The absence of obvious capillary pores seemingly makes pore-bound diffusion of "unwanted" substances impossible, whereas those "required" are specifically transferred (possibly by means of specific "transfer sites" in the membranes of the endothelial cells?)— but along the concentration gradient. The lipid-soluble O_2 and CO_2 pass readily, as does water, but acids do not: on the contrary, many waste

I. LIPOPHILIC SUBSTANCES	Passive diffusion	No barrier effect
II. HYDROPHILIC SUBSTANCES		
1. "Nutrients" (glucose, amino acids, etc.)	Specific transfer* Blood →CNS	Barrier effect above max. transport capacity
2. "Waste products," organic ions (conjugates, indicator dyes, PAH, etc.)	Specific transfer* CNS →Blood	Barrier effect linked to "counter transport."
3. Non-metabolizable and non-charged solutes (inulin, sucrose, mannitol, etc.)	No specific transfer	Barrier effect "passive"

*Carrier mediated—saturable (limited transport capacity)—inhibitable by competitive overloading or by toxic influences.

Fig. 24-2. Model of the blood-brain barrier system. (From Broman and Steinwall, 1967. By permission.)

products are actively transferred from the brain to the blood or from the cerebrospinal fluid to the blood, usually by "carrier" systems of a nature similar to those in the renal tubules (e.g. Pappenheimer et al., 1961).

Several blood-borne vasoactive substances, especially the catecholamines, are hindered from passing the endothelium, so they have little access to the smooth muscle of the cerebral vessels. The catecholamines and some of their precursors actually accumulate within the endothelial cells of the *cerebral* capillaries, whereas they pass freely across the capillary walls elsewhere without there being any intra-endothelial accumulation (Bertler *et al.*, 1963). The brain capillary walls, moreover, contain DOPA-decarboxylase and monoamine oxidase, which break down such accumulated vasoactive amines. This is yet another aspect of the complex "blood brain barrier" function, which thus comprises several different mechanisms.

Similarly, cerebrospinal fluid that communicates with the very narrow "interstitial spaces" has a unique composition (see Pappenheimer, 1967). Lymphatic vessels of conventional type are absent.

Vascular Dimensions and Normal Flow Range

As it supplies both the cell-rich grey matter and the cell-poor white matter, the cerebral vascular bed should be considered as a multicompartment circuit. The oxygen usage of mammalian peripheral axons is only 0.3 ml/100 g/min, whereas that of the whole brain is 3.3 ml/100 g/min. If the white matter comprises 60% of the brain weight, and has an oxygen consumption of about the same order of magnitude as peripheral nerves, or somewhat higher, then in 100 g brain the white matter would use perhaps 0.3 to 0.5 ml and the grey matter would use close to 3 ml of oxygen/min. Grey matter would then use 6 to 7 ml O_2 per 100 g/min. With such an allocation (60% white, 40% grey) this means that 600 g of grey matter use some 40 ml of O_2 per min, or almost 20% of the basal oxygen usage of the whole body. The heart itself uses about 20 to 25 ml/min—equal to about 10% of the total oxygen consumption in the basal state. Grey matter thus has a very high oxygen usage.

In accordance with this, the cortex and some parts of the grey matter of the brain stem have a very rich blood supply—approximately 300 to 400 ml/min/100 g at *maximal* dilatation (e.g. Häggendal and Johansson, 1965)—and the number of capillaries/mm³ tissue is 3000 to 4000. White matter, however, receives a maximal supply only some 20 to 25% of that of grey matter.

In anaesthetized animals (dog) the "resting" flow values for the two tissue compartments are some 60 to 80 and 15 to 20 ml/min/100 g, respectively. In conscious animals the levels are presumably higher, especially in the grey matter, as most types of anaesthesia lower both the cerebral metabolism and the cerebral blood flow. The resting mean value of 50 to 60 ml/min/100 g for man's brain thus probably implies a cortical flow of some 100 ml/min/100 g and perhaps 20 to 25 ml/min/100 g for white matter. Comparison of these "resting" values with those during maximal dilatation, which are 3 to 4 times higher, shows that the cerebral resistance vessels display a considerable basal tone.

Regulation of Cerebral Blood Flow

Nervous Factors

The vasoconstrictor fibre influence on cerebral blood flow is normally quite small, as regional sympathetic blockade usually does not significantly decrease cerebral flow resistance. Further, even supramaximal vasoconstrictor fibre stimulation (15 impulses/sec) increases cerebral flow resistance only some 20 to 30% in the cat (Ingvar, 1958), and the same holds true for man (Fig. 24-3) (Krog, 1964)—trifling effects considering the fact that the vasoconstrictor fibres may produce resistance increases of 500 to 600% e.g. in muscle. The histochemical methods show that the adrenergic vasoconstrictor fibres are distributed only to the *larger* cerebral arteries *outside* the brain proper, with few or no axon ramifications along the true resistance vessels (Falck *et al.*, 1968). Hence the slight neurogenic increase in flow resistance mentioned above must mainly reflect luminal reductions of these larger arterial vessels (unless some myogenic spread of excitation takes place towards the smaller vessels).

Teleologically, it can be argued that the relative lack of vasoconstrictor nerves in the brain, as in the myocardium, is "A Good Thing". Elsewhere in the body elaborate adjustments by baroreceptor reflexes adjust cardiac output and vascular resistance to secure a fairly stable arterial pressure in the face of postural changes, etc., ultimately aimed at maintaining the supply to the vitally important cerebral and myocardial tissues. Thus the fall of cardiac output and arterial pressure on assuming the upright position is offset by sympathetic venoconstriction and arteriolar constriction in splanchnic, renal, muscle, and skin circuits, together with sympathetic stimulation of the heart. If the brain vessels were themselves richly innervated by constrictor nerves which participated in such reflexes, any advantage gained elsewhere in bolstering the perfusion pressure head would, of course, be lost by the increase in cerebral vascular resistance. In fact, when blood pressure falls after a severe blood loss, where an increasingly intense peripheral vasoconstriction takes place, the cerebral vessels *dilate*, thanks to their "autoregulation", so that cerebral blood flow remains nearly constant even down to pressures of 50 to 60 mm Hg. However, once they have reached maximal dilatation in the course

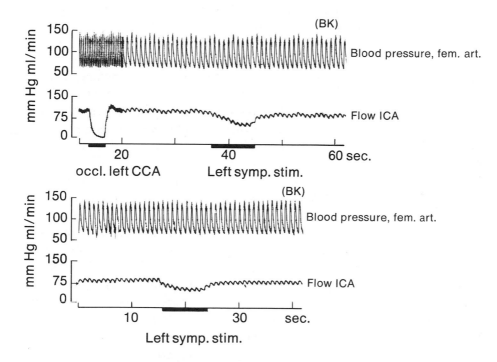

Fig. 24-3. Effect of cervical sympathetic stimulation (15 imp/sec.) on blood flow through the internal carotid artery in anaesthetized man, recorded by means of an electromagnetic flowmeter probe placed on the internal carotid artery. (From Krog, 1964. By permission.)

of this autoregulatory process, a further drop in pressure abruptly reduces flow and loss of consciousness ensues.

As stated in Chapter 16, the pial vessels are supplied with dilator fibres, but the range of action and the functional significance of these is as yet unknown.

Local Control

The remarkable power of autoregulation of cerebral vessels was first shown in 1934 by Fog (see Fog, 1938) and has more recently been studied in detail (see e.g. Häggendal and Johansson, 1965). As elsewhere, this autoregulation seems to result from the combined effects of changes in the transmural pressure and in the local chemical environment on vascular smooth muscle activity (Chapter 16).

An increase in cerebral metabolism, a fall in the perfusion pressure head, or a change of the perfusing blood—hypercapnia and/or anoxia— all cause cerebral vasodilatation. The cerebral precapillary smooth muscles are highly sensitive, not only to stretch, but especially to shifts in their immediate chemical environment. Until recently it was assumed that pCO_2 was the *prime* "chemical" regulator of cerebral blood flow, just as it was believed that hypoxia itself determined coronary vascular resistance (Chapter 22).

However, it has become increasingly clear that it is the *hydrogen ion concentration of the "interstitial fluid"* (Severinghaus et al., 1966; Fencl et al., 1968) which predominantly serves as the "negative feedback" to counter-balance the myogenic tone of the cerebral resistance vessels. Thus, the profound vasodilator action of CO_2 inhalation (Fig. 24-4A) depends mainly on the fact that the lipid-soluble CO_2 readily crosses the blood brain barrier and affects the local extravascular $[H^+]$ by influencing the balance between CO_2 and HCO_3 (for details see Ingvar et al., 1968). It should be stressed that it is the *extravascular* $[H^+]$ (*not* that of the blood, which, be-cause of the blood brain barrier, has no direct access to the vascular smooth muscles) that regulates cerebral vascular tone. Thus, non-gaseous acid-aemia (e.g. lactacidaemia) *constricts*, if anything, the cerebral vessels, probably by causing hyperventilation, which lowers the arterial pCO_2 and thus reduces the interstitial $[H^+]$ of the brain.

For these reasons, intense voluntary hyperventilation produces cerebral vasoconstriction, dizziness, and even loss of consciousness: the lowering of arterial pCO_2 leads to a decrease in hydrogen ion concentration within the brain, which enhances the regional precapillary vascular tone by reducing the environmental inhibitory influence on myogenic activity. Cerebral blood flow may be reduced to some 50% of normal. Further, the associated blood alkalosis shifts the oxygen dissociation curve to the left (Bohr effect), rendering the unloading of oxygen from the blood HbO_2

more difficult and, lastly, the perfusion pressure falls. All these factors reduce the delivery of oxygen to the cerebral neurones.

The cerebral vessels, besides altering their calibre in response to changes in the interstitial [H^+], also respond to changes in blood pO_2, dilating at low pO_2 values and constricting when exposed to high pO_2 values. Thus, the ventilation of oxygen-rich gas mixtures causes cerebral vasoconstriction. Lambertsen et al. (1953) found that men breathing oxygen at 3.5 atmospheres had an arterial pO_2 of 2300 mm Hg, but that the cerebral venous pO_2 was only 75 mm Hg, which indicated that cerebral vasoconstriction had occurred. The addition of 2% CO_2 to the inspired gas mixture increased the cerebral venous pO_2 to 1000 mm Hg by increasing cerebral blood flow.

These results indicate the importance of avoiding the use of any anaesthetic agent which may act as a cerebral vasodilator during hyperoxic operations. Paradoxically, high oxygen pressures inactivate oxidative cellular metabolism by oxidizing the co-factor α-lipoic acid (a sulphydryl compound) which is responsible for the conversion of pyruvic acid to acetyl coenzyme A and the conversion of α-ketoglutaric acid to succinyl coenzyme A (Haugaard, 1964). In a way, the vasoconstrictor response to high pO_2 helps to protect the cells from such disturbances, by normalizing the balance between oxygen delivery and oxygen usage.

This remarkable biological effect of high oxygen pressures on cell metabolism reached its grimmest human result when premature babies treated in oxygen tents developed retrolental fibroplasia and became blind. The condition begins with an abnormal and profuse growth of the retinal vessels and finally results in retinal detachment (Ashton et al., 1954).

Relation between Cerebral Activity and Blood Flow

Schmidt showed that illumination of one retina by repeated flashes of light caused an increase in the blood flow only in the visual cortex (registered by a thermocouple). Kety and co-workers injected solutions containing radioactive inert gases intravenously and demonstrated by radioautography of histological sections that some areas contained more of the radioactive material than others. In unanaesthetized animals, motor, somatic, sensory, visual, and auditory cortical areas showed a much higher concentration than elsewhere; thiopentone anaesthesia reduced these concentrations to values similar to that of the remainder. Radioautographs of the lateral geniculate bodies and visual cortex of cats, subjected to 5 minutes photic stimulation and then sacrificed, showed a far greater density than did those of animals sacrificed after being kept in the dark (see Kety, 1960). An example of cerebral functional hyperaemia is shown in Fig. 24-4B.

By using a similar approach, but utilizing external recordings of γ scintillation (Krypton method) over different parts of the cerebral cortex, Ingvar and co-workers traced regional vasodilator responses in conscious man in connection with various types of sensory, emotional, and intellectual stimuli. Such manifestations of regional functional hyperaemia may be utilized for identifying the cortical area that is predominantly engaged in different types of stimuli or in psychomotor activities (e.g. see Ingvar and Risberg, 1967).

Increased Intracranial Pressure

The cerebral blood volume, and eventually flow, is of course affected by intracranial extravascular factors. Cushing showed that an acute rise of intracranial pressure was accompanied by the development of arterial hypertension (the "Cushing reflex") and attributed the cause of this to bulbar ischaemia affecting and stimulating the medullary cardiovascular centres. The development of bradycardia in patients with intracranial neoplasms, etc., is considered to be an alarming sign. It is induced reflexly from the baroreceptors as a consequence of the centrally elicited pressor response.

Fig. 24-4. A. Effect of a brief period of 10% CO_2 inhalation (1-5) on cortical blood flow in the lightly anaesthetized cat (venous outflow from superior sagittal sinus measured by drop recorder).
B. Effect of an "arousal reaction" (induced by topical stimulation of the mesencephalic reticular formation) on cortical blood flow and EEG in an "encéphale isolé" preparation of the cat. Note the vasodilator response and the disappearance of EEG spindles during the stimulation period. (From Ingvar, 1958. By permission.)

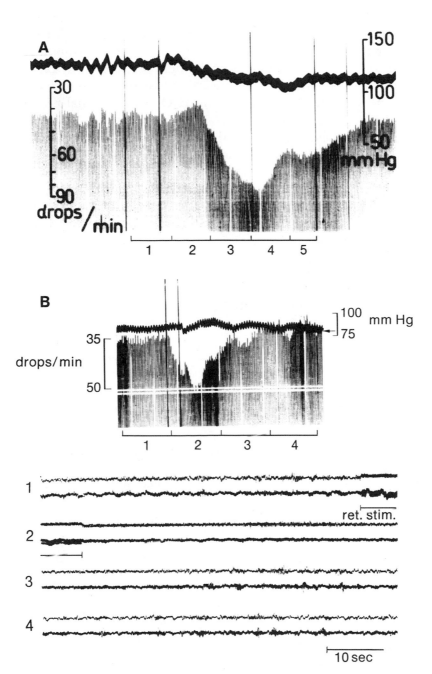

Kety investigated the effects of increased intracranial pressure caused by brain tumours on the cerebral blood flow, using the N_2O technique. Normally the cerebrospinal fluid pressure in a recumbent subject is some 10 cm H_2O. With rises of cerebrospinal fluid pressure up to some 50 cm H_2O the arterial pressure rose linearly while the cerebral blood flow remained constant. Above some 50 cm H_2O of intracranial pressure the cerebral blood flow tended to fall progressively. As the arterial pressure usually does not increase any further, the situation implies a gradually falling effective pressure head and transmural pressure for the cerebral vessels. Both these factors lead to an "autoregulatory" vasodilation which will tend to maintain the cerebral blood flow. Ultimately, with further increases of intracranial pressure, the cerebral blood flow diminishes to such low levels (below some 40 ml/min/100 g) that the patient becomes comatose.

References

Ashton, N., B. Ward, and G. Serpell (1954). "Effects of oxygen on developing retinal vessels with particular reference to the problem of retrolental fibroplasia," *Brit. J. Ophthal.* **38,** 397–432.

Bertler, Å., B. Falck, and E. Rosengren (1963). "The direct demonstration of a barrier mechanism in the brain capillaries," *Acta Pharmacol. et Toxicol.* **20,** 317–21.

Brightman, M. W. (1970). "Morphology of the blood-brain barrier including studies with some electron dense larger molecules," in *Alfred Benzon symposium II on Capillary Permeability.* Copenhagen: Munksgaard Internat. Publ.

Broman, T., and O. Steinwall (1967). "Model of the blood-brain barrier system", in '*Brain Edema*' (ed. I. Klatzo and F. Seitelberger). New York: Springer-Verlag.

Crone, C. (1965). "Facilitated transfer of glucose from blood to brain," *J. Physiol.* **181,** 103–13.

Davson, H. (1963). "The cerebrospinal fluid," *Ergebn. Physiol.* **52,** 20–73.

Dobbing, J. (1963). "The blood-brain barrier: some recent developments," *Guy Hosp. Rep.* **112,** 267–86.

Falck, B., K. G. Nielsen, and C. Owman (1968). "Adrenergic innervation of the pial circulation," *Scand. J. Lab. Clin. Invest.*, Suppl., 102, VI:B.

Fencl, V., J. R. Vale, and J. R. Broch (1968). "Cerebral blood flow and pulmonary ventilation in metabolic acidosis and alkalosis," *Scand. J. Lab. Clin. Invest.*, Suppl., 102, VIII:B.

Ferris, E. B., Jr. (1941). "Objective measurement of relative intracranial blood flow in man with observations concerning the hemodynamics of the cranio-vertebral system," *Arch. Neurol. Psychiat.* **46,** 377–401. (Chicago.)

Fog, M. (1938). "Relationship between blood pressure and tonic regulation of the pial arteries," *J. Neurol. Psychiat.* **1,** 187–97.

Häggendal, E., and B. Johansson (1965). "Effects of arterial carbon dioxide tension and oxygen saturation on cerebral blood flow autoregulation in dogs," *Acta Physiol. Scand.* **66,** Suppl., 258, 27–53.

Haugaard, N. (1964). "The toxic action of oxygen on metabolism and the role of trace metals", in Frank Dickens and Eric Neil (eds.), *Oxygen in the Animal Organism*, pp. 495–505. Oxford: Pergamon Press.

Ingvar, D. H. (1958). "Cortical state of excitability and cortical circulation," in *Reticular formation of the brain*, pp. 381–408. Boston: Little, Brown.

Ingvar, D. H., and N. A. Lassen (1962). "Regional blood flow of the cerebral cortex determined by Krypton[85]," *Acta Physiol. Scand.* **54,** 325–38.

Ingvar, D. H., and J. Risberg (1967). "Increase of regional cerebral blood flow during mental effort in normals and in patients with focal brain disorders," *Exp. Brain Res.* **3,** 195–211.

Ingvar, D. H., N. A. Lassen, B. K. Siesjö, and E. Skinhøj, eds. (1968). "Third Internat. Symp. on Cerebral blood flow and Cerebro-spinal Fluid. Lund-Copenhagen, May 9–11," *Scand. J. Clin. Lab. Invest.*, Suppl., 102.

Kety, S. S. (1960). "The cerebral circulation," *Handbook of Physiology*, 1, Neurophysiology **III,** 1751–60.

Kety, S. S., and C. F. Schmidt (1945). "The determination of cerebral blood flow in man by use of nitrous oxide in low concentrations," *Am. J. Physiol.* **143,** 53–66.

Kety, S. S., and C. F. Schmidt (1948). "The nitrous oxide method for the quantitative determination of cerebral blood flow in man: theory, procedure and normal values," *J. Clin. Invest.* **27,** 476–83.

Krog, J. (1964). "Autonomic nervous control of the cerebral blood flow in man," *J. Oslo City Hospital*, **14,** 25–33.

Lambertsen, C. J., R. H. Kough, D. Y. Cooper, G. L. Emmel, H. H. Loeschke, and C. F. Schmidt (1953). "Oxygen toxicity. Effects in man of oxygen inhalation at 1 and 3.5 atmospheres upon blood gas transport, cerebral circulation and cerebral metabolism," *J. Appl. Physiol.* **5,** 471–86.

Pappenheimer, J. R. (1967). "The ionic composition of cerebral extracellular fluid and its relation to control of breathing," from *The Harvey Lectures*, Series 61. New York: Academic Press.

Pappenheimer, J. R., S. R. Heisey, and E. F. Jordan (1961). "Active transport of diodrast and phenolsulfonphtalein from cerebrospinal fluid to blood," *Am. J. Physiol.* **200,** 1–10.

Severinghaus, J. W., K. Chiodi, E. I. Eger II, B. Brandstater, and T. F. Hornbein (1966). "Cerebral blood flow in man at high altitude. Role of cerebrospinal fluid pH in normalization of flow in chronic hypocapnia," *Circ. Res.* **19,** 274–82.

Sokoloff, L. (1959). "The action of drugs on the cerebral circulation," *Pharmacol. Rev.* **11,** 1–85.

25

Cutaneous Circulation

General Considerations

The skin provides a waterproof protective cover for the body. No other tissue is so exposed to trauma and to extensive variations of temperature. About 1 to 1.5 mm thick and with a total body surface area of 1.7 to 1.8 m², the skin weighs some 2 kg in all. Skin and subcutaneous adipose tissue (which varies greatly in thickness) serve as an efficient heat insulator when cutaneous blood flow is kept minimal.

Homeothermic animals without fur, such as man, depend heavily for their heat regulation on control of the skin circulation. The *total* skin blood flow in man exposed to cold may be reduced by sympathetic vaso-constriction to 20 ml/min or even less, so that almost the full heat-insulating power of the skin and fat is realized. Conversely, during maximal heat stress the skin blood flow may be some 3 litres/min, improving radiation and convection and also delivering the raw material for sweat secretion (which itself may reach 1 to 2 litres/hour). Evaporation, convection, and radiation then ensure a huge heat loss, hindered only when the environment is moist and close to body temperature.

The cutaneous vascular circuit is tailored for levels of flow which can far exceed the local metabolic needs and, moreover, functions under a central nervous control which dominates its adjustment. There are many specific A-V shunts in the cutaneous circulation, which is perhaps unique

449

in this respect. These are situated in the fingers, toes, ears, etc.—sites in which the tissue mass is small in relation to the surface area—thus they favour heat loss when patent. Such capillary "bypasses" allow a huge blood flow and a free transfer of heat which, in contrast to solute exchange, does not necessitate specific exchange membranes.

There is an extensive network of superficial cutaneous veins; these relax fully during heat load, as is evident on inspecting the forearm veins in subjects submitted to heat stress. This venous relaxation greatly favours the loss of heat from the skin.

While naked man is heat-insulated only by means of his skin and sub-cutaneous fat, with thermoreceptors at the very surface which signal any drop in the skin temperature, his comfortable environmental temperature during rest is about $+27°$ C (Fig. 25-1). His physiological protection against cold is poor—he provides himself with an artificial "tropical microclimate" (clothing and warmed houses). He can, however, tolerate heat stress well by means of sweating, etc. Man is thus designed for tropical-subtropical climates, in which he probably originated.

Quite different problems, reflected also in the organization of the cutaneous circulation, are met with in furry animals (Scholander et al., 1950; reviewed by Irving, 1967). For example, the polar fox is so excellently heat-insulated that he remains in comfortable thermal equilibrium down

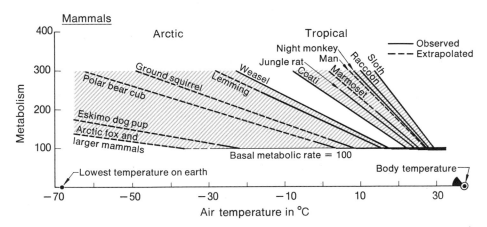

Fig. 25-1. Heat regulation and temperature sensitivity of some arctic and tropical animals in relation to man. (From Scholander et al., 1950. By permission.)

to environmental temperatures of -30 to $-40°C$ (Fig. 25-1). The problem here is not how to keep warm, but rather how to get rid of heat excess in exercise. Cutaneous vasodilatation provides little amelioration of this heat load, for the heat is trapped by the insulation provided by the fur; even sweat glands would be of little use. Such animals lose their excess heat by panting—an excessive dead space ventilation which exposes the blood in the respiratory tract and mouth to efficient cooling.

Whales live in cold sea water and must conserve heat. Thick layers of subcutaneous blubber subserve the main insulating function in these creatures. Vasoconstriction reduces their cutaneous-subcutaneous circulation to a minimum, allowing the realization of almost the full heat insulating power of the blubber. The thin, wide flippers and tail would favour heat loss, but such parts possess an efficient heat exchange system in which the veins break up into fine branches closely surrounding the arteries at the roots of the extremities (Fig. 25-2; Scholander and Schevill, 1955). Thus, the heat of the arterial stream passing to the periphery is here short-circuited to the blood returning; venous blood "pre-cools" the

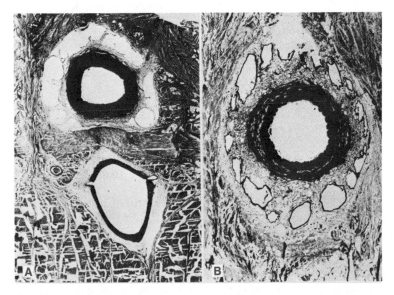

Fig. 25-2. Arrangement of artery and veins in the tail (A) and the dorsal fin of a small whale (Tursiops truncatus). Note that the arteries are closely surrounded by thin-walled veins, an arrangement that greatly favours countercurrent heat exchange. (From Scholander and Schevill, 1955. By permission.)

arterial blood, minimizing heat losses from the body core. During positive heat balance a greatly increased blood flow through the blubber layer to the skin allows efficient cooling. In the flippers and tail, blood flow is also increased and thus reduces the efficiency of the heat exchanger; moreover, the venous return now seems to be directed mainly through widened superficial veins, thereby minimizing countercurrent exchange and improving heat loss to the surrounding water.

Man shows a similar mechanism, but it is far less well developed. During cold the skin vessels and superficial veins are strongly constricted. Blood flow to the extremities is thus directed more to the deeper tissues and returns mainly by venae comites situated close to the main arteries, thereby favouring heat exchange and cooling of the arterial blood. During heat load the skin circuit and the superficial veins open widely and a plentiful supply of blood reaches outer skin layers to return via the dilated superficial veins, which offer less resistance than do the deep venae comites and allow for prolongation of blood cooling.

These general considerations show that the cutaneous circulation may differ markedly from species to species. But as man commands our particular interest, most of this chapter is concerned with the special problems in man. Excellent reviews exist (Burton and Edholm, 1955; Hertzman, 1959; Barcroft, 1960; Ström, 1960; Hardy, 1961; and Greenfield, 1963).

Local Control Mechanisms

"Resting" Flow Levels and Basal Vascular Tone

The "resting" blood flow of the skin is determined, not primarily by local metabolic requirements, but by those of thermal homeostasis of the body as a whole. The hypothalamic temperature regulating centres, exerting their control of the skin vessels by means of selective adjustments of their sympathetic supply (see Ström 1960), do not affect all parts of the cutaneous circuit to the same extent. In delicate adjustments of heat loss they primarily involve vessels in the skin of the face, hands, and feet—and then especially the A-V shunts in such regions. These thick walled vessels respond vividly to even slight shifts in constrictor fibre discharge.

If one defines the "resting" equilibrium for the cutaneous circuit as that in which resting man is in comfortable thermoequilibrium—i.e. when naked exposed to an environmental temperature of 25 to 30°C—his *average* skin blood flow is around 20 ml/min/100 g (there being considerable regional differences). In such circumstances the vasoconstrictor discharge is low and the skin blood flow is approximately doubled by blocking the sympathetic nerves.

Expressed in flow per 100 g of *hand* tissue—the hand is commonly used in studies of cutaneous blood flow in man (only some 30 to 35% skin, but with many A-V shunts in the fingers)—the flow through the acutely denervated hand vessels is 25 to 30 ml/min at local temperatures of 25 to 30°C. As the blood flow in muscle, tendons, and bone (65 to 70% of the weight of the hand) is well below 10 ml/min/100 g in this situation, it follows that the average skin blood flow of the acutely denervated hand may be as high as some 60 to 80 ml/min/100 g. However, most of this probably passes through the A-V anastomoses, which on acute sympathetic blockade are almost maximally dilated at such an environmental temperature.

The patency of the A-V anastomoses may be varied from that of complete closure to that of maximal dilatation by only small changes in sympathetic discharge (Fig. 25-3). Their smooth muscles are entirely dominated by neurogenic control and display little of inherent activity or basal tone, at least at such local temperature levels as may be deemed "comfortable" in man.

Skin sections, both in the hand and in most other regions, which contain few or no A-V shunts, appear to have a blood flow of some 25 to 30 ml/min/100 g skin on sympathetic blockade at local temperatures around 25 to 30°C. This is far below the level of maximal dilatation (see below), showing that the resistance and precapillary sphincter sections of the skin vessels in man display a considerable basal tone, while the venous capacitance side is far more dominated by the vasoconstrictor fibres.

As in other circuits, the precapillary resistance and sphincter sections of the skin display autoregulatory adjustments to changes in transmural pressure (Greenfield, 1963; Mellander *et al.*, 1964) and this is important for counteracting edema formation in the feet, for instance (Chapter 16). Skin vessels are thus quite sensitive to mechanical stimuli, as exhibited also by the so-called "white reaction" (Lewis, 1927). If the skin is stroked lightly, a localized vasoconstrictor response can be seen within 15 sec. It lasts about a minute. This response is independent of nerve connections.

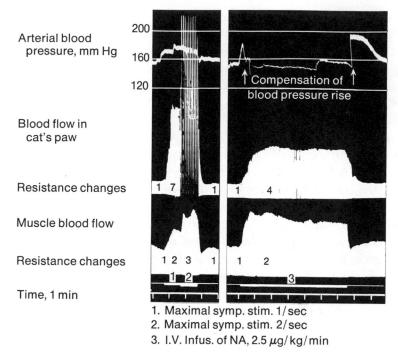

Arterial blood
pressure, mm Hg

Blood flow in
cat's paw

Resistance changes

Muscle blood flow

Resistance changes

Time, 1 min

1. Maximal symp. stim. 1/sec
2. Maximal symp. stim. 2/sec
3. I.V. Infus. of NA, 2.5 µg/kg/min

Fig. 25-3. The effect of low-frequency sympathetic stimulation on A-V anastomoses in the cat's paw, as compared with the effect on muscle resistance vessels (left panel). Drop recorder technique, height of ordinates being *inversely* proportional to flow. Note the far more extensive neurogenic constriction of the A-V anastomoses. This is partly due to more powerful innervation, partly to bigger luminal reduction to a given noradrenaline concentration (right panel). (From Celander and Folkow, 1953a. By permission.)

Tissue pressure appears to be subatmospheric in the skin and subcutaneous tissues (Guyton, 1963). At least in part, this seems to result from the high level of precapillary tone and autoregulatory ability of the small precapillary vessels, so that the mean capillary pressure is appreciably lower than that of the colloid osmotic pressure gradient (see Chapter 8). It may help to explain why the skin and the subcutaneous tissues so closely follow even concave body contours such as in the axilla.

Thus, constrictor fibres operate upon a pronounced level of basal tone in most of the skin and an increase of their discharge, when intense, may reduce flow to 1 ml/min/100 g or less. The hyperaemia seen during thermal stress requires, however, an "active" dilator mechanism which can inhibit this basal tone. Flow may then reach 150 ml/min/100 g skin or more, as in the forearm skin (Edholm et al., 1956). This vasodilatation, accomplished by the release of bradykinin (or perhaps Kallidin) (Fox and Hilton, 1958), is secondary to the neurogenic sweat gland activation (compare salivary glands, Chapter 26). Specific vasodilator fibres to skin vessels have not been convincingly shown. This may seem curious when one considers that emotional blushing in man is one of the best known and most vivid responses of the skin, but such responses are not so easily analysed as one might expect. Man, for example, is the only species that blushes with shame (and for solid reasons, according to authorities on human nature); a cat couldn't care less. Unfortunately, it is not so easy to provoke a habitual blusher to behave properly when suitable recording instruments and circumstances for regional nerve fibre blockade are at hand (we have tried; insults, jokes, even dirty ones; nothing worked. When, after hours, we had given up and thanked the kind subject for brave co-operation, she blushed violently). It is, after all, not impossible that these vivid but transient vasodilator responses are also the result of kinin release, secondary to a phasic activation of sweat glands in the face.

Local Responses to Environmental Temperature

The skin may be exposed to a great range of temperatures, from 0°C up to some 45°C, without there being significant tissue damage upon brief exposures. Beyond these wide limits cold injury and burn, respectively, occur; in fact, cold lesions may occur even well above temperatures where tissue freezing occurs, if cold exposure is prolonged and accompanied by moisture (e.g. "trench foot", Burton and Edholm, 1955; Greenfield, 1963).

Skin is a "poikilothermic" tissue, as is subcutaneous adipose tissue and even some of the skeletal muscles of the limbs to a lesser degree. Only the *body core* is truly homeothermic, and it is so at the expense of the more superficial tissues, which serve as an insulating shield. Skin is usually exposed to environmental temperatures below that of the body and even intense sympathetic vasoconstriction can be well tolerated, because the tissue cooling that ensues upon such flow restriction itself reduces tissue metabolism. Thus, the vasoconstriction reduces the rate of production of vasodilator metabolites in the skin, factors which efficiently counteract neurogenic flow restrictions elsewhere in the body (Chapter 16). Hence the vasoconstrictor effects in the skin are usually well sustained.

These variations of skin metabolism and temperature greatly affect regional vascular tone and blood flow (Fig. 25-4), whether the constrictor activity is abolished or pronounced. The lowest levels of flow in the steady-state situation occur at regional temperatures of 10 to 15°C. These reductions of flow with a fall in local temperature are due not only to an increase of vascular tone, but also to increased blood viscosity on cooling; viscosity is more than doubled when the blood temperature falls from 37°C to below 10°C (Chapter 4).

Skin temperatures below 6 to 10°C and above 43 to 45°C are associated with the sensation of pain. Concomitantly, "protective" local vascular responses in the form of "cold vasodilatation" and "inflammatory vaso-

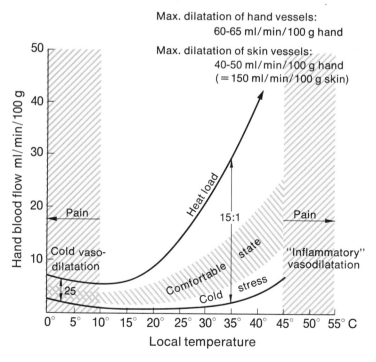

Fig. 25-4. Approximate levels of blood flow in the hand when immersed in water at temperatures between 0° and 45°C and when vasoconstrictor fibre activity is inhibited ("heat load"), moderate ("comfortable"), and intense ("cold stress"). (Modified from Greenfield, 1963. By permission.)

dilatation" are induced (Fig. 25-4). In most respects these reactions are in all likelihood identical with those of the "triple response" of Lewis (1927), seen when the skin is damaged—mechanically, chemically, or thermally—or when allergic manifestations occur (see below).

Cold vasodilatation is preceded by an initial phase of 6 to 10 min of intense vasoconstriction (both local and reflex in origin) when the skin is

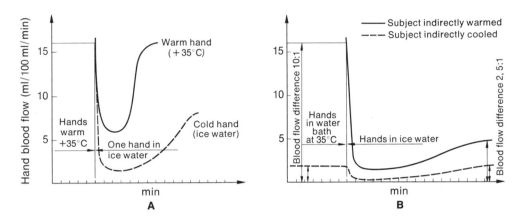

Fig. 25-5A. Diagram illustrating blood flow changes in the two hands when one hand is suddenly exposed to ice water. Note transient reflex constriction in the "warm" hand and the more intense (both reflex and local) constriction in the "cold" hand, later on followed by cold vasodilatation.

Fig. 25-5B. Diagram illustrating the relationship between extent of cold vasodilatation and prevailing vasoconstrictor fibre discharge. The constrictor fibre influence is still noticeable during cold vasodilatation, though greatly reduced compared with the situation before local cooling. (From Folkow et al., 1963. By permission.)

in contact with ice water, for example (see Fig. 25-5A, B). Cold vasodilatation preferentially, but probably not exclusively, involves the A-V anastomoses and its background is complex. Thus, "axon reflexes", i.e. axon collaterals from unmyelinated nociceptive fibres to nearby arterioles, are involved. These fibre collaterals liberate a transmitter of unknown identity and this induces a surprisingly long-lasting vasodilatation whenever these cutaneous nociceptive fibres are excited. In addition, chemical vasodilator factors may be released locally in this situation, when tissue damage is imminent. However, cold also causes what might be called a partial "cold suppression" of vascular smooth muscle activity (Keatinge, 1958) and, lastly, reduces the sensitivity of the vessels to vasoconstrictor fibre discharge (Folkow *et al.*, 1963; Gaskell and Hoeppner, 1966).

Cold vasodilatation in the hands of men subjected to *general* cooling gives a flow of 2 to 3 ml/min/100 g—a value well below that seen in warm subjects (5 to 7 ml/min/100 g) (Krog *et al.*, 1960; Folkow *et al.*, 1963). This implies that the effect of the vasoconstrictor fibre discharge on the dilating vessels, is still present, though greatly reduced (Fig. 25-5B). However, as the blood viscosity is much higher in these situations the extent of vasodilatation must be more marked than the figures for flow suggest. If the flow in muscle, bone, and joints in the cooled hand is only about 1 to 2 ml/min/100 g, and skin constitutes 30% of the tissue volume, then in a subject submitted to *general* warming this would mean an average blood flow in the skin of the cooled hand of some 15 to 20 ml/min/100 g skin. The apparent blood viscosity at these low temperatures is perhaps three times that at 37°C. Then the average degree of cutaneous vascular relaxation during cold vasodilatation may be equivalent to that seen in the warm hand when the flow is of the order of 40 to 60 ml/min/100 g skin. As most of the increase of flow in cold vasodilatation occurs in the A-V shunts of the fingers, these vessels are probably almost maximally widened in this situation.

As is well known, temperatures above 45°C cause redness and swelling— a first-degree burn (Fig. 25-6). Higher temperatures cause tissue destruction.

External Pressure

Pressure causes ischaemia of the skin. The skin tolerates such temporary ischaemia well, but the accumulation of metabolites ultimately results in the excitation of nociceptive fibres and this induces reflex or voluntary shifts in position with a consequent restoration of nutritional blood flow. The colour of the skin thereupon reveals that the accumulated metabolites are vasodilator and cause reactive hyperaemia. The cooler the skin the lower is its metabolism and the less pronounced are both the subjective discomfort of pressure and the subsequent hyperaemia. A prolonged complete interruption flow for several hours causes tissue damage and even necrosis, exemplified by the bed sores often elicited in debilitated uncon-

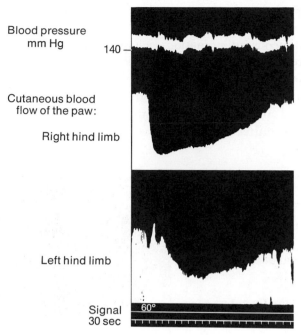

Fig. 25-6. Difference in extent of cutaneous vasodilator response to brief immersion in hot water (60°C) in the cat's hind paws, where the "axon reflexes" connected to the pain fibres of the left paw had been eliminated by total afferent fibre degeneration. Same techniques for blood flow recording as in Fig. 25-3. Note the more prompt and pronounced vasodilator response in the right paw, where all the elements of the triple response are present, while "the flare" is lacking in the left paw. (From Celander and Folkow, 1953b. By permission.)

scious patients or paraplegic patients. During normal sleep, frequent shifts in body position occur which eliminate such risks.

Tissue Trauma

Lewis (1927) described the "triple response" of skin vessels to cutaneous trauma or allergic manifestations. Vasodilator factors, like histamine, bradykinin-like polypeptides, etc., cause, successively, a localized vaso-dilatation ("red reaction") and an inflammatory oedema (the "wheal"). These are surrounded by a more widespread dilatation (the "flare"), mediated via local axon reflex pathways of the nociceptive fibres. These three elements constitute the classical "triple response" that occurs in all types of cutaneous inflammations, whatever their cause.

If the nociceptive fibres are blocked by local anaesthesia, or have degenerated following section, the "flare" is abolished but the "red reaction" and the closely connected "wheal" still occur (Fig. 25-6), causing a more circumscribed and less intense vasodilatation and local oedema. As the unknown transmitter released has a very prolonged action, it requires only

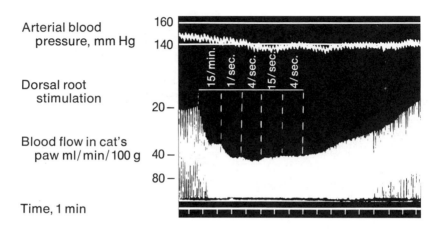

Fig. 25-7. Relationship between frequency of antidromic stimulation of unmyelinated pain fibres and extent of cutaneous vasodilatation in the cat's paw. Same technique for blood flow recording as in Fig. 25-3. Note that almost maximal vasodilatation is achieved already at one impulse per second and that regain of vascular tone is very slow. (From Celander and Folkow, 1953. By permission.)

a very sparse impulse discharge in the nociceptive fibres to induce a pronounced vasodilatation (Fig. 25-7). Thus, a marked "flare" may result from skin damage so trivial as not to cause significant pain.

Widespread and intense cutaneous vasodilatation is seen in certain serious dermatological diseases, where allergic and toxic factors produce generalized erythrodermia. Thermoregulation of the patient may be seriously threatened, for vasoconstrictor fibre discharge cannot reduce the skin flow adequately.

Central and Reflex Nervous Control

Two sets of cutaneous vascular pathways—the "specialized" A-V anastomoses, which are mainly confined to skin areas in the face, hands, and feet and dominated by sympathetic vasoconstrictor fibres, and the "regular" cutaneous vessels, which are present everywhere and display a pronounced basal tone—subserve the thermoregulatory function. Reduction of flow in these latter cutaneous vessels are induced by vasoconstrictor discharge, whereas "active" dilatation beyond the basal level is secondary mainly, if not only, to the release of bradykinin (or kallidin) which occurs when sweat glands are excited (Chapter 16).

The threshold of vasodilatation achieved by reducing constrictor fibre discharge is much lower than that of sweat gland activation. However, the hypothalamic centres command these two efferent links involved in the heat loss mechanism of man in a geographically characteristic pattern. With a gradual increase of heat load, first the A-V anastomoses of, e.g. the ears and hands dilate, owing to inhibition of discharge of the vasoconstrictor fibres which supply them; they also respond more strongly to a given neurogenic discharge than do the "ordinary" skin vessels. Then the anastomoses of the feet dilate, and gradually the vasoconstrictor fibres to the more proximal skin areas begin to reduce *their* discharge. Much the same order is seen during gradually increased cooling of the body.

If the increase of flow due to reduction of vasoconstrictor discharge— which allows almost maximal dilatation of the A-V anastomoses, but only moderate dilatation elsewhere in the skin—is insufficient to restore heat balance, then the sweat glands become active. (Again, this shows a similar geographical pattern, sweating usually starting in the forehead.) Now the vasodilatation becomes greatly intensified in skin sections that lack A-V shunts and whose basal vascular tone is high in resting conditions. This increased dilatation is, as mentioned, induced by kinin formation and serves the dual purpose of delivering enough blood flow to the sweat glands to provide the fluid they secrete and providing a sufficient delivery of heat to the skin to warm it, thereby rendering the evaporative loss of heat (0.58K cal/gm) more efficient in terms of heat elimination.

In intense generalized sweating the total blood supply of the skin in man may approach 3 to 4 l/min, which provides efficient cooling of the body by these mechanisms except when the environment is both hot and damp.

If, in such a situation, heavy exercise is performed, the heart may be faced with an impossible task, trying to supply simultaneously the wide-open muscle and skin circuits. Exercise has to be reduced or acute circulatory collapse may ensue.

Thermoregulatory hypothalamic centres usually dominate the calibre of the cutaneous vascular circuit (see Ström, 1960). The exigencies of temperature homeostasis usually take precedence even over those of salt/water equilibrium and circulatory balance. Thus, in hot climates man succumbs rather from fluid loss and circulatory collapse before the heat-loss mechanisms of cutaneous hyperaemia and sweating are suppressed.

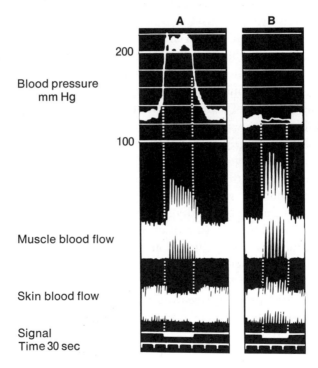

Fig. 25-8. Difference in extent of reflex increase of blood flow resistance in skeletal muscle as compared with skin (paw vessels) produced by carotid occlusion in the vagotomized cat. Panels A and B show the same reflex response, but in B the perfusion pressure to muscle and skin is kept constant, so that the height of the ordinates (drop recorder technique) directly reflects the extent of reflex resistance increase. Note the comparatively insignificant reflex engagement of the cutaneous circuit; here dominated by the A-V anastomoses of the pads. (Courtesy of Dr. B. Löfving, Göteborg, Sweden.)

Skin vessels, especially the A-V shunts (Fig. 25-8), though enjoying an unusually powerful sympathetic constrictor fibre control, are relatively insensitive to baroreceptor and chemoreceptor reflexes (Roddie *et al.*, 1958; Löfving, 1961). After severe blood loss, however, subjects in normal thermoequilibrium do show marked reflex vasoconstriction of their skin vessels. The exposure of such a subject to a heat load is dangerous because "thermally" enforced cutaneous vasodilatation tends to overcome this reflex vasoconstriction (Chapter 30).

On a warm day, soldiers in thick uniforms who are standing to attention—a posture which minimizes muscle pumping of the venous return—may faint. Their cutaneous vessels are widely dilated and perhaps up towards one litre of blood may be "pooled" in the relaxed cutaneous veins, especially those below heart level which become well distended. Baroreceptor reflexes provide little reflex command over the skin vessels in the face of the heat load. Central venous pressure and cardiac filling decline and cardiac output falls, eventually provoking a vasovagal syncope where the efferent pattern seems to be identical with that induced in emotional fainting (Chapter 19).

Emotional stimuli exert profound, but usually transient, effects on skin vessels, especially those in the face, hands and feet. As mentioned, the emotional blushing of the face in man may or may not involve specific dilator fibres. The slightest "alerting response" is usually accompanied by a transient constriction especially of the cutaneous A-V anastomoses, in the hands, for instance. However, if emotional sweating is induced as well, a vasodilator response, probably due to kinin release, may partly mask the neurogenic constriction and cause a "cold sweat". These responses may be very pronounced in fully developed defence reactions. Authors through the ages have done full justice to the infinitely variegated appearance of the facial skin in circumstances of emotion. Our own favourite, culled from a paperback novel (presumably subjected to slovenly proofreading) is, "A rosy slush dismantled her features".

References

Barcroft, H. (1960). "Sympathetic control of vessels in the hand and forearm skin," *Physiol. Rev.* **40,** Suppl., 4, 80–99.

Burton, A. C., and O. G. Edholm (1955). *Man in cold environment*. London: Arnold.

Edholm, O. G., R. H. Fox, and R. K. Macpherson (1956). "Effect of body heating on the circulation in skin and muscle," *J. Physiol.* **134,** 612–19. (London.)

Folkow, B., and O. Celander (1953a). "A comparison of the sympathetic vasomotor fibre control of the vessels within the skin and the muscles," *Acta Physiol. Scand.* **29,** 241–50.

Folkow, B., and O. Celander (1953b). "The nature and the distribution of afferent fibres provided with the axon reflex arrangement," *Acta Physiol. Scand.* **29,** 359–70.

Folkow, B., and O. Celander (1953c). "The correlation between the stimulation frequency and the dilator response evoked by 'antidromic' excitation of the thin afferent fibres in the dorsal roots," *Acta Physiol. Scand.* **29,** 371–76.

Folkow, B., R. H. Fox, J. Krog, H. Odelram, and O. Thorén (1963). "Studies on the reactions of the cutaneous vessels to cold exposure," *Acta Physiol. Scand.* **58,** 342–54.

Fox, R. H., and S. M. Hilton (1958). "Bradykinin formation in human skin as a factor in heat vasodilatation," *J. Physiol.* **142,** 219–32.

Gaskell, P., and D. L. Hoeppner (1966). "The relative influence of nervous control and of local warming on arteriolar muscle during indirect vasodilatation," *Can. J. Physiol. Pharmacol.* **45,** 83–91.

Greenfield, A. D. M. (1963). "The circulation through the skin," *Handbook of Physiology*, 2, Circulation **II,** 1324–51.

Guyton, A. (1963). "A concept of negative interstitial pressure based on pressures in implanted perforated capsules," *Circ. Res.* **XII,** 399–414.

Hardy, J. D. (1961). "Physiology of temperature regulation," *Physiol. Rev.* **41,** 521–606.

Hertzman, A. B. (1959). "Vasomotor regulation of cutaneous circulation," *Physiol. Rev.* **39,** 280–306.

Irving, L. (1967). "Ecology and thermoregulation," *Les consepts de Claude Bernard sur le milieu intérieur*. Fond. Singer-Polignac, 381–92. Paris: Masson & Cié.

Keatinge, W. R. (1958). "The effect of low temperatures on the responses of arteries to constrictor drugs," *J. Physiol.* **142,** 395–405.

Krog, J., B. Folkow, R. H. Fox, and K. L. Andersen (1960). "Hand circulation in the cold of Lapps and north Norwegian fishermen," *J. Appl. Physiol.* **15,** 654–58.

Lewis, T. (1927). *The blood vessels of the human skin and their responses.* London: Shaw.

Löfving, B. (1961). "Differentiated vascular adjustments reflexly induced by changes in the carotid baro- and chemoreceptor activity and by asphyxia," *Med. Exp.* **4,** 307–12. (Basel.)

Mellander, S., B. Öberg, and H. Odelram (1964). "Vascular adjustments to increased transmural pressure in cat and man with special reference to shifts in capillary fluid transfers," *Acta Physiol. Scand.* **61,** 34–48.

Roddie, I. C., J. T. Shepherd, and R. F. Whelan (1958). "Reflex changes in human skeletal muscle blood flow, associated with intrathoracic pressure changes," *Circ. Res.* **6,** 232–38.

Scholander, P. F., and W. E. Schevill (1955). "Counter-current vascular heat exchange in the fins of whales," *J. Appl. Physiol.* **8,** 279–82.

Scholander, P. F., R. Hock, V. Walters, F. Johnson, and L. Irving (1950). "Heat regulation in some arctic and tropical mammals and birds," *Biol. Bull.* **2,** 237–58.

Ström, G. (1960). "Central nervous regulation of body temperature," *Handbook of Physiology*, 1, Neurophysiology **II**, 1173–96.

26

Gastrointestinal and Liver Circulations

General Considerations

The gastrointestinal (G.I.) tract is designed for the intake and mechanical-chemical treatment of food which, when mixed with secreted juices, is split into basic constituents by enzymes. These constituents are absorbed into the bloodstream; non-digested material is ultimately expelled. Most of the absorbed material is carried via the portal vein to the liver; the bulk of lipid material, however, enters the lymphatics and reaches the general circulation by this route. The liver may immediately burn the food products, may store them, or may, when necessary, transform them into more suitable molecular forms and pass them on via the hepatic vein to the general blood stream.

The G.I. system therefore displays (1) a variety of specialized motility functions, effected in the main by *smooth muscle*; (2) a daily secretion (a total of 6 to 8 litres in man) of digestive juices (saliva, gastric, intestinal, pancreatic secretions, bile) by various *gland cells*; and (3) an efficient and differentiated absorption of nutritional material, effected both actively and passively across a huge surface of *epithelial cells*.

Such functions require a highly organized vascular bed which debouches finally upon the liver. The liver is coupled in series with the G.I. tract by means of the portal vein, which drains essentially all abdominal sections

466

of the gut. The liver is the main chemical factory of the body and its oxygen usage is nearly 20% of that of the whole body in a man at rest. Its oxygen supply is reinforced by the hepatic artery, which provides 25 to 30% of its blood flow and 40 to 50% of the oxygen used. Portal venous and hepatic arterial blood mix in the so-called hepatic sinusoids, from which the hepatic vein returns the blood to the inferior caval vein. Thus, the vascular bed of the liver is coupled both *in series with* and *in parallel to* the G.I. tract.

The combined vascular beds of liver and gut are often called the *splanchnic circulation*, and in a 70-kg man it approaches 4 kg in tissue bulk, excluding the mesenteries and their highly varying fat deposits. The liver weighs about 1.5 kg. The G.I. tract and pancreas (60 to 80 g) amounts to about 2 kg of tissue, of which perhaps half is smooth muscle and the other half mainly glandular and mucosal structures. The spleen is a small organ (200 g) in man, but in some animals it serves as an important blood depot and may contain as much as 10 to 20% of the blood volume. The splenic vein joins the portal vein.

At rest, the splanchnic vascular bed receives some 25% of cardiac output, nearly 1500 ml/min in a 70-kg man, and of this, 25 to 30% is provided by the hepatic artery. Thus, during rest the liver has the richest blood supply of the major organs in the splanchnic region, while in the G.I. tract itself the duodenum has the largest blood flow when calculated per unit weight (Steiner and Mueller, 1961).

If all the splanchnic vessels were maximally dilated simultaneously, their total blood flow would probably be about 4 to 5 l/min. However, even during intense hyperaemia seen during digestion of a large meal, the G.I. compartments are not involved together, but rather in a *sequential* fashion, so that the actual flow increase at any one time is only some 50% above that at rest. Possibly the highest blood flow to the gut occurs in violent gastrointestinal infections.

Some recent reviews, covering various aspects of the G.I. and liver circulations, are available and should be consulted for details and references (Brauer, 1963; Bradley, 1963; Grim, 1963; Grayson and Mendel, 1965; Texter, 1963; and a recent symposium on G.I. circulation, Jacobson, 1967). This chapter deals mainly with the general principles of splanchnic vascular control; aspects of the reflex and central involvement of the splanchnic circulation in over-all cardiovascular control are presented in Chapter 18 and 19.

The G.I. Tract

Vascular Dimensions and Local Vascular Control of Various G.I. Compartments

Salivary and Pancreatic Glands

The vascular bed of the salivary and pancreatic glands is more uniform than that of stomach and gut wall, although the small but important pancreatic islets provide an exception to this statement. Both glands are composed of secretory cells (of course of different character) each capable of an abundant production of its particular secretion (Burgen and Emmelin, 1961).

Salivary glands, when maximally excited, produce nearly their own weight of saliva per min; for this reason it is clear that their vascular beds must allow for very high blood flows and a huge capillary exchange surface, which is of the fenestrated type. The demand for delivery of the raw material by the plasma for the formation of the secretion often far exceeds the nutritional demands for oxygen. As the extraction of a substantial portion of the plasma would greatly increase viscosity and plasma oncotic pressure, maximal blood flow capacity must far exceed the maximal secretory volume.

A maximal blood flow near 700 ml/min/100 g has been recorded at a pressure head of 100 mm Hg, together with a maximal secretion of 70 ml within the cat's salivary gland. The average "extraction" from the plasma is then of the order of 15 to 20%, but it may reach 30% (Martinsson and Odelram, 1968). It seems likely that the vascular bed of the pancreas has nearly as great a flow capacity, though for functional reasons there is not the same demand for creating abrupt or massive increases in pancreatic secretion. Resting blood flow, however, is only of the order of 20 to 25 ml/min/100 g. This means that basal vascular tone is high and the establishment of functional hyperaemia dramatic.

Parasympathetic nerves supply and stimulate the salivary glands and, closely coupled to this activation, hyperaemia is induced (Burgen and Emmelin, 1961). Not only does relaxation of the resistance and sphincter sections occur, but there is also a considerable increase in capillary permeability, presumably allowing for the huge transfer of fluid and solutes. Häggendal and Sivertsson (1967) have recently shown that this increase of flow passes only through the capillary bed and not partly through A-V shunts, as was earlier often believed.

Following the introduction of the concept of specific vasodilator fibres by Claude Bernard (1858), it has been generally assumed that such fibres were mainly responsible for the functional vasodilatation in the salivary glands. This appeared likely, both because atropine suppressed the secretion of the gland, although leaving the dilatation almost unchanged, and because the neurogenically induced hyperaemia far exceeded the increased O_2 consumption and production of conventional vasodilator metabolites. Likewise, it was thought that vagal stimulation elicits pancreatic vasodilatation. However, Kraut *et al.* (1930), by extraction of pancreatic tissue, discovered *kallikrein*, which on intravenous injection produced intense vasodilatation. Hilton and Lewis (1956) showed that the activation of both salivary and pancreatic gland cells release a specific proteolytic enzyme, identical with kallikrein, into the tissue spaces, which splits off a vasodilator polypeptide from a plasma and tissue fluid globulin, *kininogen* (Fig. 26-1). This polypeptide was first thought to be the nonapeptide *bradykinin* but is now considered to be the decapeptide *kallidin* (lysin-bradykinin; Webster and Pierce, 1963; see also Chapter 16). Plasma and tissue fluid enzymes appear to rapidly transform kallidin into bradykinin. These substances are the most powerful vasodilator agents known and their vasodilator action appears to be accompanied by an increase of capillary permeability.

This type of specialized vasodilator mechanism—of a nature intermediate between specific dilator fibres and conventional vasodilator metabolites—appears to be the *main* cause of the remarkable increase of blood flow and capillary permeability which furnishes the raw material for the profuse secretion of these glands. Release of these polypeptides is also involved in the potentiated cutaneous vasodilatation which occurs when sweat glands are activated and in the hyperaemia which takes place when the pancreas is stimulated. It may be important in the hyperaemia which accompanies secretory activity of the G.I. mucosa (see below). This does not deny that specific vasodilator fibres also play a role in the establishment of functional hyperaemia in the salivary glands (Schachter and Beilenson, 1967). Recent experiments strongly suggest that *both* mechanisms are involved. It might be that the larger resistance vessels are controlled by such fibres and that the kinin mechanism mainly affects the smallest resistance vessels and the capillaries (Gautvik, 1970).

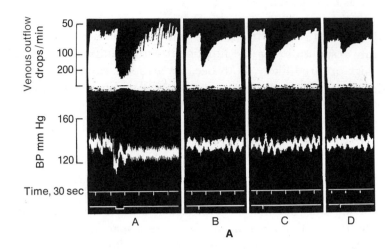

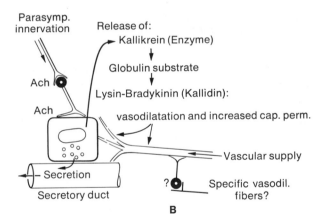

Fig. 26-1. A. The effect of stimulation of the submandibular gland on its blood flow (a). In (b) and (c) 0.2 ml of 0.1% saliva and 0.2% saliva, respectively, were injected intra-arterially. Note the pronounced vasodilatation due to the presence of kallikrein in the saliva. The injection of saline (d) causes only a slight transient increase of blood flow presumably by lowering blood viscosity. (From Hilton and Lewis, 1956. By permission.)

B. The vasodilatation is due to the presence of kallikrein in the saliva which acts as an enzyme to split off from a globulin the powerful vasodilator lysin-bradykinin (kallidin). This, in turn, can be rapidly transformed into bradykinin.

The sympathetic innervation of the vessels in salivary glands allows for a rather powerful vasoconstrictor effect, but it can also, at least in some species and glands, induce a relatively sparse production of mucus-rich secretion. This type of secretory response is also accompanied by a transient but moderate hyperaemia, possibly due to the kinin mechanism and to the production of "conventional" vasodilator metabolites.

The Stomach

The wall of the stomach, like that of the intestine, is composed of smooth muscle, an intramural nerve cell plexus, glandular structures, and a specialized surface epithelium. For these reasons the gastric vascular bed, like that of the intestines, should be considered as comprising a set of parallel-coupled circuits, specialized for the requirements of these different

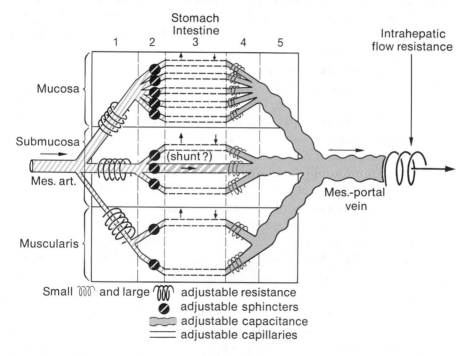

Fig. 26-2. Schematic illustration of the different tissue compartments in the stomach and intestines, with their specialized parallel-coupled vascular circuits and their consecutive sections (1. precapillary resistance vessels, 2. "sphincter" sections, 3. capillaries, 4. postcapillary resistance vessels, and 5. capacitance vessels.) (Modified from Folkow, 1967. By permission.)

tissue compartments (see Jacobson, 1967) (Fig. 26-2). During resting conditions gastric blood flow is some 20 to 40 ml/min/100 g and during maximal dilatation it may increase to some 150 ml/min/100 g. However, as
several tissue compartments are present, measurements of the net arterial
or venous blood flow in the stomach (or intestine) may conceal, for instance, an increased mucosal blood flow which occurs perhaps together
with a reduction of the flow to the smooth muscle part of the wall. The use
of techniques like the clearance of ^{85}Kr, etc. (Chapter 7) has shed new
light on such problems.

Flow in different wall compartments: The *smooth muscle component* of the
gastric wall (and that of the small and large intestine) may receive up to
40 ml/min/100 g tissue during maximal vasodilatation—a figure which is
not very different from that of phasic skeletal muscles. However, it seems
likely that the difference between "resting" and maximal metabolism is
far less in smooth muscle than in skeletal muscle, and that the blood supply
to smooth muscle suffices to cover metabolic demands aerobically.
Mechanical interferences with flow, as produced by very intense gastrointestinal contractions, might occasionally interfere with the blood supply.
The blood supply of the smooth muscle compartment is 10 to 15 ml/min/
100 g during basal conditions. The blood supply of the *intramural ganglionic
plexus* is likely to be rich but no measurements exist concerning this small
tissue compartment.

The *mucosal-glandular compartment* of the stomach seems to have a maximal blood flow of some 300 to 400 ml/min/100 g, while the blood supply
to the glandular crypts might reach figures as high as those for the salivary
glands, if parallels can be drawn from studies in the intestine. Under
"resting" conditions gastric mucosal blood flow is 50 to 80 ml (Delaney
and Grim, 1964; Jansson *et al.*, 1966). It has been suggested (Walder,
1952) that the stomach wall contains specific submucosal A-V anastomoses
(so possibly does the duodenum), but the functional significance of these
pathways remains obscure.

Functional Hyperaemia: Vagal stimulation causes hyperaemia, primarily
confined to the mucosa and its glandular section. Gastric vagi contain two
groups of efferent fibres. Low-threshold motor fibres evoke increased gastric
motility; stimulation of the high-threshold group elicits a pattern of corpus-
fundus relaxation (responsible for reflex "receptive relaxation" of the
stomach), gastric secretion, and increased mucosal blood flow (Martinson,
1965). (See Fig. 26-3.) Whether this mucosal vasodilatation is due to "con-

ventional" vasodilator metabolites, to specific vasodilator fibre endings, to kinin release; and/or to the local release of histamine, which seems to form a link in the complex events leading to acid secretion, is not yet known.

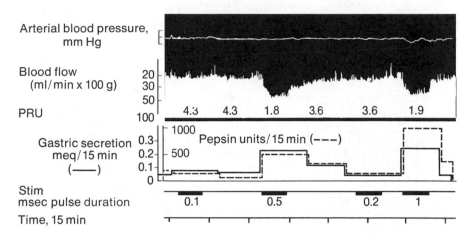

Fig. 26-3. Effect of stimulation of the high-threshold vagal fibres on gastric blood flow and secretion. First when the threshold of these fibres is reached (pulse duration at least 0.5 msec at 5 volts) the secretory and vasodilator responses appear together with a profound relaxation of the corpus-fundus region. The vasodilatation is primarily confined to the mucosa, to judge from studies of [85]Kr clearance. (From Martinson, 1965. By permission.)

The Small Intestine

Here again the same types of tissue compartments exist, but a new functional element is added by the huge villous surface specialized for absorption. During resting equilibrium, and at low or negligible vasoconstrictor fibre discharge, the total blood supply of the small intestine of the cat is 20 to 40 ml/min/100 g. This increases to 250 to 300 ml/min/100 g on maximal dilatation. There is little evidence that a capillary bypass by means of specific A-V shunts in submucosal part, as suggested earlier (Spanner 1932), is of any functional importance.

The intestinal vascular bed characteristically displays a marked autoregulation of flow (Johnson, 1964; see also Chapter 16), as do most of the other parts of the G.I. tract. Thus, if the arterial pressure is lowered from high levels down to 35 to 40 mm Hg, the blood flow and the capillary pressure change but little. This constancy of the capillary pressure as a result of the autoregulation is functionally important, for the huge fenestrated capillary surface area of the mucosa would otherwise imply a considerable risk of rapid oedema formation.

Flow in different wall compartments: The blood supply to the *smooth muscle* portion of the small intestine is of the same order as in the stomach. In the *mucosa* (Fig. 26-4) there is an especially rich vascularization of the secretory crypts, where maximal blood flow figures rivalling those in the

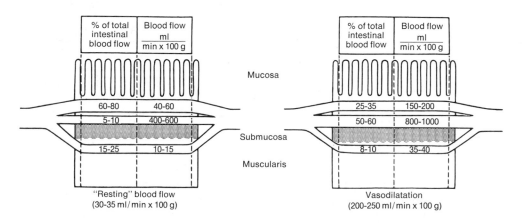

Fig. 26-4. Blood flow distribution in the small intenstine of the cat at "rest" and intense vasodilatation. The three vascular pathways depict in essence the villous mucosal circulation, the submucosal circulation, especially that of the secretory crypts, and the muscularis circulation. Note the huge flows in the submucosa, presumably reflecting the rich vascularization of the secretory crypts. (From Lundgren, 1967. By permission.)

salivary glands seem to be reached (700 ml/min/100 g and more). In the cat the maximal blood flow capacity in the "absorptive", villous part of the intestinal mucosa may reach 150–200 ml/min/100 g from a resting value of 40–60 ml (Lundgren, 1967).

The total capillary surface area of the mucosa, as measured by determinations of PS and CFC (Chapter 8), is correspondingly large (Fig. 26-5). Both techniques give values for the intestine as a whole which are ten times higher than those of skeletal muscle (Wallentin, 1966). If the muscularis compartment has a capillary surface area per unit weight similar to that of skeletal muscle, it follows that the mucosa has an enormous capillary surface area available for pore-bound secretion and absorption. However, since the mucosal capillaries are fenestrated (Chapter 8), and especially suited for such processes, the presence of a dense population of such larger pores helps to explain the large values for PS and CFC.

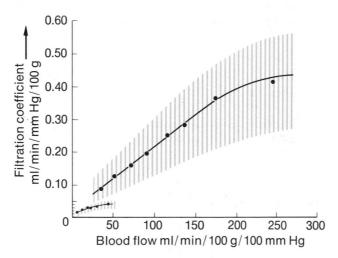

Fig. 26-5. The correlation between blood flow and capillary filtration coefficient (CFC, reflecting the perfused capillary surface area) when the basal vascular tone of the intestinal circuit in the cat is gradually reduced until maximal dilatation is reached. As a comparison the same correlation for phasic skeletal muscle is given (curve in lower left corner). (From Folkow *et al.*, 1963. By permission.)

The exact mechanisms involved in the creation of mucosal functional hyperaemia in the small intestine are not known. There is no evidence that specific parasympathetic dilator fibres exist. Intestinal secretion is governed more by hormonal and local mechanisms than by extrinsic nerves, but this does not, of course, exclude the possibility of a local formation of kinins. An increased production of vasodilator metabolites probably contributes to the establishment of functional hyperaemia in the mucosa and also in the muscularis.

Villous countercurrent mechanism: An especially interesting and functionally important phenomenon is met within the intestinal villi, where the vessels are arranged in the form of complex hairpin loops. Strong evidence (Lundgren, 1967) has been presented for *a countercurrent exchange* in the villi (Fig. 26-6). Such a mechanism would imply an automatic "damping" of the entrance into the general bloodstream of rapidly absorbed materials, particularly of small lipid-soluble particles which can pass across the entire exchange surface, but probably also for molecules like water, which relatively freely penetrates cell membranes. When such substances are carried with the bloodstream in the descending limbs of the hairpin loop they will pass very close to the ascending bloodstream, and the concentration difference will lead to their entrance into the ascending bloodstream by means of cross-diffusion. Consequently, high concentrations of absorbed substances will be reached in outer parts of the villi in the steady-state

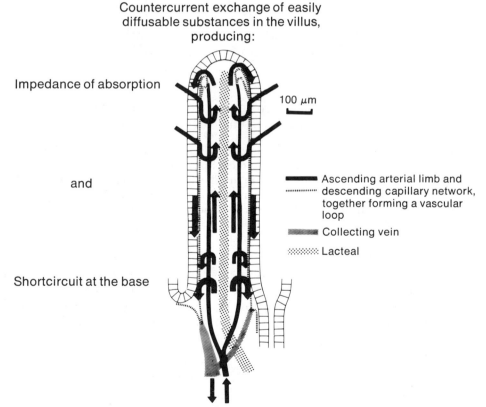

Fig. 26-6. Principles of the countercurrent exchange in the villus "hairpin loops" of the small intestine. (From Lundgren, 1967. By permission.)

situation and they will leave the villi by the venous drainage relatively slowly. Thus, the entrance of the highly diffusible ^{85}Kr from the lumen into the venous effluent is so slow that it is fully equilibrated with only 10 to 15% of the intestinal bloodstream, while some 70% of this bloodstream reaches the mucosa. Molecules or ions which are less diffusible are less affected by such a countercurrent mechanism (Lundgren and Svanvik, 1968).

Conversely, rapidly diffusing molecules in the arterial blood stream, such as oxygen, will tend to leave the arterial ascending limbs of the villi, and by such cross-diffusion become "short-circuited" over to the venous descending limbs. Thus, the O_2 tension at the tip of the villi will be lower than that at their base. Such a consequence of the countercurrent system may be one reason for the rapid turnover of epithelial cells at the tip of the villi, where oxygen delivery is probably poor. It is known that there is a steady and considerable production of new epithelial cells from basal parts of the villi which are gradually displaced towards the tip. There may be other important functional consequences of the hairpin arrangement of the blood flow in the villi which are still unknown. In any case, when the villous bloodstream becomes rapid, such as in very intense dilatation, less time is available for cross-diffusion and countercurrent "trapping" may then be less efficient. It is, however, premature to discuss the importance of the villous countercurrent exchange in intestinal absorption in more detail.

The arrangement of the vascular tree in the intestinal wall also favours the occurrence of "plasma skimming". There is evidence that the blood reaching the villous part of the mucosa has a decidedly lower haematocrit than that going to, for example, the muscularis. The functional importance of this arrangement is not known.

The Large Intestine

Essentially the same tissue compartments are present in the large intestine as in the small, but as the colonic mucosa has no villi, its mucosal vessels show no hairpin loops, and its powers of absorption are normally limited to the transference of water and electrolytes. The colonic mucosa produces a mucous secretion.

Flow in different wall compartments: The blood supply of the muscularis shows the same general characteristics as that of the stomach and small intestine. The mucosa is well vascularized, showing a maximal blood flow level of 200 to 250 ml/min/100 g, with an especially rich supply at the bases of the secretory crypts. During "rest" total blood flow to the colonic wall is of the order of 15 to 25 ml/min/100 g, but the mucosal flow (30 to 35 ml/min/100 g) is about three times larger than that of the muscularis, which is some 10 ml/min/100 g (Hultén, 1969).

Functional hyperaemia: Stimulation of the sacral parasympathetic supply causes increased motility, mucosal secretion, and a virtually maximal, though usually transient, increase of the mucosal blood flow only, which seems to be accompanied by an increased capillary permeability. This mucosal vasodilatation in response to parasympathetic stimulation, like that in the salivary glands, is hardly affected by atropine. The secreted mucus, like saliva, possesses a strong vasodilator action. It is therefore possible that this "neurogenic" hyperaemia, closely coupled not only with an increased motility but also with a secretory response, is mainly, perhaps entirely, due to a local production of vasodilator kinins, linked to the primary neurogenic activation of the secretory cells (Hultén, 1969).

Vasoconstrictor Fibre Control of the G.I. Tract

The entire G.I. tract and its associated glands are richly supplied with vasoconstrictor fibres which affect both the precapillary and postcapillary sections.

Precapillary Nervous Control

The resistance response to sustained sympathetic stimulation of the small intestine is very characteristic. An initial, often marked, increase of resistance occurs, but this is usually followed by a rapid decline ("autoregulatory escape") within 1 to 2 min, after which a steady-state situation is reached, in which resistance is only moderately higher than that of the control value, despite the continuation of sympathetic stimulation (Fig. 26-7). This "autoregulatory escape" from the constrictor fibre influence is not solely, or even mainly, a consequence of the accumulation of local vasodilator metabolites, secondary to the reduced flow, for it occurs even at *constant-flow* perfusion. It seems rather to reflect an intramural flow redistribution of a purely local origin, since the capillary filtration coefficient

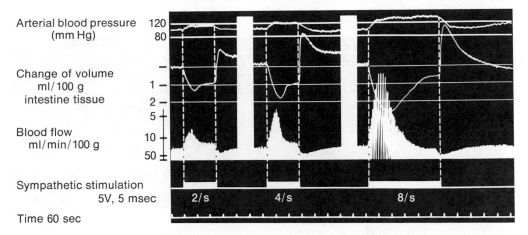

Arterial blood pressure
(mm Hg)

Change of volume
ml/100 g
intestine tissue

Blood flow
ml/min/100 g

Sympathetic stimulation
5V, 5 msec

Time 60 sec

Fig. 26-7. Effect of sympathetic vasoconstrictor fibre stimulation on intestinal blood flow (drop recorder technique) and tissue volume (reflecting regional blood volume) in the cat. Note the gradually increasing vasoconstrictor responses as stimulation frequency is increased but also the increasingly powerful "autoregulatory escape". Upon cessation of the stimulation a reactive hyperaemia ensues. (From Folkow *et al.*, 1964. By permission.)

(CFC) and the PS values remain reduced throughout constrictor fibre stimulation (Fig. 26-8).

The combined evidence suggests that the constrictor fibres produce a sustained reduction of outer mucosal blood flow, which probably is the reason why CFC is reduced, since considerable parts of the mucosal capillary flow appear to be obstructed. This means, then, that blood flow increases elsewhere, and probably in deeper parts of the mucosa-submucosa, but evidently this does not involve passage of the blood through non-nutritional A-V shunts (Wallentin, 1966) as has sometimes been assumed in the past. Possibly this secondary flow increase takes place around the secretory crypts and/or it may involve the peculiar sinusoidal "Venenbällchen" arrangements in the submucosa, which appear to be supplied by small arterioles with longitudinal smooth muscle (Spanner, 1932). In any case, it seems clear that these neurogenic intramural flow adjustments cannot be irrelevant for intestinal function with respect to absorptive and secretory events, for example.

One of the consequences of the precapillary autoregulatory escape is that neurogenic vasoconstriction in the G.I. tract causes no significant

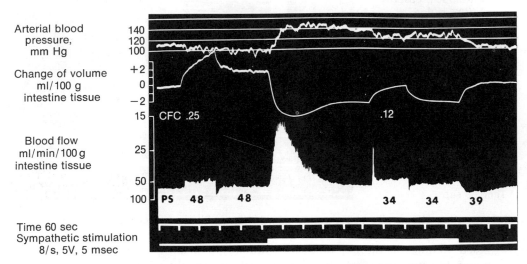

Arterial blood pressure, mm Hg

140
120
100

Change of volume ml/100 g intestine tissue

+2
0
−2

Blood flow ml/min/100 g intestine tissue

CFC .25   .12

15
25
50
100

PS   48   48   34   34   39

Time 60 sec
Sympathetic stimulation
8/s, 5V, 5 msec

Fig. 26-8. Sympathetic vasoconstrictor fibre stimulation and its effects on blood flow, regional blood volume, and CFC and PS values in the small intestine of the cat. Note that regional blood volume, CFC and PS remain low throughout the period of stimulation whereas the resistance response displays a marked "autoregulatory escape" after its initial increase. (From Dresel *et al.*, 1966. By permission.)

shifts in mean capillary pressure, as is obvious from the isovolumetric state shown in Fig. 26-8. This is in striking contrast to the situation in the skeletal muscle (Chapter 20). Hence, the reflex adjustments in the G.I. circuit, which has an enormous capillary surface but a relatively small amount of interstitial fluid, do not normally serve as significant regulators of plasma volume in the same way as they do in the muscle circuit. The G.I. circuit has little to "give" of fluid and has little accommodation for extra tissue fluid, since, in this rather small tissue mass with a huge, highly porous capillary surface, increases of capillary pressure might rapidly lead to oedema, especially in the mucosa. In fact, part of the importance of the "autoregulatory escape" is that, in one way or the other, it balances off any neurogenic shifts in mean capillary pressure within the G.I. tract.

The characteristic neurogenic redistribution of flow in the intestine might suggest a differentiated fibre distribution to the different vascular compartments. However, since intra-arterial infusion of noradrenaline produces much the same type of response, it would then follow that not only the nerve ramifications but also the location of the α-receptors show a differentiated distribution. No doubt, therefore, interesting but so far poorly understood blood flow adjustments occur in the intestinal wall upon vasoconstrictor fibre activation, and largely similar, though not quite so extensive, local adjustments of the primary constrictor fibre effect are seen also in the stomach and colon. Detailed analyses of compartmental blood flow changes in the intestinal wall during vasoconstrictor fibre activation, using ^{85}Kr clearance, have confirmed such intramural flow redistributions (Lundgren, 1968).

Occasionally no "autoregulatory escape" is seen, so that the vasoconstrictor fibre reductions of flow are then sustained, perhaps indicating that the secondary increases in deep mucosal-submucosal blood flow may fail to appear, for unknown reasons.

Postcapillary Nervous Control

The constrictor fibre effect on the *venous* side of the G.I. tract is usually well sustained and powerful (Fig. 26-8). Apparently there is also a postcapillary "escape", but this can be shown to be a passive-elastic phenomenon and venous smooth muscle contraction remains stable. Up to 40% of the regional blood content can be "mobilized" at discharge rates in the higher physiological range. Since the blood content of the G.I. tract proper is high, up to 7 to 8% of tissue weight, and still higher if the mesenteric vessels are included in the measurement, substantial mobilizations of blood may be achieved within the splanchnic area by means of the constrictor fibre control of the veins. Thus, it appears that about one litre of blood is present in the splanchnic area in resting man and, if 40% of this can be expelled, it would mean a mobilization of nearly half a litre of blood.

Resting sympathetic discharge to the G.I. tract has much less impact on the total resistance to flow in the splanchnic vascular bed than has often been assumed. In cats, elimination of the constrictor fibre effect by means of splanchnic nerve section usually causes less than a 20 to 30% reduction of regional flow resistance. This, in turn, means only a 5 to 7% fall in total resistance, provided that 25% of the cardiac output goes to the splanchnic circuit. Therefore, the often profound fall in blood pressure seen upon splanchnic nerve section is probably not so much a consequence of a reduction in flow resistance but is rather due to *venous pooling* within the splanchnic area, with a reduced cardiac output as a result. Even considerable reflex increases of sympathetic discharge do not usually produce more extensive increases of G.I. flow resistance, once the steady-state equilibrium is reached. *Potentially*, the effect is strong, however, and this becomes apparent if the "autoregulatory escape" does not occur, as occasionally is the case (for unknown reasons). The neurogenic responses to reflex and central autonomic activations and during shock are dealt with elsewhere (see Chapters 18, 19, 30).

The Spleen

The vascular bed of the spleen empties via the portal vein into the liver. In many animals (dog, cat) the spleen is an important blood depot which, thanks to extensive amounts of smooth muscle in the capsule and trabeculae, can greatly change its blood content. In man, the splenic capsule contains only little muscle and is small (some 200 g), and its role as a blood depot is therefore negligible.

The spleen acts as an important "RES sieve" for the blood, among other things disposing of dying erythrocytes, exerting a general phagocytotic function, and participating in the production of lymphocytes—this mainly in the Malphigian bodies ("white pulp"). Arterial follicular branches give off an extensive wide-pore capillary network in the Malphigian bodies, possibly allowing for free entrance of lymphocytes to the blood. Then the follicular arteries enter the "red pulp" while branching out into precapillary arterioles ("penicilli"), which open up in a complex network of wide-pore sinusoids which seem to be in rather free communication with the reticular meshwork of the red pulp.

It has been suggested that there should be some sphincter-like arrangements at the arteriolar and venular ends of the sinusoid-reticular meshwork which probably constitutes the "storage system" for high haematocrit blood. This is emptied by neurogenic contraction of the capsular-trabecular smooth muscle, presumably associated with relaxation of the suggested sphincterlike arrangements, even though the arterial inflow channels become constricted. However, the exact arrangements are still much debated (Grayson and Mendel, 1965).

The splenic vessels, and especially the splenic capsule and trabeculae in animals, in which the spleen serves as a reservoir, are richly supplied with adrenergic fibres, and these produce a virtually maximal emptying of blood at 3 to 4 impulses/sec (Celander, 1954). During resting conditions there seems to be virtually no discharge in these fibres (Shepherd, 1968). This is one of several examples of the differentiation of sympathetic discharge, since in the same situation there is a definite discharge, though of

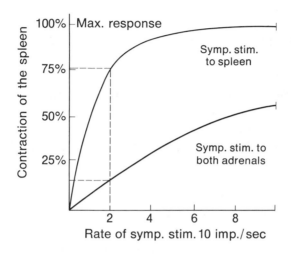

Fig. 26-9. Frequency-response characteristics for the sympathetic vaso-constrictor fibre effect on the spleen of the cat. As a comparison the effects of adrenal medullary hormones, released at similar frequencies of discharge, are shown. Note the dominating influence of the direct nervous control, also characterizing the G. I. vascular bed and most other cardiovascular effector systems. (From Celander, 1954. By permission.)

low frequency, to the skeletal muscles, for example. Blood loss, hypoxia, defence reactions, etc., induce powerful splenic contractions, but this requires only moderate sympathetic discharge in this particular organ. In dogs, this may cause a 10 to 20% increase of blood volume with a considerable rise of haematocrit, since far more cells than plasma are stored in the spleen. Circulating catecholamines exert similar but much weaker effects (Fig. 26-9).

The Liver

Vascular Arrangements and Dimensions

The influx of an arterial and a venous bloodstream, ultimately mixed in the liver sinusoids and commonly drained via the hepatic veins, imposes many intricate problems (Brauer, 1963). For example, where and how do the two influx pathways merge, how is the smooth muscle control arranged in the vessels proximal to their confluence so that no complications arise because one is a high-pressure influx, the other a low-pressure one, etc.?

Inflow Pathways

The painstaking stereographic reconstructions by Elias (1949a, b) have allowed a better understanding of the arrangements of the liver tissue and its vessels (Fig. 26-10). The liver is a very homogenous tissue and so is, in one sense of the word, its vascular bed, despite the complexity inherent in mixing an arterial and a venous inflow. Blood enters the hepatic arterial branches at a pressure close to that in the aorta. In the portal vein, on the other hand, pressure is only 10 to 12 mm Hg. Nevertheless, the two streams join and equalize their pressures as they enter the sinusoids. This necessitates a marked pressure drop along the muscular hepatic arteriolar sections, whereas the wide portal arborizations normally offer vary scant resistance to flow. Thus, the two systems meet at the proximal ends of the sinusoids at a pressure of 8 to 9 mm Hg. The pressure drop profile along the portal tree is steepest near the sinusoids, which suggests that active adjustments of flow and flow distribution may be made here (Brauer, 1963).

It is still not clear how the details of the arterial and portal inlets into the sinusoids are arranged. The most distal arteriolar branches appear to contain sphincter-like portions, as do the precapillary sections of other vascular beds. This suggests that myogenic activity occurs here and hence some "autoregulation" and rhythmicity of the influx into the peribiliary capillary plexus, via which at least part of the arterial bloodstream appears to enter the wide sinusoids. The exact details of this arrangement are, however, still debated. True shunts, which bypass the sinusoids, apparently do not exist in the liver, though "functional shunting" (Chapter 8) may occur to some extent.

The Sinusoids

The sinusoids—the specialized wide-pore capillaries of the liver—fill out the wide lacunae between the one-cell thick "plates" of liver cells, which form a complex and richly anastomosing system, almost like the walls in a building. These plates of liver cells tend to converge towards a centre with the sinusoids placed in between. The sinusoids empty into the central vein, from which debouch the tributaries of the hepatic venous system. This type of "tissue-vascular unit" constitutes what is often called the liver *lobulus*, but the entire organ features such a fairly uniform syncytial

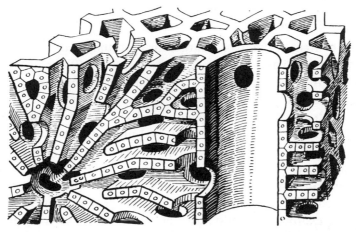

Fig. 26-10. Stereogram of a part of an hepatic lobule, with the central vein to the lower left, portal venous branch to the right, and the sinusoids in between, interconnecting through "holes" in the liver cell labyrinth. (From Elias, 1949. By permission.)

labyrinth, allowing for such free communications throughout the blood spaces, that the concept of such special subunits has sometimes been questioned (Fig. 26-10).

The endothelial cells of the sinusoids, the so-called littoral cells, some of which exhibit phagocytosis (Kupffer cells), overlap to a degree. The littoral cells are perforated and allow an almost free exchange even of macromolecules between the blood and the narrow perisinusoidal spaces. Thus, liver lymph, which emerges from these perisinusoidal spaces, contains nearly as much protein as plasma. It has sometimes been suggested that the sinusoids are able to contract actively, but here, as in other vascular circuits, it seems likely that active control of blood flow and volume is essentially dependent on the precapillary and postcapillary smooth muscles. It is true that the sinusoidal flow patterns can vary markedly, but as the sinusoids constitute a wide, freely communicating system, dependent on inflow, outflow, and regional transmural pressures, quite minor adjustments of smooth muscle tone upstream and downstream would result in considerable shifts in sinusoidal blood flow distribution. Bulging and swelling of the endothelial cells may occur: such phenomena might affect the sinusoidal lumina, but are not credited with much importance normally.

Capacitance Function

The blood content of the liver is large, for both the portal and the hepatic venous systems are voluminous, as are the sinusoids. Older figures quoted in the literature (one litre or even more) are, however, probably greatly exaggerated except, perhaps, in severe cases of liver stasis.

The entire splanchnic circuit contains slightly more than one fifth of the total blood volume in resting man, and probably not more than 30 to 40% of this fraction is normally confined to the liver. Even this means that 350 to 500 ml are present in a 1500 g organ, corresponding to a blood content per unit tissue of as much as 20 to 30%. This considerable intrahepatic "blood depot in circulation" can be drawn upon. The hepatic veins, which exhibit very little resistance to flow, are further only lightly "scaffolded" and this facilitates their passive-elastic recoil when their transmural pressure falls, as caused, for instance, by upstream constriction.

Due to complex phasic changes in the pressure gradient between the hepatic and inferior caval veins, in turn related to the respiratory movements, the hepatic outflow exhibits considerable rhythmic shifts during the phases of the respiratory cycle. Two factors are involved during inspiration: (1) mechanical compression of the G.I. bed augments portal inflow, but (2) an increase in resistance in the hepatic bed prevents the portal flow from passing on to the hepatic vein. This increases portal pooling, while at the same time, hepatic sinusoids are squeezed out and augment hepatic venous outflow. The reverse happens during expiration.

In some species, e.g. in the dog and especially in diving animals, the hepatic vein has a sphincter-like arrangement under nervous control. This may lead to considerable pooling of blood upstream and is one of the mechanisms involved in the integration of the diving reflex (Chapter 19).

Local Control of the Liver Vessels

In resting man the total blood supply to the liver averages some 100 ml/min/100 g, of which 25 to 30% is supplied by the hepatic artery. However, this arterial inflow evidently may vary to a great extent depending on the current level of basal tone of the arterial resistance vessels. This basal tone is usually high, for the resting arterial inflow of some 25 to 30 ml/min/100 g tissue may reach 100 to 150 ml/min/100 g at maximal hepatic artery dilatation.

The myogenic arterial tone is counterbalanced by the influence of the local chemical environment ("vasodilator metabolites", which in the liver might be somewhat different from those in other tissues) and as elsewhere, is influenced by vasoconstrictor fibres and blood-borne hormones (see below). Flow autoregulation is well displayed by the liver arteries (Brauer, 1964) and this is in line with the existence of an efficient local vascular control, similar to that of most other circuits. Increases in liver metabolism cause an increase of the arterial flow. Portal flow probably rises after a meal because of the functional hyperaemia in the gut: the relative changes in the two liver inflows may then be difficult to predict.

The evidently sensitive interplay between arterial myogenic tone and local chemical environment in the liver may explain why the hepatic arterial flow tends to increase if the portal inflow is reduced, and vice versa. Any reduction in the portal blood supply would probably cause an accumulation of "vasodilator metabolites", tending to dilate the arterial vessels. Such a situation resembles that in a skeletal muscle with two major arterial supply routes, where closure of the one will lead to compensatory dilatation of the other. Hence, the control of the vascular bed of the gut does not only determine, in a sense, the amount of portal blood that the liver will receive. It also thereby indirectly influences the hepatic arterial supply as well. Taken from another angle, it may be that the liver, by means of the sensitive local control of its arterial inflow, can secure a suitable oxygen supply for itself. If some G.I. adjustment reduces portal inflow, the liver appears to release the smooth muscle "throttle" on its arterial inflow by an automatic inhibition of the inherent tone of the arterial resistance vessels.

Marked dilatation of the hepatic arterial branches would, a priori, *increase* sinusoidal pressure, unless a "waterfall phenomenon" occurs at the site where these arterial channels empty into the sinusoids. If arterial dilation were to increase the sinusoidal pressure this would decrease the small gradient for portal flow and even raise the portal pressure, thereby greatly affecting the pattern of intrahepatic flow distribution. Many intricate interactions between these two inflows may exist; they are still poorly understood.

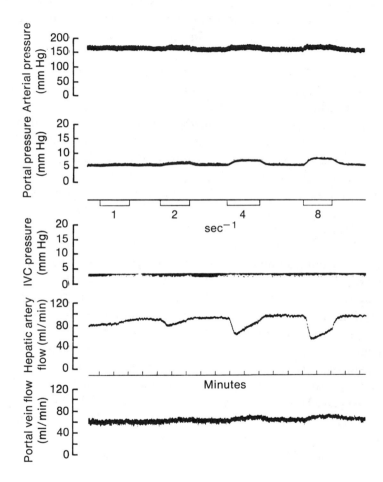

Fig. 26-11A. The response of the hepatic arterial vessels and the portal venous vessels to increasing frequencies of sympathetic vasoconstrictor fibres. Note the rather pronounced effects on the arterial inflow to the liver which, however, soon decline due to autoregulatory escape. In contrast, the portal vein responses, though fairly weak, are sustained throughout the period of stimulation. (From Greenway *et al.*, 1967. By permission.)

Nervous Control of Liver Vessels

Local control of the tone of the hepatic arterial vessels seems to dominate even the vasoconstrictor fibre influence. Thus, during sustained constrictor fibre stimulation the arterial flow to the liver approaches or returns to normal after a peak constrictor effect, which may imply an increase of resistance up to fivefold, at a high rate of discharge, but which usually lasts only about a minute. Interestingly enough, such an "escape" from the constrictor fibre influence occurs even when the liver is supplied by a *constant* arterial inflow (pump perfusion) (Greenway *et al.*, 1967). Such a response is similar, then, to that seen in the small intestine, and it suggests either that the vasoconstrictor fibre effect induces some redistribution of intrahepatic flow or that some other type of smooth muscle adjustment is induced secondarily. Further, it is conceivable that the adrenergic fibres may themselves induce metabolic changes in the liver cells, which may secondarily affect vascular tone. There is no evidence of any dilator fibres to the liver vessels.

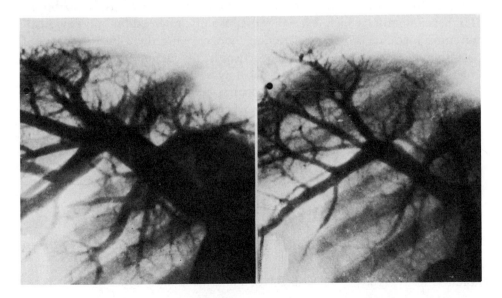

Fig. 26-11B. The effect of sympathetic vasoconstrictor fibre stimulation on the "capacitance" function of the portal tree. Left: before stimulation; right: during stimulation. (From Daniel and Prichard, 1951. By permission.)

The vasoconstrictor fibres also affect the portal vessels, raising their low resistance to flow, and causing a moderate rise in the portal pressure if there is not simultaneously a reduced portal flow, secondary to a G.I. vasoconstriction. In contrast to those on the arterial inflow, the effects of sympathetic vasoconstrictor stimulation on the portal vessels are well sustained.

In keeping with their influence on the portal flow resistance the vaso-constrictor stimulation causes a relatively marked reduction of the blood content within the portal tree (Daniel and Pritchard, 1951). Thus, sym-pathetic control of hepatic capacitance, directly and indirectly affecting the hepatic venous tree as well, is relatively marked. Perhaps as much as 30 to 40% of the liver blood content may be expelled by active constriction and passive-elastic recoil, if parallels may be drawn with the extent of capacitance responses in other tissues.

The hormonal output of the adrenal medulla—mainly adrenaline in man—causes liver *vasodilatation* when administered in amounts comparable to those normally released by the adrenal glands in life. This may be due either to a dominant presence of β-receptors in the vascular smooth mus-cles, or to metabolic effects of adrenaline on the liver cells, or to both. Higher amounts, which exceed those usually released in physiological circumstances, cause vasoconstriction by occupying the α-receptors.

Other hormones (insulin, glucocorticoids, glucagon, etc.) which cause metabolic changes in the liver cells may secondarily affect liver blood flow as well. Whether they exert any primary effects on the liver vasculature is not known. The infusion of amino acids causes increased liver blood flow (Brauer, 1964), possibly as a result of increased liver cell metabolism in connection with the imposed intermediary metabolic turnover.

References

Bradley, S. E. (1963). "The hepatic circulation," *Handbook of Physiology*, 2, Circulation **II**, 1387–1438.

Brauer, R. W. (1963). "Liver circulation and function," *Physiol. Rev.* **43**, 115–213.

Brauer, R. W. (1964). "Autoregulation of blood flow in the liver," *Circ. Res.* **XIV, XV,** Suppl., 1, 213–53.

Burgen, A. S. V., and N. G. Emmelin (1961). *Physiology of the salivary glands.* London: Edward Arnold Ltd.

Celander, O. (1954). "The range of control exercised by the 'sympathico-adrenal system,'" *Acta Physiol. Scand.* **32,** Suppl., 116.

Daniel, P. M., and M. M. L. Prichard (1951). "Effects of stimulation of the hepatic nerves and of adrenaline upon the circulation of the portal venous blood within the liver," *J. Physiol.* **114,** 538–48.

Delaney, J., and E. Grim (1964). "Canine gastric blood flow and its distribution," *Am. J. Physiol.* **207,** 1195–1202.

Dresel, P., B. Folkow, and I. Wallentin (1966). "Rubidium[86] clearance during neurogenic redistribution of intestinal blood flow," *Acta Physiol. Scand.* **67,** 173–84.

Elias, H. (1949). "A re-examination of the structure of the mammalian liver, I. Parenchymal architecture," *Am. J. Anat.* **84,** 311–27; "A re-examination of the structure of the mammalian liver, II. The hepatic lobule and its relation to the vascular and biliary systems," *Am. J. Anat.* **85,** 379–456.

Folkow, B. (1967). "Regional adjustments of intestinal blood flow," *Gastroenterology,* **52,** 423–32.

Folkow, B., O. Lundgren, and I. Wallentin (1963). "Studies on the relationship between flow resistance, capillary filtration coefficient and regional blood volume in the intestine of the cat," *Acta Physiol. Scand.* **57,** 270–83.

Folkow, B., D. H. Lewis, O. Lundgren, S. Mellander, and I. Wallentin (1964). "The effect of graded vasoconstrictor fibre stimulation on the intestinal resistance and capacitance vessels," *Acta Physiol. Scand.* **61,** 445–57.

Gautvik, K. (1970). "The interaction of two different vasodilator mechanisms in the chorda-tympani activated submandibular salivary gland," *Acta Physiol. Scand.,* **79,** 188–203.

Grayson, J., and D. Mendel (1965) *Physiology of the splanchnic circulation.* London: Edward Arnold Ltd.

Greenway, C. V., A. E. Lawson, and S. Mellander (1967). "The effects of stimulation of the hepatic nerves, infusions of noradrenaline and occlusion of the carotid arteries on liver blood flow in the anaesthetized cat," *J. Physiol.* **192,** 21–41.

Grim, E. (1963). "The flow of blood in the mesenteric vessels," *Handbook of Physiology,* 2, Circulation **II,** 1439–56.

Häggendal, E., and R. Sivertsson (1967). "About arterio-venous shunts in salivary glands," *Acta Physiol. Scand.* **71,** 85–88.

Hilton, S. M., and G. P. Lewis (1956). "The relationship between glandular activity, bradykinin formation and functional vasodilatation in the submandibular salivary gland," *J. Physiol.* **134,** 471–83.

Hultén, L. (1969). "Extrinsic nervous control of colonic motility and blood flow," *Acta Physiol. Scand.*, Suppl., 335.

Jacobson, E. D. ed. (1967) "The gastrointestinal circulation" (symposium), *Gastroenterology*, **52,** 332–471.

Jansson, G., M. Kampp, O. Lundgren, and J. Martinson (1966). "Studies on the circulation of the stomach," *Acta Physiol. Scand.* **68,** Suppl. 277, 91.

Johnson, P. C. (1964). "Origin, localization, and homeostatic significance of autoregulation in the intestine," *Circ. Res.* **XIV, XV,** Suppl., 1, 225–32.

Kraut, H., E. K. Frey, and E. Werle (1930). "Der Nachweiss eines Kreislaufhormons in der Pankreasdrüse," *Hoppe-Seyl.* **189,** 97–106.

Lundgren, O. (1967). "Studies on blood flow distribution and countercurrent exchange in the small intestine," *Acta Physiol. Scand.*, Suppl., 303.

Lundgren, O. (1968). Personal communication.

Lundgren, O., and J. Svanvik (1968). "Uptake of Kr^{85} from the lumen of the small intestine to the intestinal blood in the cat," *Acta Physiol. Scand.* **74,** 20A–21A.

Martinson, J. (1965). "The effect of graded vagal stimulation on gastric motility, secretion and blood flow in the cat," *Acta Physiol. Scand.* **65,** 300–309.

Martinson, J., and H. Odelram (1968). Personal communication.

Schachter, M., and S. Beilenson (1967). "Kallikrein and vasodilation in the submaxillary gland," *Gastroenterology*, **52,** 401–5.

Shepherd, J. T. (1968). Personal communication.

Spanner, R. (1932). "Neue Befunde über die Blutwege der Darmwand und ihre funktionelle Bedeutung," *Morph. Jb.* **69,** 394–454.

Steiner, S. S., and C. E. Mueller (1961). "Distribution of blood flow in the digestive tract of the rat," *Circ. Res.* **14,** 99–102.

Texter, E. C., Jr. (1963). "Small intestinal blood flow," *Am. J. Digestive Diseases*, **8,** 567–613.

Walder, D. N. (1952). "Arteriovenous anastomoses of the human stomach,"
    Clin. Sci. **11,** 59–71.

Wallentin, I. (1966). "Studies on intestinal circulation." *Acta Physiol. Scand.* **69,**
    Suppl. 279.

Webster, M. E., and J. V. Pierce (1963). "The nature of the kallidins released
    from human plasma by kallikreins and other enzymes," *Ann. N. Y. Acad.*
    Sci. **104,** 91–107.

27

Renal Circulation

General Considerations

The functional unit of the kidney is the nephron (Fig. 27-1A), of which there are a million or so in each kidney in man. The nephron comprises: (1) *The Malpighian body*, which consists of Bowman's capsule invaginated by a knot of specialized capillaries—the *glomerulus*. An ultrafiltrate of plasma is transuded across these capillaries into the capsular space. From the capsule this fluid passes successively through various parts of the nephric tubular system in which the tubular cells exercise active absorptive and secretory functions. The glomeruli lie in the *cortex* of the kidney. (2) *The tubular system*, which drains the ultrafiltrate. This system can be conveniently divided into (a) the proximal convoluted tubule (PCT); (b) the descending limb, the thin segment, and the ascending limb of the loop of Henle; (c) the distal convoluted tubule (DCT); and (d) the collecting tubule. As Fig. 27-1B shows, the tubular system dips first from the cortex into the medulla and then turns, in the loop of Henle, back towards the cortex. The DCT lies closely approximate to the glomerulus in part of its length (macula densa). Finally the DCT gives place to the collecting tubule, which passes from the cortex through the medulla to empty into the pelvic calyces, whence the ureter eventually debouches.

The mechanism of urine formation in the mammal is, at first sight, improbable. Although only some 1.5 litres of urine, containing waste

494

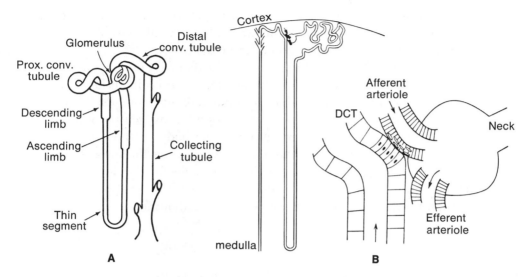

Fig. 27-1A. The nephron (diagrammatic). (From Keele and Neil, 1965. By permission.)

Fig. 27-1B. Schematic drawing of the anatomical arrangements of the individual nephron unit and the juxtaglomerular apparatus. At lower right: point of contact between the ascending limb of Henle's loop and the vascular pole. The tubular cells whose nuclei are shown are the macula densa cells. (Thurau *et al.*, 1967. By permission.)

products of metabolism such as nitrogenous constituents, hydronium ions, potassium ions, etc., are formed in one day by a man living in a temperate climate, this is achieved initially by the ultrafiltration of about 170 litres of plasma, from which subsequently all the "essential" constituents (e.g. glucose and sodium) and water are reabsorbed. The reabsorption of solutes requires active chemical work by the tubular cells. In addition, chemical work by the tubular cells is required for the secretion of ions, such as those of potassium and hydronium, for example.

Clearly, the oxygen usage of the kidney will be closely related to the chemical work of the tubules, for filtration itself is a passive physical process. On the other hand, the enormous filtered bulk required presupposes a filtration pressure higher than elsewhere in the body, and such indeed is the case. The ultrafiltration of 170 litres/day requires a renal plasma flow (RPF) far in excess of this and measurements of RPF indeed reveal that some 900 litres of plasma and hence about 1750 litres of blood traverse the two kidneys in 24 hours. In man the two kidneys weigh only 300 grams, so the renal blood flow is some 400 ml/min/100 g.

The arteriovenous oxygen difference is only about 1.3 ml/100 ml—renal venous blood is bright red in colour as the blood flow is dimensional to the huge filtrate production rather than to the metabolic demands. This in a way disguises the fact that the kidneys use 15 ml of oxygen per minute— i.e. 6% of the total resting oxygen usage of the body—although they represent less than one-200th of the total body weight. It is the fantastic blood bath that the kidneys enjoy which is responsible for the low A-V O_2 difference, but which at the same time ensures that the renal tissue pO_2 is kept high for the purposes of active cellular metabolism.

Arrangement of the Vascular Bed

Each kidney is supplied by a single renal artery which takes origin from the abdominal aorta. After entering the hilus the artery subdivides into a number of branches which radiate from the hilus. These interlobar arteries pass between the calyces to the junction between the cortex and medulla. Here they branch and form the misleadingly named arcuate arteries, which run parallel to the surface of the kidney along the cortico-medullary region. The arcuate arteries do not form arches; they end by bending into the cortex to form interlobular arteries which once more run radially towards the cortical surface (Fig. 27-2A). These interlobular arteries give rise to short lateral branches—the so-called afferent arterioles —each of which supplies a glomerulus (Fig. 27-2B). The preglomerular vessels, especially the interlobular and afferent arterioles in the outer cortex, are richly supplied with adrenergic vasoconstrictor fibres.

Just before the afferent arteriole joins the glomerulus, the media cells become swollen and afibrillar ("Polkissen"). They contain secretory granules, thought to be renin or its precursor. This *juxtaglomerular apparatus* (JGA), which is especially well developed in outer cortical parts, is of great importance. The JGA cells, normally exposed to the continuous stretch of the blood pressure, appear to function as "stretch receptors" which *increase* their renin release when unloaded, whether the unloading is due to a pressure fall or a neurogenic arteriolar constriction. It is further

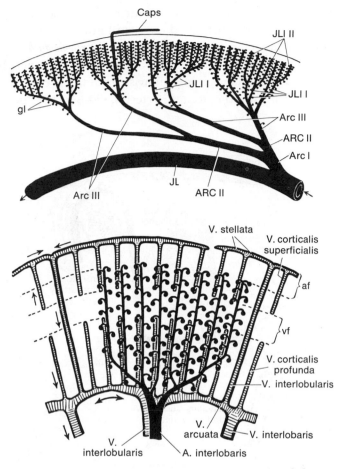

Fig. 27-2. Arrangement of the arterial and venous supply of the renal cortex. (From Selkurt, 1963. By permission.)

interesting that part of the distal convoluted tubule regularly makes close contact with JGA, forming the characteristic *macula densa* arrangement. It is here that the final, "facultative" sodium reabsorption takes place; it is known that the JGA release of renin is also affected by the sodium content. It has been suggested, originally by Goormaghtigh (1945), that the macula densa, involved in the final sodium reabsorbtion, might in some way influence the JGA cells (see below). In any case, the JGA–macula densa complex is a remarkable arrangement, evidently of great importance for renal circulation and function, though still not fully understood.

The glomeruli are classified as *cortical* and *juxta-medullary*, the latter constituting some 15 to 20% of the total of one million glomeruli in man's kidney. The juxta-medullary glomeruli arise from the very first part of the interlobular or even from the arcuate arteries, close to the cortico-medul-

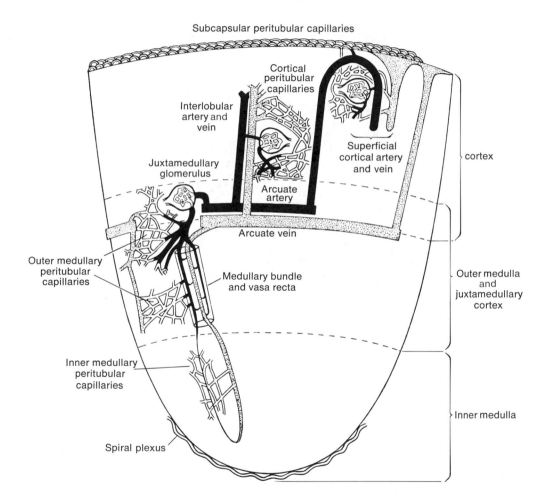

Fig. 27-3. Schematic diagram of the vascular architecture of the normal kidney. (From Pomeranz *et al.*, 1968. By permission.)

lary junction (Fig. 27-3). As it enters Bowman's capsule the afferent arteriole widens and branches, forming six or more trunks from which further subdivisions occur to constitute a separate glomerular lobule. Each glomerulus contains about six lobules, each of which in turn consists of 3 to 6 capillary loops—approximately 20 to 40 capillary loops in all (Fig. 27-4A). Many anastomoses occur between the capillary loops within one lobule.

The wide pores (diameter about 0.1 μ) of the *fenestrated glomerular endothelium* ("lamina fenestra") do not hinder the passage of plasma macromolecules and therefore cannot alone constitute the "ultrafilter". However, there are two other major wall components in the glomerular capillaries: the relatively thick *basement membrane* ("lamina densa") and the *visceral cell layer* (the "podocytes") of the Bowman capsule. At their borders the podocytes form interdigitated pedicles (Fig. 27-4B), separated by narrow slits, some 90 to 100 Å wide. It has been suggested that these slits constitute the "slit pores" that restrain plasma proteins from passing the glomerular capillary walls. The size of these morphologically defined slit pores corresponds well with functional estimations of the porosity in the glomerular capillaries (see also Chapter 8; Selkurt, 1963).

The glomerular capillaries rejoin to form the efferent arteriole of the relevent glomerulus. In contrast to the afferent arterioles, the efferent ones —from which all the blood supply to the tubules originates—are *not* controlled by any vasoconstrictor fibres, and their further arrangement depends on whether they originate from *cortical* or *juxta-medullary* glomeruli. The cortical efferent arterioles, which are smaller than the corresponding afferent ones, supply a plexus of fenestrated capillaries which surrounds the tubules beneath the renal capsule and between the interlobular vessels (Fig. 27-3).

The juxta-medullary efferent arterioles, on the other hand, which are often equal to or even wider than the corresponding afferent vessels, supply the subcortical and medullary zones, as well as the medullary rays. These efferent arterioles divide in the outer medulla to form two types of arrangements, where again the capillary sections are provided with the fenestrated type of endothelium. The more frequent type of arrange-ment (80%) forms a leash of straight *vasa recta*, which course through the medulla so that some even reach the tip of the renal papillae. They return as the ascending limbs of a hairpin loop. Using a double injection tech-nipue, Moffat and Fourman (1963) have shown that all vasa recta break into capillary loops which have to be traversed by the blood before it reaches the venous side of the system.

The other, less frequent type of arrangement takes off either directly from the juxta-medullary efferent arteriole, or from the proximal vasa recta, and forms a capillary network, distributed especially in the juxta-medullary cortex and the outer medulla, but also to some extent penetrating the inner medulla (Fig. 27-3).

Veins show an arrangement which varies from species to species. In the dog and in man, blood from the cortical capillaries is partly drained via superficial veins, partly by deep ones, which are interconnected by means of relatively sparse interlobular veins but which in the end all empty into the arcuate, and thence by interlobar veins (Fig. 27-2B). Numerous wide venous channels drain the subcortical zone and medulla. They open into the arcuate veins or into the proximal part of the interlobular veins, either directly or via collecting veins.

The renal lymphatics contain one section which originates in subcapsular parts of the cortex, and another which starts beneath the papillary mucosa draining the medulla. They usually follow the vessels, which means that the medullary lymphatics run parallel to the vasa recta, draining the protein from the tissue spaces around these capillary hairpin loops.

The kidneys have an unusually rich supply of sympathetic fibres, mainly emanating from T_{10}–T_{12} and destined only for the vascular bed. The outer cortical preglomerular vessels, particularly, are densely innervated, up to the point where the afferent arteriole enters the glomerulus. The efferent arterioles, on the other hand, are devoid of constrictor fibres. The vessels of the juxta-medullary nephrons are similarly innervated, but whether the *extent* of this innervation is the same as in the outer cortex is not known.

Fig. 27-4A. Bowman's capsule and the glomerular capillary loops.

Fig. 27-4B. A schematic illustration of a glomerular capillary. At the upper right, parts of three epithelial cells (ep.) are shown with terminal processes interdigitating upon the capillary surface (layer 1). The appearance of these feet in cross section is indicated at the left, and in the insert at the lower right. The epithelial feet are slightly embedded in a cement layer (2), which in turn rests upon the dense structural portion of the basement membrane (layer 3). An inner cement layer (4) provides a bed for the endothelium (layer 5). The holes are a little over 0.1 μ in diameter, as may be seen in surface view to the right of the figure, and in the transverse section to the left, and in the insert. (From Pease, 1955. By permission.)

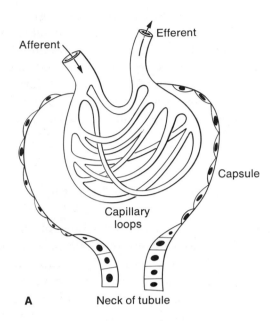

A Neck of tubule

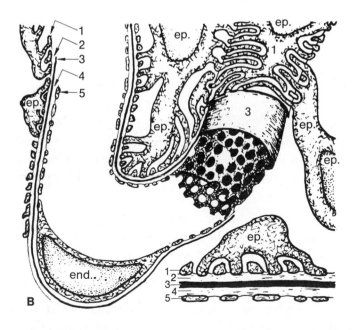

B

Further, some adrenergic fibres, but also cholinergic ones (vasodilator?), are distributed to the vasa recta of the outer medulla, and these may be important in the control of medullary blood flow and function. Inner parts of the medulla lack adrenergic fibres (McKenna and Angelakos, 1968a, b).

The kidneys are supplied with some nociceptive fibres, running with the sympathetic ones which are excited by capsular distension. Possibly more "specific" afferents may exist, too, but little is known about these.

Renal Blood Flow and Its Regulation

The kidney is steadily active. Flow restrictions of any magnitude occur only episodically, such as in heavy exercise, alarm situations or when over-all cardiovascular performance is seriously threatened. The renal blood supply in resting man is not far below that at maximal renal vasodilatation (400 ml compared with 500 to 600 ml/min/100 g), which indicates that the basal tone of the renal resistance vessels is low.

Blood Flow Measurements

Because of the complexity of the renal circuit, measurements of total and regional blood flows deserve to be outlined in more detail in this context (see also Chapter 7). Renal blood flow is intimately connected to glomerular filtration, and it is usually desirable to measure both these parameters simultaneously. This proved difficult until the *clearance* technique was introduced. The clearance of a substance from the plasma may be defined in terms of the minimal or virtual volume of plasma which during the course of one minute would provide that amount of the substance which appears in the urine.

If U = urinary concentration of the substance
P = plasma concentration of the substance
V = volume of urine formed in 1 minute

then   Clearance rate = UV/P

Obviously, if a substance is filtered and is not absorbed or secreted by the renal tubules, then its clearance rate must equal that of the glomerular ultra-filtration. The clearance rate of such a substance must be independent of its plasma concentration. Inulin satisfies this criterion and its clearance rate, which equals the glomerular filtration rate (GFR), is of the order of 125 ml/min in man.

It is obvious, in turn, that the renal plasma flow (RPF) must greatly exceed the GFR, as only a fraction of the plasma can be filtered in the glomeruli. Renal plasma flow can only be measured by the clearance technique if the substance used is *completely* cleared from the plasma during its renal transit, and this presupposes that tubular *secretory* activity (in addition to glomerular filtration) is exerted with respect to the substance employed. Organic iodine compounds (diodrast) and, better, para-amino-hippuric acid (PAH) are nearly completely cleared during their passage through the kidney and their clearance rate, 650 ml/min or so, gives a measure of the RPF. The filtration fraction is thus 125/650, or about 0.2. As the haematocrit is about 45%, the renal blood flow in man is 650 × 100/ 55, approximately 1200 ml/min; i.e. almost a quarter of the cardiac output of man at rest.

In animals, different types of direct recorders have additionally been used, which have been of considerable value for studies of flow autoregulation. Further, the electromagnetic flow-meter can be used for continuous recordings even in chronic experiments in conscious animals.

^{85}Krypton has been used in man in a modified Kety method. Only arterial and venous blood samples are required, which is an obvious advantage when renal blood flow measurements are made in patients with anuria or oliguria.

The intrarenal distribution of blood flow has also been investigated in conscious, trained animals by placing a scintillation probe over the kidney and recording the disappearance curve following a single injection of ^{85}Kr into the renal artery. Such a technique reveals that the "renal decay curve" is non-exponential and can be described by three or even four components (see Chapter 7). Different experimental controls, including autoradiography, indicate that these three (or four) components reflect the flow through (1) cortex, (2) juxta-medullary cortex and outer medulla, (3) inner medulla, and (4), when present, hilar and perirenal fat (e.g. Thorburn *et al.*, 1963). Such an approach, together with regional measurements of transit times for injected dyes (Fig. 27-5) by Kramer *et al.* (1960), has been important in studies of *intrarenal* blood flow distribution and renal function.

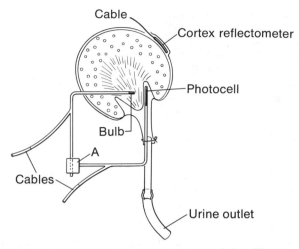

Fig. 27-5. Schematic drawing of the method used by Kramer's group for measurements of cortical and medullary circulatory transit times. (From Kramer *et al.*, 1960. By permission.)

Regional Blood Flows

It is the renal cortex, especially perhaps its outer sections, which receives the extraordinary flow figure of 450 to 500 ml/min/100 g. The outer medulla gets 120 to 140 ml/min/100 g and the inner medulla some 25 ml/min/100 g. The ^{85}Kr clearance method actually somewhat *underestimates* the blood flow in the inner medulla due to "trapping" of the indicator by its "cross-diffusion" in the hairpin loop of the vasa recta. Also, oxygen diffuses readily from the arterial to the venous segment at this site (Levy and Sauceda, 1959). In the kidney, the inner medullary blood flow—though low compared with that of the renal cortex—is nevertheless half that enjoyed by the brain itself per unit weight. About 75% of renal tissue is cortex, so the total cortical weight is $3/4 \times 300 = 225$ g in man. Thus, 225 g renal cortex receives 500×225, or more than one litre of blood each minute, i.e. 90% or more of the total renal flow. This means that 0.3% of the body weight receives about 20% of the resting cardiac output; a profuse blood supply indeed.

The whole renal medulla actually receives only some 7% of the total renal blood flow, the inner medulla only 1%. However, per unit tissue weight this is still quite a substantial blood supply. This lower flow is not due to a poor vascular bed. But the great length (40 mm in the dog) and the narrow lumina—especially in the descending limb—of the many parallel vasa recta implies a high flow resistance for each of them and the pressure head is rather low.

Kramer, Thurau, and their colleagues used a photoelectric method (Fig. 27-5) to study medullary blood flow and its influence on renal medullary function. Increases of this flow, though small in comparison with the total flow, can easily "wash out" the osmotic gradients in the long vasa recta loops and the accompanying loops of Henle. By such increases of blood flow urine osmolarity could even be reduced to values below that of the plasma (Thurau and Deetjen, 1962). In other words, adjustments of the blood flow in the vasa recta (note the presence of adrenergic and cholinergic fibre supply of these vessels; constrictor and dilator fibres?) may markedly adjust the mechanism for urine concentration, as first outlined by Wirz et al. (1951) and such adjustments are of paramount importance in understanding renal function (see Selkurt, 1963). Water diuresis causes medullary vasodilatation, whereas ADH administration appears to constrict the medullary vessels, judging by the increased transit time for the injected dye. If so, ADH might influence the concentration process by a strategically localized medullary vasoconstriction as well as by its effect on tubular permeability to water.

Table 27-1 summarizes mean circulation times calculated from results obtained by Kramer's group. Blood flows were calculated from regional blood volumes, and circulation times were obtained for cortex, outer medulla, and inner medulla. On the whole, the flow figures deduced from the ^{85}Kr clearance are in good agreement with this more direct approach, though the krypton method tends to understimate flow wherever countercurrent loops are present, i.e. in the medulla.

Intrarenal Vascular Pressures

The total renal resistance to flow is normally furnished almost entirely by the afferent and efferent arterioles related to the glomeruli. No one has measured the glomerular *capillary* pressure directly, but it has been calculated to be of the order of 70 mm Hg. Micropuncture of the peritubular capillaries in the rat has revealed that the pressure falls from 20 mm Hg to about 15 mm Hg along these capillaries, indicating only a small resistance to flow in this segment (Thurau and Wober, 1962).

Table 27-1

Source	Weight % of total kidney	Intrarenal circulation times	Vascular volume		Blood flow rates		
			ml/100 g tissue	ml/100 g kidney	ml/100 g tissue	ml/100 g kidney	% of Total renal blood flow
Cortex	70	0.02	19.2	13.5	458	321	92.5
Outer medulla	20	0.086	19.2	3.9	112	22.4	6.5
Inner medulla	10	0.75	22.0	2.2	29	2.9	1.0

From K. Thurau (1964). By permission.

With a mean arterial pressure of 100 mm, the pressure at the end of the afferent arteriole is 70 mm and the postglomerular pressure drops from 70 mm to about 20 mm Hg at the end of the efferent vessel. An interesting —and complicating—factor in considerations of renal haemodynamics is the rather high tissue pressure (up to 15 mm Hg or so; see Fig. 27-6). Thus, the *transmural* pressure in the tubular capillaries is quite low, favouring fluid absorption, particularly as the oncotic pressure of the blood is here

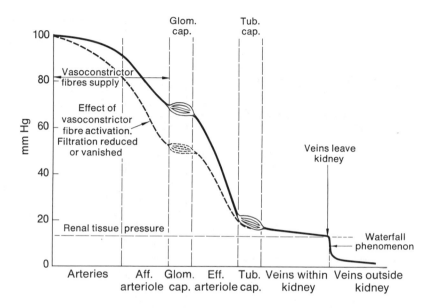

Fig. 27-6. Diagram illustrating the pressure drop profile of the renal vascular circuit with the effect of vasoconstrictor fibre activation.

especially high. Where the veins emerge from the renal capsule a "waterfall phenomenon" occurs (Swann *et al.*, 1952) because of the sudden change from a section of high tissue pressure to one of low pressure.

   The high intrarenal pressure is largely due to the enclosure of the organ in a fairly rigid capsule and the distension of the large vascular bed by the blood pressure transmits part of the pressure to the whole organ, almost as if it were a cavernous tissue. Thus, arterial occlusion or intense renal vasoconstriction causes a substantial shrinkage of the kidney.

Autoregulation of Blood Flow

Rein (1931) noted that the renal blood flow remains remarkably constant between arterial pressures of 80 and 200 mm Hg (Fig. 27-7A, B), as, indeed, does GFR. As GFR does not alter and, moreover, as renal tissue pressure and volume, as well as tubular capillary pressure, remain largely the same, it appears that the resistance changes responsible for this constancy of flow occur in the *preglomerular* vessels. Denervation of the

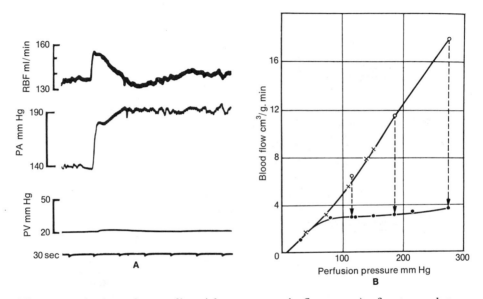

Fig. 27-7. A. Actual recording (electromagnetic flowmeter) of autoregulatory adjustment of renal blood flow in response to a primary pressure rise. (From Semple and De Wardener, 1959. By permission.)
B. Immediate and stabilized pressure—flow relationship for the renal vascular bed. (From Thurau and Kramer, 1959. By permission.)

kidney or blockade of intrarenal ganglia does not affect autoregulation, but it is abolished by addition of drugs that paralyse smooth muscle and transform the renal circuit into a passive-elastic tube system (see Selkurt, 1963). Autoregulation can also be abolished or greatly reduced by *intense* constrictor fibre stimulation; presumably the strong extrinsic activation of the preglomerular smooth muscles so dominates them that purely local adjustments are then masked.

Drugs that paralyse smooth muscle have no effect on renal blood flow at pressures below 80 mm Hg, which indicates that the myogenic "basal" tone of the renal resistance vessels is negligible at low arterial pressures, fairly slight at the normal pressure level, and pronounced only when the arterial pressure is substantially raised.

It appears that these local reactions of the preglomerular vessels are brought about by changes in the tension of the vessel wall of the afferent arterioles—if so, this is a specific example of the myogenic reaction, first suggested by Bayliss in 1902 (see Chapter 16). Although this remains an unproved hypothesis for the kidney, many favour the view that the tangential wall tension is the major determinant of renal myogenic vascular tone and is responsible for the constancy of GFR and of RPF.

Other hypotheses advanced to explain autoregulation in the kidney include that of Pappenheimer and Kinter (1956), which suggested that the plasma skimming of red cells in the interlobar arteries was basically responsible for autoregulation. Though there is evidence of plasma skimming in the kidney (Ulfendal, 1962), it is now thought to provide only a minor factor in autoregulation.

Thus, autoregulation of renal flow is a matter of preglomerular vascular adjustments, but from this it does not follow that Bayliss's myogenic effect is necessarily the only, or even the most important, factor. It should be recalled that renal oxygen consumption is proportional to sodium reabsorption (Kramer and Deetjen, 1961). In skeletal muscle or in cardiac muscle, metabolism governs the local control of the blood flow, but the kidney is unique in the sense that blood flow governs the metabolism of renal tissue as the filtered load of sodium is normally *determined* by the renal blood flow. For such reasons it is unlikely that any "conventional" metabolic autoregulation, caused by vasodilator metabolites (Chapter 16), is involved in the kidney, as here a rise of pressure provokes vasoconstriction but *raises* the metabolism, and vice versa.

However, the possibility remains that the filtered sodium load in some other, more specific way affects the preglomerular vascular tone and hence the blood flow which determines filtration. If so, the work load would itself provide a specific servocontrol, keeping renal function within narrow limits, except when overridden by powerful extrinsic mechanisms. In this context the close structural relationship between the macula densa and the JGA should be recalled—Goorghmagtigh suggested a functional relationship between the two in 1945. Over recent years there has been much debate as to whether this arrangement might be the site of some specific chemical (osmotic, ionic, etc.) control for the preglomerular smooth muscles, instead of—or in addition to—the less specific myogenic stretch response which occurs in most systemic resistance vessels (Chapter 16).

On the basis of micropuncture studies, Thurau *et al.* (1967) suggested that an *increased* sodium content in the macula densa, secondary to an increased blood flow and filtration, might trigger a local renin release, and vice versa. This renin, arriving in the tissue spaces, would promptly split off angiotensin from available globulin (compare kallikrein-kallidin-bradykinin in glands!) and constrict the corresponding afferent arteriole, perhaps long before renin-angiotensin leaked out in traceable amounts in the blood.

This hypothesis, implying that a pressure *rise* (indirectly, via the tubular sodium load) causes renin release, is apparently in sharp conflict with the well-established fact that *lowering* the blood pressure is one of the surest ways to provoke renin release. Arguments, both vigorous and protracted, continue (see Page and McCubbin, 1968). This contradiction might, after all, not be so definite as it may first seem; it is possible that the peculiar JGA cells are made to secrete by *two* different types of stimuli, i.e. increased sodium and reduced stretch.

However, if high pressure in this way should provoke a renin release large enough as to constrict the renal vessels strongly, though little renin appears in the blood, why does not *low* blood pressure (which causes a much greater release of renin into the blood) cause a still more intense renal vasoconstriction? Instead, a lowered blood pressure causes renal vasodilatation unless reflex vasoconstriction "compensates". Thurau's results strongly suggest that renal vasoconstriction does occur when the macula densa is exposed to an increased sodium load. Thus, mannitol diuresis, which lowers the distal tubule [Na^+], is accompanied by renal vasodilatation. Mercurial diuretics, which deliver more sodium to the macula densa region, cause renal vasoconstriction. Another, more indirect argument is that dogs fed on a high sodium diet for months exhibit a less prominent renal autoregulation; high sodium diets do deplete the renin content of the JGA. Still, however, many contest the hypothesis. It may after all be that the increased sodium load in the macula densa induces preglomerular constriction by means of some excitatory influence that is not due to the renin mechanism.

Whichever the case, the macula densa–JGA complex seems to be implicated in a type of "specific" servocontrol related to the sodium load. This, perhaps together with the "unspecific" myogenic response, may underlie the autoregulation of renal blood flow and GFR.

This lengthy survey of renal autoregulation may appear to be "much ado about nothing" for readers struck by the normal *constancy* of arterial pressure and the prompt interference of neurogenic, usually contrary-directed, adjustments whenever this pressure falls; there seems to be little room in the intact organism for the beautiful pressure-flow curves illustrated in Fig. 27-7B. The point is, of course, that experimental studies of pressure-flow curves—even over a range far removed from normal—provide evidence of the behaviour of the local control mechanisms which normally govern the blood vessels and the tissue blood supply.

With respect to the juxtamedullary–vasa recta systems, it has generally been assumed that these vessels display little or no flow autoregulation. Birtch *et al.* (1967), however, have suggested that the blood flow in the outer medulla may remain constant when the renal artery pressure is decreased and that this effect is abolished by small amounts of intrarenal atropine. It is possible that the cholinergic fibres along the vasa recta referred to previously may be involved here in an *intrarenal* neurogenic adjustment, which tends to stabilize the medullary circulation. A relatively constant blood flow in the vasa recta loops is desirable for the equilibrium of the medullary countercurrent exchange—which itself is so important for the production of hypertonic urine (see Selkurt, 1963).

Nervous Control of Renal Blood Flow

The kidneys are not subjected to much sympathetic restriction of their *total* blood supply during resting conditions, though there is no question that the potential power of the renal vasoconstrictor fibres is formidable (Fig. 27-8). The medullary cardiovascular centre is so "organized" as to leave the kidneys, and to some extent the skin (especially the A-V anastomoses), relatively unaffected in over-all cardiovascular homeostatic adjustments, except when these become pronounced (see Chapter 17). This seems reasonable, considering the fact that both the renal and cutaneous circuits are steadily involved in the equally important homeostatic mechanisms of salt/water-balance and temperature equilibrium, respectively. Nevertheless, striking renal vasoconstriction may occur

Blood pressure
mm Hg

Renal blood flow

Signal
Time, 30 sec

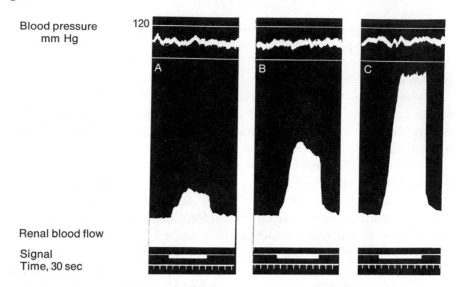

Fig. 27-8. Effects of graded sympathetic stimulation at 3, 6, and 12 imp/sec on renal blood flow resistance in the cat. The ordinates for blood flow recording (drop recorder) are directly proportional to the flow resistance. (From Celander, 1954. By permission.)

episodically, in alarm situations, heavy exercise, and severe blood loss, for example (see Chapters 17–20). The defence reaction (Chapter 19) may be accompanied by a very powerful neurogenic renal vasoconstriction (Fig. 27-9). Curiously, however, in most situations of intense constrictor fibre discharge to the kidneys, the renal vessels soon tend to "escape" from the neurogenic influence (Fig. 27-9). The background of this local "escape" (compare that of the intestinal or liver vessels; Chapter 26) is not known; it might be due in part to an intrarenal redistribution of blood flow.

The relatively trivial neurogenic vasoconstrictor effects on *total* renal blood flow during rest, or in moderate cardiovascular adjustments, by no means imply that these sympathetic influences play no part in renal function. Sympathetic vasoconstriction is more pronounced in the outer renal cortex, as has already been suggested by the studies of Trueta *et al.* (1947). The highest renin contents are usually found in the JGA cells of the outer cortex.

Moreover, weak vasoconstrictor fibre stimulation, insufficient to alter total renal blood flow, nevertheless provokes a substantial renin release

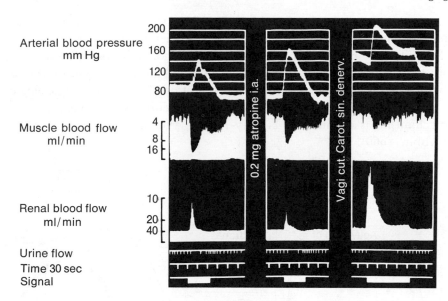

Fig. 27-9. The effect of hypothalamic defence area stimulation on blood pressure, muscle and renal blood flows (drop recorder technique), and on urine flow. Between first and second panel the sympathetic vasodilator fibres to the muscles are blocked by atropine; between the second and third panel all baroreceptor reflexes are eliminated. Renal flow resistance increases initially 4–5 times and especially in the last panel. (From Feigl *et al.*, 1964. By permission.)

(Bunag *et al.*, 1966). This is possibly the result of an especially strong constrictor fibre effect in the outermost cortex, here unloading JGA "stretch receptors" that have an especially rich renin content; these cells are perhaps even *directly* excited by adrenergic nerve endings. In any case, such a finding has important consequences for the understanding not only of renal nervous control but also of the interconnections between nervous and hormonal regulation of renal function in general—particularly with respect to the water/salt equilibrium—and is of great relevance also in patho-physiological situations such as shock and hypertension. Thus a minor increase of constrictor fibre discharge, due to a slight sodium-fluid loss, may leave renal blood flow, ultrafiltration, and the over-all "rinsing" of the body fluids largely undisturbed, but may still increase renin release and angiotensin formation substantially. This, in turn, increases aldosterone secretion, and consequently tubular sodium (and water) reabsorption is enhanced and the sodium loss is compensated for. In other words, a slight reflex constrictor fibre activation may "amplify" the effect on the JGA cells of a minor fluid loss without necessitating restrictions of other aspects of renal function, thus selectively bolstering the adequate sodium-water retention (Chapter 20). The elegant but complex control of the JGA release of renin by nervous and other mechanisms is outlined in Fig. 27-10 (see Wood, 1967; Page and McCubbin, 1968).

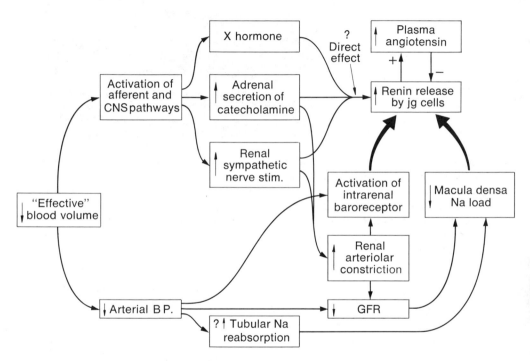

Fig. 27-10. Diagram illustrating the control of renin release. (From Page and McCubbin, 1968. By permission.)

The nervous control of intrarenal flow distribution is still obscure. Since Trueta's days it has been vividly debated whether medullary and juxtamedullary blood flow is *increased* in connection with a neurogenic restriction of cortical blood flow. There is certainly no easy answer to this question, and some conflicting points of view, which merely reflect the utmost difficulties involved in this field, will be briefly mentioned.

Pomeranz *et al.* (1968) claimed that weak sympathetic stimulation reduced outer cortical flow but *increased* that of the outer medulla; both regional flows were decreased by strong sympathetic stimulation. McKenna and Angelakos (1968b) found that cholinergic fibres (vasodilator?) were distributed to the vasa recta of the outer medulla; it is possible that such fibres in some situations of sympathetic activity might *increase* medullary blood flow. Aukland (1968), however, found no evidence of an alteration of the pattern of intrarenal circulation during *direct* sympathetic stimulation. Whether the situation is a different one when reflex and central response pattern are induced (which might be differentiated with respect to the extent of involvement of the intrarenal constrictor fibre supply) is not known.

References

Aukland, K. (1968). "Effect of adrenaline, noradrenaline, angiotensin and renal nerve stimulation on intrarenal distribution of blood flow in dogs," *Acta Physiol. Scand.* **72,** 498–509.

Bayliss, W. M. (1902). "On the local reactions of the arterial wall to changes of internal pressure," *J. Physiol.* **28,** 220–31. (London.)

Birtch, A. G., R. M. Zakheim, L. G. Jones, and A. C. Barger (1967). "Redistribution of renal blood flow produced by furosemide and ethacrynic acid," *Circ. Res.* **21,** 869–78.

Bunag, R. D., I. H. Page, and J. W. McCubbin (1966). "Neural stimulation of release of renin," *Circ. Res.* **19,** 851–58.

Celander, O. (1954). "The range of control exercised by the 'sympathico-adrenal system,' " *Acta Physiol. Scand.*, Suppl, 116, 1–132.

Feigl, E., B. Johansson, and B. Löfving (1964). "Renal vasoconstriction and the 'defence reaction,' " *Acta Physiol. Scand.* **62,** 429–35.

Goormaghtigh, N. (1945). "Facts in favour of an endocrine function of the renal arterioles," *J. Path. and Bact.* **57,** 392–405.

Kramer, K., and P. Deetjen (1961). "Sodium reabsorption and oxygen consumption in the mammalian kidney," *Proc. 1st Intern. Cong. Nephrol.*, Geneve et Evian, 687.

Kramer, K., K. Thurau, and P. Deetjen (1960). "Hämodynamik des Nieren-marks: Capillare Passagezeit, Blutvolumen, Durchblutung, Gewebshä-matokrit and O_2-Verbrauch des Nierenmarks in situ," *Pflügers Arch. Ges. Physiol.* **270**, 251–69.

Levy, M. N., and G. Sauceda (1959). "Diffusion of oxygen from arterial to venous segments of renal capillaries," *Am. J. Physiol.* **196**, 1336–39.

McKenna, O. C., and E. T. Angelakos (1968a). "Adrenergic innervation of the canine kidney," *Circ. Res.* **22**, 345–54.

McKenna, O. C., and E. T. Angelakos (1968b). "Acetylcholinesterase-con-taining fibres in the canine kidney," *Circ. Res.* **23**, 645–51.

Moffat, S. M., and J. Fourman (1963). "The vascular pattern of the rat kidney," *J. Anat.* **97**, 543–53. (London.)

Page, I. H., and J. W. McCubbin (1968). *Renal hypertension.* Chicago: Year Book Med. Publ.

Pappenheimer, J. R., and W. B. Kinter (1956). "Hematocrit ratio of blood within mammalian kidney and its significance for renal hemodynamics," *Am. J. Physiol.* **185**, 377–90.

Pease, D. C. (1955). "Fine structures of the kidney seen by electron micro-scopy," *J. Histochem. Cytochem.* **3**, 295–308.

Pomeranz, B. H., A. G. Birtch, and A. C. Barger (1968). "Neural control of intrarenal blood flow," *Am. J. Physiol.* **215**, 1067–81.

Rein, H. (1931). "Vasomotorische Regulationen," *Ergebn. Physiol.* **32**, 28–82.

Selkurt, E. E. (1963). "The renal circulation," *Handbook of Physiology*, 2, Circulation **II**, 1457–1516.

Semple, S. J. C., and H. E. DeWardener (1959). "Effect of increased renal venous pressure on circulatory 'autoregulation' of isolated dog kidneys," *Circ. Res.* **7**, 643–48.

Swann, H. G., B. W. Hink, H. Koester, V. Moore, and J. M. Prine (1952). "The intrarenal venous pressure," *Science*, **115**, 64–65.

Thorburn, G. D., H. H. Kopald, J. A. Herd, M. Hollenberg, C. C. O'Marchoe, and A. C. Barger (1963). "Intrarenal distribution of nutrient blood flow determined with Kr[85] in the unanesthetized dog," *Circ. Res.* **13**, 290–307.

Thurau, K. (1964). "Renal haemodynamics," *Am. J. Med.* **36**, 698–719.

Thurau, K., and P. Deetjen (1962). "Die Diurese bei arteriellen Drucksteigerungen," *Pflügers Archiv*, **274,** 567–80.

Thurau, K., and K. Kramer (1959). "Weitere Untersuchungen zur myogenen Natur der Autoregulation des Nierenkreislaufes," *Pflügers Archiv*, **268,** 188–203.

Thurau, K., and E. Wober (1962). "Zur Lokalisation der autoregulativen Wiederstandsänderung in der Niere," *Pflügers Archiv*, **274,** 553–66.

Thurau, K., J. Schnermann, W. Nagel, M. Horster, and M. Wahl (1967). "Composition of tubular fluid in the macula densa segment as a factor regulating the function of the juxta-glomerular apparatus," *Circ. Res.* **21,** Suppl., II, 79–90.

Trueta, J., A. E. Barclay, P. M. Daniel, K. J. Franklin, and M. M. L. Prichard (1947). *Studies of the renal circulation.* Oxford: Blackwell.

Ulfendal, H. R. (1962). "Hematocrit and hemoglobin concentration in venous blood drained from the outer cortex of cat kidney," *Acta Physiol. Scand.* **56,** 61–69.

Wirz, H., B. Hargitay, and W. Kuhn (1951). "Localization des Konzentrierungsprozessen in der Niere durch directe Kryoskopie," *Helv. Physiol. et Pharmacol.*, *Acta*, **9,** 196–210.

Wood, J. E., ed. (1967). "Renin mechanisms and hypertension," *Circ. Res.* **21,** Suppl., 11.

28

Circulation in Bone, Bone Marrow, and Adipose Tissue

Bone and Bone Marrow

General Considerations

The skeleton is one of the largest tissue masses and weighs some 10 to 12 kg in a 70 kg man, yet is is often assumed that, from the metabolic and circulatory point of view, bone is a "dull" and in demands rather indifferent tissue. This is far from the truth, especially when the metabolism, and the blood supply, are related to the size and function of the *cell* fraction. The metabolic activity and blood supply of bone tissue are in fact considerable, particularly during growth or during fracture healing.

Further, the skeleton envelops one of the body's largest and certainly one of its most important organ systems. This is the parenchymal "red" bone marrow, where erythrocytes and most leukocytes are produced; it almost equals the liver in size and its metabolic rate is quite high. The "red" marrow is a most flexible organ system; the "yellow" bone marrow (mainly lipocytes; in adult man occupying most of the long bones) may be rapidly transformed into red marrow by hypoxia, severe blood loss, etc. In other words, the "yellow" marrow might be considered as a "dormant" variant of the "red" marrow, where the reticulum does not contain any active hematopoietic cells, but where such activity may be initiated by the proper stimuli.

Vascular Arrangements

The principal arrangement of the blood supply of bone and bone marrow is illustrated in Fig. 28-1. Even though the bone structure and the enwrapped marrow constitute two separate organ systems, their vascular beds are in many ways closely interconnected, which is natural, as the supply of the marrow has to be delivered via connections to the bone (for refs. see Root, 1963; Brånemark, 1968). Further, the vascular beds of bone and bone marrow seem to be so richly connected to surrounding vascular beds via collaterals that all the major vessels may be ligated without causing damage to either bone or marrow tissue.

Circulation in Bone

The arrangement of the bone vascular bed is such as to provide an especially rich blood supply to the growth zone in childhood and adolescence (Fig. 28-1). The small vessels and capillaries follow the Haversian canals and everywhere the capillary network seems to be so rich as to keep the diffusion distance between blood and osteocytes well below 50 microns.

The enclosure of the blood vessels in a rigid matrix in the Haversian canals—even though they are here surrounded by a film of tissue fluid—might to some extent hinder *rapid* luminal and hence flow changes, but, on the other hand, bone is hardly a tissue where rapid shifts in metabolism and demands for supply are to be expected. For obvious technical reasons very little is known about the control of the circulation in bone in man, but indirect estimations suggest that the skeleton proper may receive in all 200 to 300 ml of blood per minute, corresponding to a flow of 2 to 3 ml/min/100 g tissue. This flow figure is of the same order as that of phasic skeletal muscle during rest, but the major part of the skeleton is inorganic extracellular material, so that blood flow per unit *cell* mass is far higher. It should be realized that the blood flow in the skeleton serves not only the immediate nutritional supply of the active cells; it serves also as transport vehicle for the considerable turnover of minerals, which seems to take place continuously. Thus bone is, in a sense, quite active metabolically and its supply of blood—if related to *active cell mass*—seems to be well beyond 10 times as large as that given above, to judge from rough evaluations of the fraction of bone that is made up of cells.

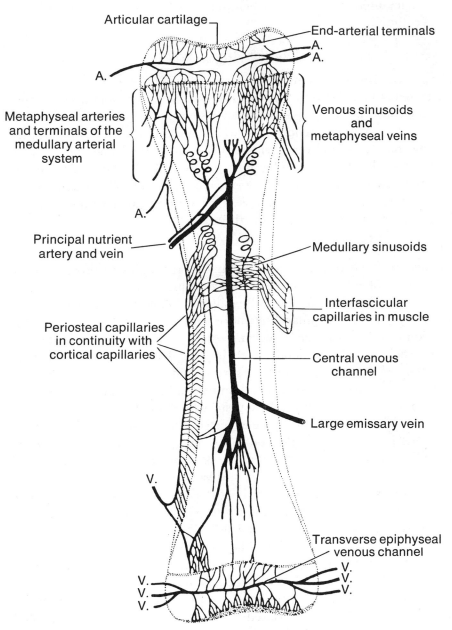

Fig. 28-1. Diagram of the vascular organization in a tubular bone. (From Root, 1963. By permission.)

It is likely that vasoconstrictor fibres exert some influence on the circulation in bone, and certainly flow can increase considerably—and new vessels may be formed—to judge from the situation during inflammation or after fractures. Obviously, much remains to be learned about this peculiar vascular bed; the problem is how to get on speaking terms with it.

Circulation in Bone Marrow

The vascular bed of the red bone marrow, and its control, exhibit many interesting and intricate peculiarities (see Brånemark, 1968; Michelsen, 1968). The principal arrangements of the major vessels are shown in Fig. 28-1 and the relationship between the small vessels and the tissue is shown in Fig. 28-2. Smooth muscles and vasoconstrictor fibres appear to be present only in the relatively thin walled arteries and the larger arterioles. There seems to be a sphincter-like arrangement just before the smooth muscle cover is lost, and from there on it is a matter of definition where the border between precapillary vessels and the true capillary section is situated. Most of these endothelial tubes enlarge into the wide and characteristic marrow sinusoids—except in the yellow marrow where few sinusoids are seen—while a few seem to make direct contacts with the venous side, bypassing the sinusoid section.

The sinusoids constitute the true "exchange section" in the marrow, where flow is often very slow due to their large transverse section area. They are extremely thin walled, and the walls are fragmented so that their lumina actually have wide-open contacts with the extravascular space surrounding the marrow reticulum, to which the hemotopoietic "stem cells" seem to be connected. There is thus an essentially free exchange between the intrasinusoidal and extrasinusoidal spaces—evident by the fact that the albumin space is almost identical with the inulin space, some 20%—with free entrance even of cells. Therefore, the passage of the newly formed blood cells into the sinusoids offers few serious problems. The extent to which this peculiar capillary bed is in open contact with the interstitial space of the marrow reticulum is clear from the fact that blood transfusions can readily be given by means of a wide needle inserted into the sternal bone marrow.

The unusually wide and thin walled veins, lacking both smooth muscles and nerves, are actually endothelial tubes with a minimum of connective tissue, and they are anchored to the surrounding marrow parenchyma.

The size of the vascular bed per se is some 8 to 10% of the tissue volume (Michelsen, 1968).

Despite the fragility of this vascular network and the exceedingly thin walls, no real problems of transmural distension, etc., are present, because the circuit is enclosed in a rigid, fluid-filled box. Thus, even though blood enters at a high pressure in the arteries, this pressure falls rapidly along the neurogenically controlled and rather narrow precapillary resistance

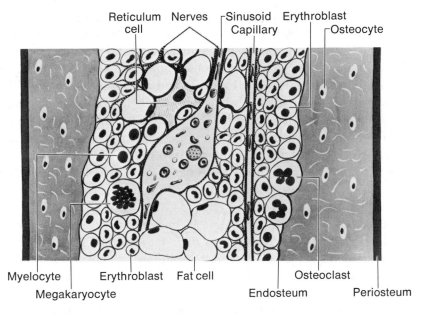

Fig. 28-2. Schematic illustration of the tissue components of the red bone marrow and their relation to the sinusoids. (From Brånemark, 1968. By permission.)

vessels. When blood thus enters the extremely thin walled sinusoid section at a reduced intravascular pressure, this pressure is immediately transmitted throughout almost the entire marrow cavity, even to the extent that the "tissue pressure" surrounding the capillary-venous compartments follows the intravascular pressure as if it were an almost freely communicating compartment. The veins obviously offer very little resistance to flow, except if semicollapsed, as their transverse area may be some 5 times that of the precapillary side. They may be compressed, however, if the sinusoids are distended, e.g. as a consequence to an upstream dilatation which would in such situations increase their flow resistance.

Thus, with respect to pressure it is almost as if the arteries at their distal ends open into a freely communicating two-compartment space; significant transmural pressure differences beyond the arteries are seen only occasionally. In diffusion, flow, and cellular passage, the two compartments are also in free communication at the sinusoidal level, but in these respects they again become separated as the venous compartment emerges. If the precapillary resistance vessels dilate or constrict, thus raising or lowering sinusoidal and venous pressures, it changes the tissue pressure to about the same degree, and these are reflected as changes in marrow pressure, which can be recorded via an inserted needle. Normally this marrow pressure seems to be below some 15 mm Hg, and this pressure level therefore largely reflects the sinusoidal and venous pressures.

The blood supply of the red marrow can vary markedly (between some 10 to 150 ml/min/100 g marrow tissue), the extremes probably reflecting the situation during neurogenic restriction of flow and "functional" hyperemia, respectively; usually it is of the order of some 40 to 50 ml/min/ 100 g (rabbit), with considerably lower figures for yellow marrow. Translated to man's situation, with an over-all lower metabolic rate and blood flow per unit tissue weight than in the rabbit, a total marrow blood flow of some 200 to 300 ml (1 to 1.5 kg of tissue) might be expected. This would imply a total skeleton-marrow blood supply/min of some 400 to 600 ml, i.e. 8 to 12% of resting cardiac output.

The marrow precapillary vessels appear to maintain a relatively pronounced basal tone, to judge from the ratio between "resting" and maximal flow levels. They are peculiar insofar as they hardly dilate when perfused with hypoxic blood; further, autoregulation and reactive hyperemia appear to be poorly displayed (Michelsen, 1968). If, however, the whole animal is made hypoxic, marrow blood flow increases; this is possibly a result of increased marrow metabolism as a consequence of released stimulating factors like erythropoietin and/or of a reflex neurogenic effect. Very little indeed is known about the reflex patterns displayed by the vasoconstrictor fibre supply of the marrow vascular bed and what these fibres imply for the hematopoietic activity. In any case, the highest flow values are met with when an animal is exposed to severe hypoxia or anemia such as after blood loss.

Adipose Tissue

General Considerations

No other tissue shows such remarkable variations in total mass as does adipose tissue. However, it appears that these variations are primarily, if not solely due to the size of the lipid store per lipocyte rather than due to the number of lipocytes. In other words, "lean" tissue mass for adipose tissue probably does not vary too much among individuals. The total amount of adipose tissue—stored fat of course included—in the average man is of the order of 6 to 10 kg, but in extreme cases the adipose depots may exceed the rest of the individual in total mass, placing a burden on cardiovascular performance.

There is much to indicate that adipose tissue in different body parts, and in different species, varies considerably with respect to storage and mobilization of the lipids, and hence in type of control, in metabolism, and in range of blood supply. This is especially true for the so-called brown adipose tissue involved in temperature regulation, in which very high blood flow figures may be encountered (Heim and Hull, 1966). It further appears that subcutaneous adipose tissue exhibits more striking changes in turnover of free fatty acids (FFA), in metabolism, and in blood flow than does mesenteric fat, for instance (see Rosell, 1969). Adipose tissue is therefore neither a uniform nor a "silent" depot tissue; it is steadily active because of the continuous processes of storage and mobilization of lipids, as controlled by the sympathetic nervous system and by a number of hormones (insulin, adrenaline, growth hormone, corticoids, etc.).

Even when the lipocytes are moderately filled with stored lipids, true cell mass constitutes only a tiny fraction of total cell volume. The cell surrounding the lipid store is like a thin shell—except where the nucleus is placed. Morphological studies have shown that each lipocyte has direct access to blood capillaries, suggesting that adipose tissue, especially when related to "lean" cell mass, is richly vascularized, which is also obvious from the blood flows recorded (see below). It is, however, only recently that the metabolism and blood supply of adipose tissue have been studied with quantitative methods *in vivo* and our knowledge about this important tissue and its vascular circuit is still fragmentary.

Vascular Dimensions and Resting Blood Flow

Practically all studies of vascular control in adipose tissue have been performed on dogs (Rosell, 1966, Öberg and Rosell, 1967) with scattered measurements in rabbits (Heim and Hull, 1966) and in man, here using the clearance method (Larsen *et al.*, 1966). In dogs with an average sized adipose tissue, i.e. where the lipocytes are moderately filled with lipids, the blood flow in subcutaneous fat during *maximal* dilatation is as high as 25 to 30 ml/min/100 g tissue. As only a small fraction of the tissue volume is made up by the metabolically active cells, this implies a rich blood supply indeed; this is also evident from the high capillary filtration coefficient (CFC) values (up to 0.08 to 0.1, twice as high as in phasic skeletal muscle; see Chapter 22). Probably the maximal flow figures for mesenteric adipose tissue, for example, are somewhat lower, but if the situation is similar in man, it is clear that in some situations quite substantial fractions of the cardiac output may be distributed to the fat depots.

In the average "resting" situation the blood supply to subcutaneous fat in the dog is 3 to 10 ml/min/100 g, with a CFC of 0.02 to 0.035. The relationship between blood flow and CFC during "rest" and maximal dilatation suggests that the basal tone of the precapillary vessels is—as in most other vascular circuits—considerable. In the adipose tissue of a lean subject the blood supply appears to be relatively higher, suggesting that both the vascular dimensions and the current blood flow are related to the number of cells rather than to the tissue volume, i.e. to the metabolically active mass. Further, the vascular bed of this tissue must be tailored for *transport* purposes, considering the fact that the albumin molecules of the blood serve as the vehicle for the mobilized free fatty acids (FFA). As the binding sites between the albumin molecules and FFA are limited, a substantial plasma volume is needed whenever larger amounts of FFA are released, if they are not to accumulate locally.

Nervous and Hormonal Control

Nervous Control

The exact arrangement of the adrenergic nerve ramifications in adipose tissue is not known, but these fibres are doubtless able to affect both the lipocytes and their vascular bed. Thus, even low-frequency sympathetic

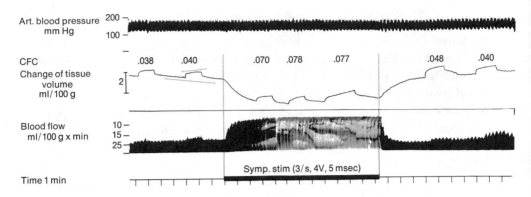

Fig. 28-3. Effects of low frequency sympathetic stimulation on blood flow, tissue volume (reflecting the change of regional blood volume) and CFC in the subcutaneous adipose tissue of the dog. (From Öberg and Rosell, 1967. By permission.)

stimulation produces a marked FFA release, which is blocked by β-receptor blocking agents (Rosell, 1966). With respect to the vascular bed, such direct nerve stimulation produces constriction of both resistance and capacitance vessels while CFC *increases* twofold or threefold (Fig. 28-3). The neurogenic constrictions may be so profound as virtually to stop the blood flow, as occurs after blood loss (Kovách and Rosell, 1968). These constrictor effects, as well as the CFC increase, are, however, blocked by α-blocking agents.

Paradoxically, this neurogenic increase of CFC is combined with a *reduced* PS value, and the reason for these opposite changes is unknown. Theoretically, however, they may be explained by a contraction of capillary sphincters, reducing the number of patent capillaries, combined with an increased capillary permeability. It should be stressed that filtration increases with the fourth power of the pore radius increase but diffusion increases only with the second power. To take an arbitrary example, suppose the pore radius were doubled but at the same time the perfused capillary surface area were reduced eight times. The PS value for water-soluble molecules would then be halved while the CFC value would be doubled (see Chapter 8).

Still it may appear surprising that an α-adrenergic mechanism produces an *increased* permeability, and, further, that it markedly delays the β-

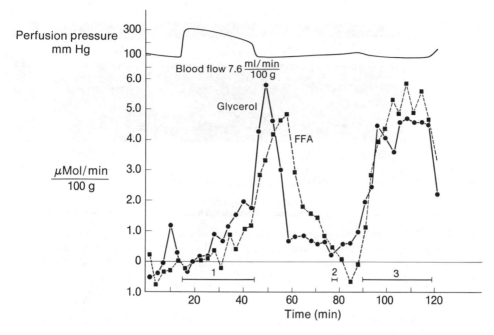

Fig. 28-4. Constant flow perfusion of subcutaneous adipose tissue in the dog. At signals 1 and 3 30 min of sympathetic stimulation at 10 imp/sec, at signal 2 i.a. administration of 100 μg dihydroergotamine. (From Fredholm and Rosell, 1968. By permission.)

adrenergic mobilization of FFA, which appears immediately upon sympathetic stimulation if α-adrenergic blocking drugs have been given (Fig. 28-4). It is possible that "local hormones" may play the role of modifying interlinks here. Thus, adipose tissue contains 5-HT and histaminc (which increases permeability) and prostaglandins (which dilate the vessels but counteract the lipolytic effect of sympathetic stimulation) and such factors might be partly responsible for these peculiar effects to sympathetic stimulation. The vascular control in adipose tissue certainly poses many problems of great interest such as these (see Rosell, 1969).

After complete α-blockade, sympathetic stimulation may produce maximal dilatation and an immediate and profound FFA release, but it causes only a moderate CFC increase (Fig. 28-5); these effects are eliminated by β-blocking drugs. Probably this dilator response represents a "functional hyperemia" secondary to a β-adrenergic stimulation of the

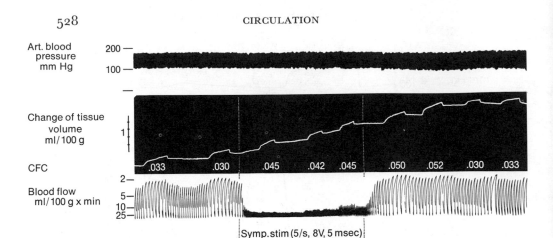

Fig. 28-5. Effects of sympathetic stimulation on blood flow, tissue volume, and CFC in the subcutaneous adipose tissue of the dog after i.a. administration of 100 μg of dihydroergotamine (α-receptor blockade). (From Rosell and Öberg, 1967. By permission.)

lipocytes; possibly it represents a direct β-adrenergic nervous effect on the vessels, and, if so, it is a rather extraordinary neurogenic mechanism.

Another question of great interest is whether the lipocytes and the vessels are controlled by the same or by different neurones. If they are separate and only the lipocyte-controlling link is activated, FFA mobilization should be more prompt in onset and not hampered by any flow restriction but rather facilitated by functional hyperemia. Such questions call for more work on the reflex and central nervous mechanisms controlling adipose tissue.

Hormonal Effects

Adrenaline produces much the same effect on FFA release as does sympathetic nerve stimulation, but with respect to the vascular bed the β-adrenergic effect might be more prominent than the α-adrenergic one, implying that blood supply is better maintained during FFA mobilization.

Adipose tissue also contains histamine and 5-HT, probably stored in mast cells, and these substances produce vasodilatation and increased CFC. Moreover, histamine causes a marked increase in FFA mobilization. Little is known, however, about the situations in which such "local hormone" mechanisms are involved. It has also been proposed that prostaglandins play a similar role; as mentioned they are powerful vasodilators in this tissue, but they counteract the lipolytic effect of sympathetic stimulation (see Rosell, 1969).

Whether hormones, like insulin, growth hormone, etc., exert any significant *direct* effects on the vascular bed of adipose tissue is not known. It seems likely that such hormones, by affecting the metabolism of the lipocytes, will produce secondary and parallel changes in blood supply, according to the inverse relationship that usually exists between tissue metabolism and regional vascular tone, other factors being unchanged.

References

Brånemark, P. J. (1968). "Bone marrow, microvascular structure and function," *Advances in Microcirculation* **1**, 1–65.

Fredholm, B., and S. Rosell (1968). "Effects of adrenergic blocking agents on lipid mobilization from canine subcutaneous adipose tissue after sympathetic nerve stimulation," *J. Pharm. Exp. Ther.* **159**, 1–7.

Heim, T., and D. Hull (1966). "The blood flow and oxygen consumption of brown adipose tissue in the new-born rabbit," *J. Physiol.* **186**, 42–55.

Kovách, A., and S. Rosell (1968). Personal communication.

Larsen, O. A., N. A. Lassen, and F. Quaade (1966). "Blood flow through human adipose tissue determined with radioactive xenon," *Acta Physiol. Scand.* **66**, 337–45.

Michelsen, K. (1968). "Hemodynamics of the bone marrow circulation," *Acta Physiol. Scand.* **73**, 264–80.

Öberg, B., and S. Rosell (1967). "Sympathetic control of consecutive vascular sections in canine subcutaneous adipose tissue," *Acta Physiol. Scand.* **71**, 47–56.

Root, W. S. (1963). "The flow of blood through bones and joints," *Handbook of Physiology*, 2, Circulation **II**, 1651–66.

Rosell, S. (1966). "Release of free fatty acids from subcutaneous adipose tissue in dogs following sympathetic nerve stimulation," *Acta Physiol. Scand.* **67**, 343–51.

Rosell, S. (1969). "Nervous and pharmacological regulation of vascular reactions in adipose tissue," *Third international symposium on drugs affecting lipid metabolism* (ed. W. L. Holmes, L. A. Carlsson, and R. Paoletti). New York: Plenum Press.

29

Uterine and Foetal Circulations

Uterine Blood Flow

The uterus possesses three layers—the superficial serosal layer, the myometrium, and the endometrium. It weighs 50 to 70 g in the nulligravid woman, but by the end of pregnancy it can have increased in bulk to about 1 kg (excluding its content of conceptus, placenta, and amniotic fluid) owing to hyperplasia and hypertrophy of the myometrium. The burden of pregnancy is associated with an increase of blood flow from one quantitatively trivial—10 to 20 ml—in the nulliparous woman, to one of the order of 750 ml.

The important features of the uterine circulation then are entirely different, according to whether the uterus is gravid or not. The literature is reviewed by Reynolds (1963).

Non-gravid Uterus (After Puberty)

The important changes in the non-gravid, postpubertal uterus involve the endometrium. The blood supply of the endometrium is derived from radial branches of the arcuate arteries. The arcuate arteries lie in the myometrium, parallel to the serosal circumference and also to the endometrium. They break up into *basal* arteries, which are straight and which supply only basal parts of the endometrium, and spiral arteries, which

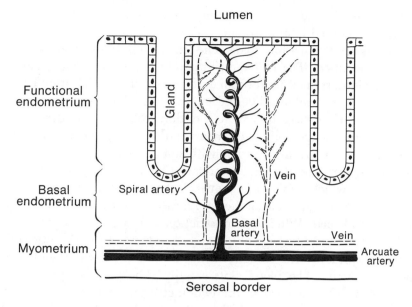

Fig. 29-1. Scheme of blood supply to endometrium.

nourish the superficial third of the endometrium (Fig. 29-1). It is this superficial layer which undergoes cyclical changes of bulk and vascularity with the menstrual cycle in the primate.

The menstrual cycle is described as beginning with the first day of bleeding. Bleeding lasts about four days and is followed by a short stage of repair (of the endometrial surface) which lasts a day or so. From the fifth or sixth day of the cycle the endometrium shows the changes of the "proliferative stage", and with release of the ovum from the Graafian follicle on about the fourteenth day, there supervenes the "secretory stage". If fertilization of the ovum is not achieved the secretory stage terminates about the twenty-eighth day and bleeding begins another cycle.

At the beginning of the proliferative stage the endometrium is about 2 mm thick, consisting of a ciliated columnar epithelium which dips into a loose stroma to form simple tubular glands. During the sixth to fourteenth day the mucosa thickens, the glands elongate, and the superficial layer becomes much more vascular due to the budding of capillaries from the spiral arteries. Ovulation is followed characteristically by an alteration in appearance of the endometrium during the "secretory stage". The glands become saw-toothed in appearance as they are distended with mucus and their linings are thrown into folds. The length and diameter of the glands is greatly increased. The endometrial capillaries are congested and exudations of blood stained fluid occur into the stroma, which itself contains many cells due to proliferation and enlargement. The appearance of the endometrium in this secretory stage is of diagnostic value in gynaecology.

The secretory stage ends with menstruation, in which the superficial part of the endometrium, together with some blood, is shed, leaving the basal layer intact. Menstruation is prefaced by bouts of constriction of the spiral arteries which may last for hours. Ischaemia of the superficial layer causes necrosis and the walls of the capillaries and the stroma surrounding them are weakened. When the constriction passes off, the restoration of the blood flow causes leakage of blood and oedema of the necrotic stroma and epithelium and these slough off into the uterine cavity together with blood and mucus. The blood clots rapidly. The process appears to be sequential in different parts of the endometrium, for if it were not so, a large haemorrhage would result from the sloughing of wide areas of the endometrium at once. After four days or so bleeding ceases; during this stage the destructive phase in any region is promptly followed by repair in which the surface epithelium and the simple tubular glands are restored by outgrowths from the basal parts of the glands.

These features of the endometrial changes during the menstrual cycle have been elegantly analysed by Markee (1940) who implanted pieces of endometrium into the anterior chamber of the eye of the Rhesus monkey and observed the changes directly. Markee noted that the endometrial grafts showed rhythmic vasoconstrictions and dilatations during the non-bleeding part of the cycle, and he attributed this to effects of oestrogens. Oestrogens injected caused a persistent hyperaemia, presumably due to relaxation of the precapillary resistance vessels. He and others concluded that the hyperaemia of oestrogenic and/or progesterone-like compounds were metabolically induced phenomena.

Oophorectomy in monkeys (or women) causes endometrial bleeding within a few days—whatever the phase of the cycle at which the operation is performed. This proves that the bleeding is due to the withdrawal of an ovarian factor (or factors). If, however, oestrogen injections are instituted immediately after oophorectomy this bleeding is prevented and only takes place when the injections are suspended. Curettings of the endometrium show this to be in the proliferative phase. Bleeding can thus be induced by oestrogen withdrawal. If progesterone injections are given upon the suspension of oestrogen administration, bleeding is postponed until the course of injections ceases, but bleeding follows this cessation. Endometrial curettings indicate that the secretory phase had supervened.

Such results indicate that the endometrial vessels are under the control of the sex hormones. With the development of the Graafian follicle, the oestrogen content of the blood rises and the spiral arteries and their branches proliferate together with an increase in the epithelial and stromatous cells. The rupture of the follicle is associated with a drop in the oestrogen concentration, but the subsequent formation of the corpus luteum leads to a secretion of progesterone from the lutein cells which is responsible for the further vascular, epithelial, and stromal development that characterizes the secretory phase. The degeneration of the corpus luteum (which secretes some oestrogen as well as progesterone) provokes the spasm of the spiral arteries that induces the necrosis of the superficial epithelium as the premonitory stage of menstruation.

It is unlikely that the sex hormones induce these vascular reactions directly; it is more probable that they alter the tone of the spiral arteries by affecting the local metabolism of the endometrium and thus causing the liberation of vasoactive substances. This assertion has not been proved, however, and it must be admitted that oestrogens can provoke hyperaemia of the nasal mucosa: moreover, the "hot flushes" of the menopause remain entirely unexplained. Much more work is required on the response of isolated endometrial vessels to the sex hormones.

The Pregnant Uterus

With the commencement of pregnancy, the maternal and foetal circulations are separated within the placenta. The distance between the maternal and foetal bloodstreams varies considerably, not only in different species, but also in the same species at different stages of gestation. In all cases, however, this distance greatly exceeds that of the alveolar capillary membrane of the mammalian lung. In the higher primates, the foetal villi are bathed in maternal blood which flows through the intervillous space.

The chorio-allantoic placentas of eutherian mammals are classified into four principal types according to Grosser's concept (Grosser, 1909, 1927) of the degree of erosion of the maternal placenta. Each type is designated by a term which indicates the two tissues, one maternal and one foetal, which are in immediate contact. An *epitheliochorial* placenta shows simple apposition of the uterine epithelium and the chorion; the pig and the horse are examples. A *syndesmochorial* placenta shows erosion of the uterine epithelium but not of the maternal connective tissue stroma (e.g. sheep, goat). In the *endotheliochorial* placenta both maternal epithelium and connective tissue are eroded; the cat and dog exemplify this type. Finally, the *haemochorial* placenta shows complete erosion of the uterine tissues so that the maternal blood is in direct contact with the foetal chorion; this is the case in man and monkey. The foetal chorion forms villi supplied by blood returning from the umbilical artery (deoxygenated). From these villi, more oxygenated blood passes via the umbilical vein to supply the foetal circulation.

The direction of maternal blood flow through the intervillous space is unknown. Bartels *et al.* (1962) have suggested that there may be a multi-villous stream system in which numerous foetal capillaries are encountered along the pathway of the maternal blood. However, in the arrangement suggested by Bartels *et al.*, different villi would be surrounded by blood of different gas tensions depending on their location in the intervillous space (Fig. 29-2). The foetal blood loses CO_2 (and possibly metabolic acids) to the maternal blood and this causes a displacement of the foetal oxygen

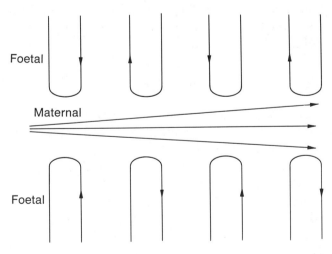

Fig. 29-2. Diagram of the suggested direction of blood flow in the multivillous placenta of woman. (From Bartels *et al.*, 1962. By permission.)

dissociation curve to the left and of the maternal blood to the right, thereby favouring the oxygen uptake by the foetal blood. Reviewing the literature, Dawes (1965) has suggested that pO_2 in the umbilical vein is of the order of 40 to 50 mm Hg—sufficient to produce a saturation in the foetal blood of 65 to 70%, as he says—the Andes, rather than Everest "in utero". Unfortunately, it is impossible to calculate the diffusion gradient because the uterine venous pO_2 is not known. Blood samples withdrawn from the intervillous space are of little use in this respect because the needle tip may be adjacent either to the arterial inflow or to the venous outflow.

Several techniques have been used for estimating the total uterine flow

Table 29-1

	Rabbit	Woman	Sheep and Goat
Uterine flow per kg foetal weight (ml/kg/min)	125	156	283
Uterine O_2 usage per kg foetal weight (ml/kg/min)	8.3	7.4	8.9

during pregnancy. In pioneer experiments Barcroft (see Barcroft, 1946) and his colleagues collected the uterine venous outflow to the common iliac for timed periods. The measurements—made in rabbits—gave figures much lower than those yielded by techniques that do not require anaesthesia and major surgical manipulation. More modern studies have been directed to the measurement of total uterine flow in sheep, goats, and women. Three main methods have been employed—direct Fick estimations, electromagnetic flow meter measurements, and the clearance of radioactive sodium injected into the intervillous space. Using a modified Fick method, Metcalfe et al. (1955, 1959) showed that the blood flow and the uterine oxygen consumption of various animals were as given in Table 29-1. It would seem that the haemochorial type of placenta (woman) is much more efficient than that of the syndesmochorial placenta of the sheep and goat.

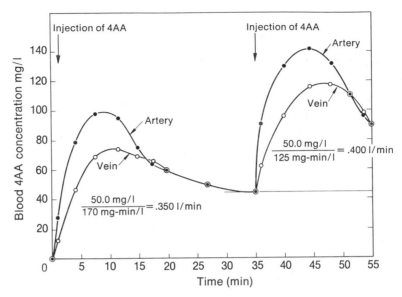

Fig. 29-3. Illustrative data from which uterine blood flows are computed after injection of 4AA in unanesthetized sheep. The calculations from these curves are typical of all diffusion-equilibration methods for regional blood flow. The time course of the second uterine blood flow determination is not shown in full. (From Huckabee *et al.*, 1961. By permission.)

Assali *et al.* (1960) compared uterine flow values obtained in women with electromagnetic flow meters and with the N_2O technique, respectively, and found that uterine blood flow increased from 50 ml/min in the 10th week of pregnancy to 190 ml/min by the 30th week. Browne and Veal (1953) injected [24]NaCl into the intervillous space in normal pregnant women and found a flow of 600 ml/min.

Huckabee (1962) used 4-amino antipyrine (4AA) to study uterine flow. This compound is injected in isotonic solution intravenously and its equilibration with the uterine tissue is studied by repeated sampling of arterial and uterine venous blood. 4AA equilibrates with the tissues of the pregnant uterus, placenta, and foetus within 20 min (Fig. 29-3). Such studies were carried out in unanaesthetized goats, or in women at caesarean section, and yielded figures of some 280 ml/kg/min uterine flow in the goat over the last half of pregnancy and a total uterine flow of 700 to 800 ml/min in women at full term. Figure 29-4 shows how variable the flow

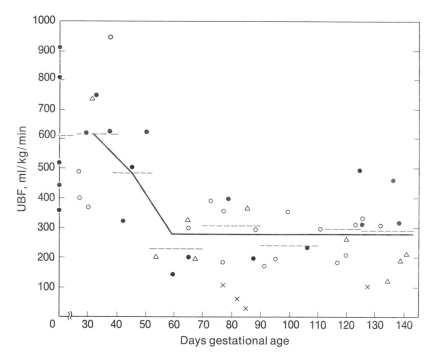

Fig. 29-4. Changes in uterine blood flow during the course of pregnancy in goats. Twin pregnancies are indicated by circles, triplets by triangles. Points shown as crosses were obtained after death of the foetus. (From Huckabee *et al.*, 1962. By permission.)

figures were in goats. It also shows the surprising result that uterine flow falls from an initial high value of 600 ml/kg/min in early pregnancy to about 300 ml/kg/min by the time term was half advanced; this lower value was maintained over the last half of pregnancy despite the fact that the majority of the increase in the weight of the conceptus occurs over this period.

Oxygen usage was calculated from flow measurements and from arterial and venous oxygen contents. Oxygen usage rose from 2 ml/kg/min in early pregnancy (while the blood flow was falling) to reach a value of 10 ml/kg/min by midpregnancy, which value was then maintained until term (Fig. 29-5). Huckabee (1962) notes that, from midpregnancy onwards, there is a definite correlation of blood flow with both size and metabolic rate of

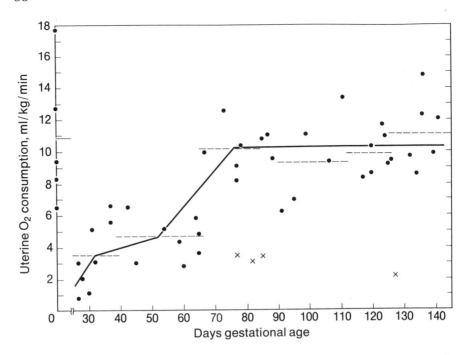

Fig. 29-5. Rate of consumption of oxygen by the pregnant uterus at various gestational ages. (From Huckabee *et al.*, 1961. By permission.)

the uterus and its contents. However, as he states, "it seems clear from the figures given that uterine blood flow does vary from one circumstance to another. It is not a fixed value".

On the other hand, hypoxaemia deliberately induced in the unaesthetized pregnant ewe caused no compensatory increase in uterine blood flow and neither did hypercapnia of the mother. Likewise, uterine blood flow and uterine vascular resistance were unaffected by spinal anaesthesia. Such apparent unresponsiveness of the uterine circulation suggests that the foetus must possess an unusual capacity for sustaining anaerobic metabolism for short periods (compare the "diving reflex"; Chapter 19). When hypoxaemia is chronic, however, uterine blood flow is increased. Thus, measurements made on pregnant ewes living at high altitude (Peruvian Andes) showed uterine flows well in excess of those recorded in pregnant ewes at sea level.

To summarize, our knowledge of the factors that *regulate* uterine blood flow during pregnancy is sparse. Many fragmentary observations have been made on the influence of contractions on uterine flow, but only by methods which do not give absolute flow rates. As might be expected, such contractions usually lower uterine flow.

Foetal Circulation

Foetal circulation is in important respects radically different from that of the extrauterine existence (for refs. see Young, 1963; Dawes, 1964, 1965, 1968); birth is accompanied by the most dramatic cardiovascular events that the individual has to face until death stops it all.

The placenta oxygenates the blood delivered to it by the umbilical artery. From the placenta, blood which is 80% saturated with oxygen travels via the umbilical vein to the liver of the foetus. Here some of the umbilical venous blood passes directly to the inferior vena cava via the ductus venosus; the remainder supplies the left two-thirds of the liver, from which the blood gains access to the inferior vena cava through the hepatic veins. The right one-third of the liver receives blood from the portal vein. Blood in the inferior vena cava is approximately 67% saturated, comprising a mixture of that from the umbilical vein (80% saturated) and that from the hepatic and systemic veins (26% saturated; see Chapter 14).

On entering the right atrium, this bloodstream from the inferior vena cava is directed two ways by the crista dividens (see Fig. 14-6, p. 246)— the bulk of the flow passes via the foramen ovale into the left atrium, and a minor flow, which is joined by blood from the superior vena cava and the coronary sinus, passes into the right ventricle. The output of the right ventricle is again divided into a bulk flow through the pulmonary trunk into the ductus arteriosus and thence into the aorta. A smaller flow passes through the lungs, for the resistance offered by the airless, collapsed lungs is high. Unlike the situation in the adult, the two ventricles act *in parallel*, not in series, and the pulmonary arterial pressure is higher than that of the aorta.

Thanks to the work of Dawes and his colleagues (Dawes, 1968) quantitative data of flows through the various parts of the foetal circulation are available (Fig. 29-6). About half of the combined output of the two

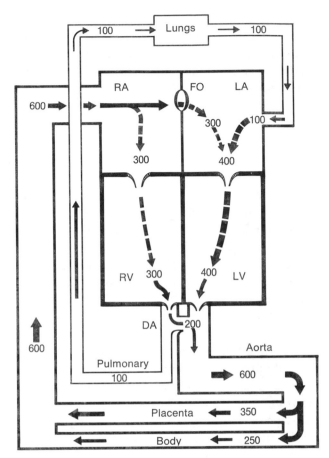

Fig. 29-6. Approximate figures for distribution of blood flow in the foetal lamb near term. DA = Ductus Arteriosus, FO = Foramen Ovale. Figures in ml/min.

ventricles is delivered to the placenta, which offers a low resistance circuit situated in parallel with the foetal tissues.

None of the foetal tissues, except the liver, is supplied by blood that exceeds 60 to 65% in saturation. Fig. 14-4 illustrates diagrammatically the results obtained in the foetal lamb. Earlier studies suggested that the arterial oxygen tension was only 30 to 35 mm Hg, compared with that of 100 mm Hg in the adult—a situation Barcroft described as the "Mount Everest in utero" which the foetus has perforce to overcome. Later work with improved methods put this pO_2 at 40 to 50 mm Hg, i.e. "the Andes in utero" (see page 535). It must be borne in mind that this low arterial pO_2 is inevitably accompanied by a higher pCO_2 and a lower arterial pH. When the arterial pO_2 of the foetus is lowered moderately umbilical blood flow increases, as do the heart rate and foetal blood pressure. Further degrees of hypoxia—resulting in a blood oxygen saturation of less than 15%—causes bradycardia and this, probably due to chemoreceptor reflexes, has long been regarded as a cardinal sign of foetal distress. The hypoxic foetus displays a "diving reflex" (see Chapter 19) and a reduced cardiac output is distributed mainly to the CNS and myocardium with considerable vasoconstriction in muscle and skin (Dawes et al., 1968).

The foetus and the new-born, unlike the adult organism, react to hypoxia with a *reduction* of metabolic rate. Even though the circulation is well maintained, when the saturation of blood in the umbilical artery falls below 50% ($pO_2 = 20$ mm Hg) the metabolic rate falls and lactate accumulation occurs, indicating that anaerobic glycolysis is at least partly supplying the metabolic requirements of the foetus.

Systemic Blood Pressure in the Foetus

As Young (1963) has pointed out, the final values recorded at term in foetuses of different species correspond well with the requirements of the newly born of the species under consideration. The helpless neonate of the rat or the rabbit is born with a mean arterial pressure of 30 mm Hg, whereas the active new-born guinea pig manifests an arterial pressure of 50 mm Hg. New-born lambs, kids, Rhesus monkeys, and humans all have a pressure of 60 to 70 mm Hg, despite their differing periods of gestation. The foetal lamb shows a blood pressure of 30 mm Hg for the first 13 weeks of gestation and this then rises to 65 mm over the remaining 7 weeks. It is not known whether the rise of arterial pressure is due solely to an increasing cardiac output or to this coupled with a rising precapillary resistance. At term the cardiac output per kg body weight is greater than that of an adult, and this indicates that the peripheral vascular resistance is low.

Foetal Heart

At term the foetal heart of the lamb expels 235 ml/min/kg body weight. The heart rate increases during the first 13 weeks of the 20-week gestation period to reach values of 150/min, and continues to increase over the latter third of pregnancy to achieve final values of 200/min—while the heart rate of the ewe is 110/min. The human foetal heart rate is highest in mid-foetal life, at 155 to 160/min, and it falls to 140 to 145 just before birth. Both sympathetic and parasympathetic innervations of the heart are established early (at the 6th week) in foetal development, but opinions are divided as to their respective influence on the heart rate of the foetus. For example, Barcroft found that bilateral vagotomy increased the foetal heart rate in the lamb, but Dawes and his colleagues could not confirm this (see Young, 1963). The foetal heart is very sensitive both to acetycholine and to adrenaline and noradrenaline, but there is little evidence that vagal or sympathetic tone contribute to the *normal* heart rate of the foetus. However, profound reflex alterations of foetal heart rate and blood pressure can undoubtedly occur in circumstances of hypoxia and asphyxia.

In early foetal life, asphyxia acts directly on the sino-atrial node to slow the heart, and the resulting reduction in cardiac output contributes to the systemic arterial hypotension which results from a temporary occlusion of the umbilical cord. Later in foetal development, umbilical cord occlusion causes a transient bradycardia, possibly due to a direct stimulation by the asphyxia of the vagal cardio-inhibitory centre. Towards the end of gestation asphyxia induces bradycardia followed by tachycardia (mediated by the cardiac sympathetic nerves), to which the adrenal output of catecholamines contribute. Bradycardia in the later stage of foetal development is reflex in origin, partly due to the asphyxial stimulation of the carotid bodies and partly due to the excitation of the sino-aortic baroreceptors by the hypertension which the asphyxia induces. When the oxygen saturation of the arterial blood falls below 15 to 20% bradycardia always supervenes. This provides an indication of foetal distress. As noted previously, this bradycardia is one manifestation of a "diving reflex" adjustment of the cardiovascular system.

Changes in the Circulation at Birth

When the foetus is delivered and the umbilical cord is tied there is an evanescent rise of blood pressure due to the increase in systemic peripheral resistance coupled with a reduction in the systemic vascular capacity. There ensues a period of partial asphyxia which provokes systemic hypertension and culminates in a succession of gasps that finally yield to the onset of breathing. Because the distensibility of the airways leading to the initially airless lungs is so high these early gasps cause dramatic swings in the intrathoracic pressure; values of 50 mm Hg or so below atmospheric pressure have been recorded. The gaseous distension of the previously collapsed lungs causes a profound reduction of the pulmonary vascular resistance, which falls to below 20% of its value in the foetal state. Consequently, pulmonary blood flow increases five or more times, although the pulmonary artery pressure falls to a value below that in the aorta.

The interruption of umbilical blood flow lowers the pressure in the inferior vena cava, and both the ductus venous and the valve of the foramen ovale close. Within a minute or two all systemic venous blood is directed only to the right atrium and ventricle, whence it is pumped out by the ventricle into the lungs. As a result of the fall of pulmonary arterial pressure, the aortic pressure now exceeds that in the pulmonary artery, and blood flow through the ductus now passes from aorta to pulmonary artery, contributing some 50% to the total pulmonary flow. This contribution of blood to the pulmonary circuit ensures that the oxygenation of the systemic blood is notably increased, and, indeed, artificial occlusion of the ductus

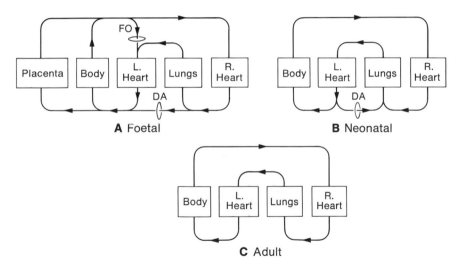

Fig. 29-7. Very simplified diagrams to illustrate the changes in the circulation at birth as described in the text. In A the two ventricles are working in parallel to drive blood from the great veins to the arteries. B is the condition reached a few minutes after birth when the cord is tied and the foramen ovale (FO) closes. When the ductus arteriosus, DA, finally closes, the adult circulation (C) is established with the two ventricles working in series. (From Born, *et al.*, 1954. By permission.)

at this stage reduces the oxygen saturation of the systemic arterial blood. The ductus arteriosus begins to close some 10 to 15 min after birth, but the process is not completed for 24 to 48 hours. During this period "retrograde" ductus flow is continuous and causes a murmur which, though continuous, reaches a crescendo with the second sound. Permanent closure of the ductus arteriosus is achieved by endothelial proliferation, which takes many weeks to complete. Fig. 29-7 shows some of the circulatory changes which occur at birth and depicts the foetal, neonatal, and adult circulations in schematic form.

Closure of the ductus arteriosus is independent of nervous connections. It occurs as a result of inflating the lungs with a high oxygen tension; conversely, the ductus dilates if the blood pO_2 is low.

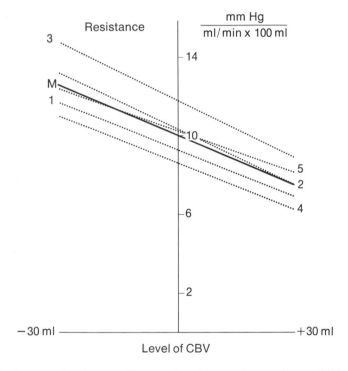

Fig. 29-8. Extent of reflex cardiovascular changes in newborn child, sleeping while circulating blood volume (CBV) is changed $\pm 12.5\%$. Note that this change of CBV changes limb flow resistance (plethysmographic recording) some 50% with only little change in mean blood pressure. (Courtesy of Dr. O. Celander, Göteborg, Sweden, 1967.)

Development of Nervous Control Mechanisms in the Neonate

The average cardiac output of the new-born human infant is 540 ml/min, which approximately corresponds to an output of 180 ml/kg/min—twice the value per unit weight shown by the adult (but fairly equal to that of the resting 3 to 4 kg cat). The heart rate is 140/min, so the stroke volume is some 4 ml. The mean arterial pressure is 60 to 65 mm at birth and rises to about 80 mm at 3 months. Peripheral resistance is therefore low, both brain and extremities receiving almost twice as much blood per unit weight as do the corresponding tissues in the adult. Baroreceptor and other cardiovascular reflexes are quite powerful in the new-born infant (see Fig. 29-8). Sympathetic circulatory responses to alteration in the thermal environment are also brisk and effective.

References

Assali, N. S., L. Rauramo, and T. Peltonen (1960). "Uterine and fetal blood flow and oxygen consumption in early human pregnancy," *Am. J. Obstet. and Gynec.* **79,** 86–98.

Barcroft, J. (1946). *Researches on prenatal life*, Vol. I. Oxford: Blackwell.

Bartels, H., W. Moll, and J. Metcalfe (1962). "Physiology of gas exchange in the human placenta," *Am. J. Obstet. and Gynec.* **84,** 1714–30.

Born, G. V. R., G. S. Dawes, J. C. Mott, and J. G. Widdicombe (1954). "Changes in the heart and lungs at birth," *Cold Spr. Harb. Symp. quant. Biol.* **19,** 102–20.

Browne, J. C. McC., and N. Veal (1953). "The maternal placental blood flow in normotensive and hypertensive women," *J. Obstet. and Gynec. Brit. Empire,* **60,** 141–47.

Celander, O., L. S. Prod'home, N. Frenck, and J. E. Sigdell (1967). "Cardio-vascular adjustments to acute hypo- and hypervolaemia during exchange transfusions in newborn infants," *Ped. Res.* **1,** 411.

Dawes, G. S. (1964). "Physiological changes in the circulation after birth," in *Circulation of the blood* (ed. A. P. Fishman and D. W. Richards), pp. 743–834. New York: Oxford University Press.

Dawes, G. S. (1965). "Oxygen supply and consumption in late fetal life and the onset of breathing at birth," *Handbook of Physiology*, 3, Respiration **II,** 1313–28.

Dawes, G. S. (1968). *Foetal and Neonatal Physiology*. Chicago: Year Book Med. Publ.

Dawes, G. S., B. V. Lewis, J. E. Milligan, M. R. Roach, and N. S. Talner (1968). "Vasomotor responses in the hind limbs of foetal and new born lambs to asphyxia and aortic chemoreceptor stimulation," *J. Physiol.* **195,** 55–81.

Grosser, O. (1909). *Vergleichende Anatomie und Entwicklingsgeschichte der Eihaute und der Placenta mit besonderer Berucksichtigung des Menschen*. Vienna: Braumüller.

Grosser, O. (1927). *Frühentwickling, Eihautbildung und Placentation des Menschen und der Säugetiere*. New York: Bergman.

Huckabee, W. E. (1962). "Uterine blood flow," *Am. J. Obstet. and Gynec.* **84,** 1623–33.

Huckabee, W. E., J. Metcalfe, H. Prystowsky, and D. H. Barron (1961). "Blood flow and oxygen consumption of the pregnant uterus," *Am. J. Physiol.* **200,** 274–78.

Markee, J. E. (1940). "Menstruation in intraocular endometrial transplants in the rhesus monkey," *Contrib. Embryol. Carnegie Inst.* **28,** 219–308.

Metcalfe, J., S. L. Romney, L. H. Ramsey, D. E. Reid, and S. C. Burwell (1955). "Estimation of uterine blood flow in normal human pregnancy at term," *J. Clin. Invest.* **34,** 1632–38.

Metcalfe, J., S. L. Romney, J. R. Swarthout, D. M. Pitcairn, A. N. Lethin, and D. H. Baum (1959). "Uterine blood flow and oxygen consumption in pregnant sheep and goats," *Am. J. Physiol.* **197,** 929–34.

Reynolds, S. R. M. (1963). "Maternal blood flow in the uterus and placenta," *Handbook of Physiology*, 2, Circulation **II,** 1585–1618.

Young, Maureen (1963). "The fetal and neonatal circulation," *Handbook of Physiology*, 2, Circulation **II,** 1619–50.

30

Shock

General Considerations

Shock is a syndrome characterized by a cardiac output that is insufficient to maintain adequate tissue nutrition. Haemorrhage, trauma, and prolonged ischaemia (caused by tourniquets) may all cause shock. Burns induce shock by provoking excessive plasma loss; dehydration, such as is caused by thermal sweating, or by prolonged diarrhoea (gastric enteritis, cholera, etc.), also leads to circulatory collapse. The essential feature of shock is a relative inadequacy of the circulatory blood volume; arterial and venous pressures are therefore low, cardiac output is subnormal, and there may be anuria.

Wiggers (1950) defined four stages in the development of shock: (1) The developing stage, in which the circulatory volume is decreased but not to the extent of causing serious symptoms; (2) the compensatory stage, in which blood volume is further reduced but reflex vasoconstriction of the skin, muscle, and splanchnic circulations permit a maintenance of e.g. arterial blood pressure and thereby allow an adequate flow to the heart and brain; (3) the progressive stage, in which the pressure inexorably falls even though vasoconstriction, tachycardia, etc., continue to increase and, as the pressure falls to 60 mm Hg, myocardial metabolism becomes prejudiced; (4) the irreversible stage, which is not relieved by transfusion, and, as a result of failure of myocardial and cerebral depression the patient dies.

The cause of shock is not known and therefore is much written about. However, some of the features of shock can be simply produced by haemorrhage; in civil or military life, trauma, burns, infections, etc., complicate the issue and must be considered separately. For reviews of various aspects of shock see Seeley and Weisiger (1961), Bock (1962), Fine (1965), Chien (1967), and Kovách (1971).

Haemorrhage

Breach of continuity of the vascular system causes blood loss. This may be rapid, and if it is too rapid it may be fatal. It is surprising, however, what the natural reactions of the body can secure in maintaining life. An individual who actually blew his arm off by discharging a shotgun into his axilla was brought into hospital unconscious two hours later with a blood pressure of 80/60 and a heart rate of 160. The severed axillary artery could be seen pulsating feebly like a moving finger in the wound, having retracted and clotted. After transfusion he recovered.

Compensatory mechanisms: Large haemorrhage, say 30% of blood volume, causes a fall of mean blood pressure and this reflexly induces sympathetic discharge. Vasoconstriction occurs in resistance and capacitance vessels; force and rate of the heart are subjected to positive stimulation by the cardiac sympathetic nerves. The pulse is rapid and less vigorous; the skin is constricted, and a patient manifests a greyish cold skin covered with "cold sweat". The sweat glands are activated, but the sweat does not evaporate readily because the skin is cold owing to the vasoconstriction. Breathing is stimulated but may be rapid and shallow.

Venoconstriction reduces the capacity of the circulation and aids the mobilization of blood to the heart. The precapillary/postcapillary resistance ratio increases reflexly, especially in the skeletal muscles (Chapter 20), so that the mean capillary pressure drops considerably, thereby favouring an uptake of tissue fluid particularly from this large tissue mass. Further, any fall in central arterial and venous pressures, other things being equal, lowers capillary pressure and therefore contributes to the uptake of tissue fluid. This tends to restore the blood volume, but does not, of course, restore plasma proteins to the circulation. Hence the plasma protein level decreases so that the force tending to draw fluid in from the tissues is reduced. Restoration of plasma proteins by their synthesis and release from the liver is a slower business—one taking days. Some restoration occurs more quickly as lymph returns some of the proteins of the interstitial space.

Renal blood flow is markedly reduced, partly due to sympathetic vasoconstriction, and partly due to the fall of pressure head. This may reduce glomerular filtration pressure to the extent that oliguria or even anuria ensues. Further, the vasoconstriction and the drop in afferent arteriolar pressure causes an increased output of renin; this forms angiotensin which, besides such concentrations that it contributes to the peripheral vasoconstriction, liberates aldosterone and hence enhances tubular sodium retention. ADH, perhaps released reflexly via cardiovascular "volume receptors" (see Chapter 20), and, in conscious subjects, as a response to the painful and emotional effects of trauma, further minimizes fluid loss in the urine. As a result of these hormonal adjustments oliguria or anuria may occur. The marked reduction of renal fluid loss is accompanied by an intense thirst (see below) which aids in the restoration of the fluid balance.

Adrenaline release induces hyperglycaemia and increases the mobilization of fatty acids. ACTH is released and liberates cortisol which causes an increase of protein catabolism and an increase of glyconeogenesis.

The depleted circulation can provide only a fraction of the normal tissue blood flow, and mixed venous blood sampled from the right ventricle shows a much smaller oxygen content than the normal value of 14 to 15 ml/100 ml. Nevertheless, the organism survives and may slowly improve on its initially disturbed conditions owing to its compensatory responses, which, by throttling the blood supply to the less essential tissues, favour those to the heart and the brain (see e.g. Gregg, 1962). These sympathetic discharges are provoked not only from the mechanoreceptor zones, but also from the chemoreceptor areas of the carotid and aortic bodies. The chemoreceptors are powerfully stimulated by a reduction in their blood flow, and their discharge further enhances the increased cardiovascular sympathetic impulse activity as well as that of the respiratory centre.

The combination of these effects is responsible for some of the signs of severe bleeding in man—rapid, shallow respiration, greyish, cool and moist skin, coupled with sunken features, dry mouth, and intense thirst.

From this brief résumé it should be clear that the increased sympathetic discharge plays a vital protective role in the immediate response to haemorrhage. Thus, Chien (1967) has shown that with an intact sympathetic nervous system 50% of a series of dogs could survive a 40% reduction of blood volume, whereas 50% of sympathectomized dogs could only tolerate a 30% reduction of blood volume. It follows that, if no fluid is available for transfusion, every effort should be made to allow this compensatory sympathetic vasoconstriction full rein.

Before World War I there was little in the way of fluid restoration for bled individuals. The war brought the use of gum-saline (which has an osmotic pressure similar to plasma), and this killed many, as it was in other respects unsuitable. There was no plasma and no blood transfusion. Treatment consisted of putting the patients in warm blankets with hot bottles and giving them hot drinks. However, H. C. Bazett made the fundamental observation in 1918 that this treatment was prejudicial to the patient's survival. Casualties at the battlefront were so frightful that medical orderly services were overburdened and many men were left in the winter cold. Bazett noted that their recovery rate was higher than that of the casualties who had been speedily withdrawn to the casualty stations and submitted to the current régime of treatment.

As stated in Chapter 19, the compensatory vasoconstriction of the skin and other regional circuits that occurs in response to circulatory depletion can be overcome by the hypothalamic response to thermal stress, which causes inhibition of sympathetic vasoconstrictor discharge to the cutaneous vascular circuit. Additionally, the metabolic rate of cold tissues rises as the temperature of the tissues increases and the provision of vasodilator metabolites contributes to the loss of tone of the precapillary vessels, e.g. in the earlier cooled extremities. The peripheral resistance falls, more blood is pooled in the cutaneous veins and the mean arterial pressure head may diminish alarmingly with consequent untoward effects on the blood supply of the heart and the brain.

One of the most characteristic symptoms of man in shock is that of insatiable thirst. Discussing the various accounts of the clinical picture of shock in the literature, Grant and Reeve (1951) draw attention to the disagreement among them in many respects. Nevertheless, nearly all accounts describe the craving of the wounded man for fluid. The recent results of Fitzsimons would seem to provide an important link in this complex chain of events. Angiotensin infused intravenously into rats in normal water balance causes the rats to drink water, although the effect is greater in nephrectomized rats (Fitzsimons and Simons, 1968). One of several possible ways in which this action might be mediated is through the direct stimulation of "drinking centres" in the hypothalamus. Epstein, Fitzsimons, and Simons (1969) investigated this by permanently implanting steel cannulae 0.5 mm in diameter in various regions of the lateral and anterior hypothalamus of rats. Intracranial doses of angiotensin (0.2μ) could be delivered through these cannulae by a remote microsyringe connected by polythene tubing. $0.2 \mu g$ angiotensin so administered (a dose some 1/25th of the smallest systemic dose required to produce an effect on water intake) provoked drinking after a latency of some seconds, and this drinking continued for 10 min without interruption. Such drinking could be induced even when a starving animal just allowed access to food received an injection—he left the food alone and drank (and drank!). Even a sleeping rat is awakened by the effects of the angiotensin injection, and subsequently displays the usual "avidity" of fluid intake.

It seems likely that these observations account for the insatiable thirst of man or animal following haemorrhage. Hypotension provokes discharge of renin, which forms angiotensin, which in turn induces the drinking reaction. The first "signals" might come from the atrial "low pressure" receptors. As stated in Chapters 18 and 20, the reflex vascular effects of these receptors appear to affect particularly the renal circuit. This, in turn, affects the renin release (Chapter 27) which may start the chain of events mentioned above.

Deterioration of the compensatory mechanisms: As described in detail in Chapter 16, sympathetic vasoconstrictor discharge increases the tone of the resistance and capacitance vessels and, by increasing the precapillary/postcapillary resistance ratio in some circuits, particularly in the muscles, lowers the capillary hydrostatic pressure, thereby favouring the uptake of tissue fluid. These reflex vasoconstrictor responses are of admirable value in the emergency situation, but as stated previously, they inevitably produce throttling of the blood supply to tissues like the muscles and the splanchnic bed. These regions correspondingly suffer inadequate nutritional supply, and if the period over which this relative ischaemia occurs is unduly prolonged secondary problems arise.

These have been analysed by Mellander and Lewis (1963), using the "hindquarters preparation" (see also Fig. 16-7, page 297). The initial responses of the resistance and capacitance vessels and the change of the precapillary/postcapillary resistance ratio caused by a standardized stimulation of the lumbar sympathetic trunks were first recorded while the arterial pressure head was normal. The arterial pressure head to the hind-limbs was then artificially reduced by 50%, either by tightening a screw-clip around the abdominal aorta or by producing a graded blood loss. The state of hypotension in the region studied was sustained for some hours while the responses of the resistance vessels, the capacitance vessels, etc., to repeated bouts of standardized sympathetic stimulation were recorded. These responses were expressed graphically as percentages of their values obtained during the control period (Fig. 30-1). The response of

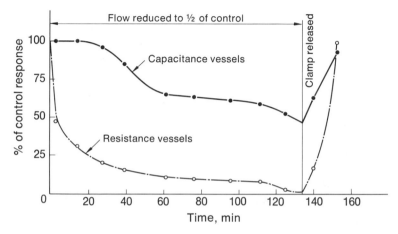

Fig. 30-1. Changes in reactivity of resistance and capacitance vessels of the cat's hindquarters to vasoconstrictor fibre stimulation during a period of hypotension and relative ischemia. Note the early and rapid decline in the resistance response which goes on to virtual abolition during the period of flow reduction (partial aortic occlusion). The decline in the capacitance response is much less pronounced. Note also recovery of both responses following release of the aortic clamp. (From Mellander and Lewis, 1963. By permission.)

the precapillary resistance vessels declined more rapidly than did that of the capacitance vessels and the deterioration was more pronounced the lower the initial blood supply (see Chapters 16, 20, and 22). However, restoration of flow to normal after the hypotensive period restored both resistance and capacitance responses to their control values fairly rapidly.

Perhaps the most important consequence of the failing precapillary response was the interference with the absorption of tissue fluid. Nerve stimulation during the control period caused a tissue fluid uptake of 0.15

ml/min/100 g. This net inward movement of fluid was reduced when the effect of sympathetic stimulation was tried at intervals during the period of reduced flow, and this reduction of uptake was progressive during this hypotensive period until, towards the end of the ischaemic episode, sympathetic stimulation caused a net *outward* movement of fluid. Such changes in net capillary fluid transfer are due to the alterations of the mean capillary

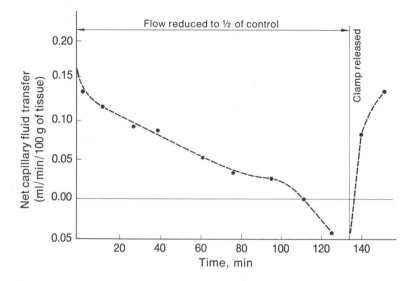

Fig. 30-2. Net capillary fluid transfer (ml/min/100 g tissue) in the cat's hindquarters during vasoconstrictor fibre stimulation (4 imp/sec). Influx of extravascular fluid occurs above the zero line (0.00) while outward movement of capillary fluid is indicated by levels below this line. Note that during the period of enforced hypotension and flow reduction the direction of transcapillary fluid movement becomes gradually changed due to the failing precapillary response. (From Mellander and Lewis, 1963. By permission.)

pressure which are produced by the sympathetic stimulation. In the first 100 min or so of ischaemia, sympathetic stimulation lowered the mean capillary pressure, although the effect became vanishingly small as the end of this period was reached. To some extent the gradual increase in CFC as a result of precapillary "sphincter" relaxation offsets the reduction in the power of the sympathetic impulses to lower the capillary hydrostatic pressure by providing an increased capillary surface area for fluid transfer.

Ultimately, however, sympathetic stimulation tended to *raise* the mean capillary pressure and correspondingly caused an egress of fluid from the capillaries into the tissues. The reason is that in this late stage only the the *postcapillary* vessels were able to respond to the vasoconstrictor fibre discharge. The precapillary resistance vessels and sphincters were then relaxed and largely unresponsive due to the excessive accumulation of vasodilator metabolites. In this situation, sympathetic discharge may lead to a *raised* capillary pressure and a fluid loss. In other words, a reflex vascular adjustment that normally is of the greatest advantage for the maintenance of the blood volume (see Chapter 20) can deteriorate to such an extent that it may ultimately cause a fluid *loss* from the vascular bed and thus have a *decompensatory* influence.

It is further likely that such an ultimate "reversal" of the constrictor fibre effect on the precapillary to postcapillary resistance ratio may be accompanied and fortified by the tendency to venular sludging of blood cells which has been noted in shocked animals and is favoured by the very low flow rate (see Knisely, 1965). Sludging at this site would tend to raise the postcapillary resistance.

In the final stages of haemorrhage hypotension even the postcapillary resistance response to sympathetic stimulation will itself disappear. Though this might ameliorate the untoward reversal of fluid movement into the tissue spaces caused by sympathetic stimulation it might more than cancel any such benefit by causing an increase in venous capacity and a reduction in venous return to the heart. In this critical situation even the slightest fluid loss, or additional venous pooling, may prove fatal.

Marked disturbances of the circulation in the gastrointestinal mucosa and the liver, for example, may also occur, leading to oedema, necrosis, and petechial bleeding, at least in some species. On the whole, all tissues suffer, and each tissue exhibits its own characteristic changes as determined by the arrangement and control of its respective circuit.

However, deterioration of the normal vascular control mechanisms, as exemplified above, is only part of the story. Thus, especially when blood loss is combined with trauma and infections disturbances of blood rheology occur (see Knisely, 1965); blood viscosity may increase markedly and add to the reduction of flow. The enhanced tendency of cell aggregation, besides the effect mentioned above, may result in extensive capillary plugging, greatly reducing the efficiency of nutritional exchange by causing "functional shunting" of the already poor supply (see also

Chapters 4 and 8). Thrombocyte aggregation, especially extensive if fragmented collagen elements accidentally enter the circulation in connection with crush injuries, contributes to the obstruction of the microvessels. It may, in the kidneys, for example, produce a situation which resembles that seen in "acute renal failure" after trauma in man (e.g. Hansson, 1965). In some cases bacterial invasions, which normally may be fairly harmless, can further deteriorate the failing cardiovascular system ("endotoxin shock"; see below).

Further, parts of the brain, perhaps especially the hypothalamus, seem to suffer badly in severe shock because the reduced blood flow is combined with an increased oxygen uptake, reducing the cerebral pO_2 to 20% of its control value, or even less. This may cause serious damage to these important centres (Kovách, 1961). Curiously enough, pretreatment with phenoxybenzamine eliminates the increase of oxygen uptake by these areas. This may in part explain the "protective" effect of phenoxybenzamine in shock.

Thus, a great number of disturbances may occur, affecting the vessels, the blood and the tissues and often establishing a vicious circuit. These disturbances probably vary from case to case in their relative importance. However, the *final* stage of irreversible shock is undoubtedly that of myocardial failure (see Bock, 1962). Once the pump gives up, despite transfusions and myocardial stimulants, the show is over.

Burns

Patients suffering from severe burns form the only group of cases of traumatic shock which manifest haemoconcentration. The burnt areas "weep" protein-rich fluid, and a progressive osmotic loss of fluid occurs from the capillaries into the interstitium. It is naïve to believe that burning necessarily causes fluid loss *only* as a result of an increased permeability of the capillary endothelium. Of considerable, often dominant, importance is the release of intracellular contents into the tissue fluids. Damaged cells liberate lysozomes; less damaged cells leak small molecule metabolites. Lysozomes contain most of the known proteolytic and hydrolytic enzymes, and when the lysozomes are disrupted these enzymes complete the digestion of the cell; if the lysozomes themselves gain access to the tissue fluid, they rapidly convert the proteins liberated into the tissue fluid to small molecule polypeptides. The consequent increase of extravascular molecular concentration exerts a powerful osmotic force attracting fluid from the capillary vascular compartment. Though, admittedly, increased capillary permeability does occur, it is of a relatively minor importance in the initial formation of oedema (Arturson and Mellander, 1964). Similar mechanisms must also be considered in crush injury.

Treatment of burns consists of giving plasma together with appropriate electrolyte solution (by mouth if possible; intravenously if necessary).

Endotoxin Shock

Sustained haemorrhagic hypotension in the dog, particularly after treatment by retransfusion, causes engorgement of the splanchnic bed with subsequent haemorrhage into the gastrointestinal tract. Fine (1965) has shown that maintaining perfusion of the portal blood supply of the liver (from a normal donor dog) in dogs subjected to sustained haemorrhagic hypotension can often prevent the development of irreversible shock. Normal, reversibly shocked, and irreversibly shocked dogs showed different powers of dealing with intravenously injected bacteria. Normal dogs cleared the blood of these bacteria within 6 hours and showed no bacteria in the liver 24 hours later. Reversibly shocked animals also cleared the blood of bacteria in 6 hours, but developed septicaemia and died in a day or two; postmortem liver cultures were bacteria-positive. Irreversibly shocked dogs were unable to clear even the bacteria from their blood. Further investigations showed that bacterial endotoxin is absorbed from the intestine and suffers destruction in the reticular-endothelial system (RES) of the liver particularly. Failure of the hepatic RES to destroy this endotoxin is progressive as hepatic blood flow deteriorates and the endotoxin itself causes irreversible collapse of the peripheral circulation.

The finding of haemorrhagic necrosis of the mucosa of the bowel, particularly that of the small bowel, which ensues upon sustained haemorrhagic hypotension in dogs, has been confirmed by Lillehei et al. (1962). They found it could be prevented by perfusing the superior mesenteric artery at normal pressure and flow, but not by perfusing the liver. They concluded that the plasma loss, haematocrit increase, and haemorrhagic necrosis of the bowel were all due to endotoxins of gram-negative bacteria. It should be recalled that the countercurrent exchange in the intestinal villi (Chapter 26) implies a reduced pO_2 at the villous tips. This is aggravated in shock and may lead to tissue necrosis.

Man subjected to haemorrhagic hypotension usually does not show splanchnic engorgement and secondary intestinal haemorrhage, and such patients have not shown anaerobic bacterial overgrowth of the liver. There may be considerable species differences; we should be wary of too facile an interpretation of haemorrhagic and/or wound shock in *man* in terms of endotoxin factors.

The Treatment of Shock

All investigators are agreed that in states of hypotension resulting from fluid loss, prompt replacement of the fluid lost is the best treatment. Thus haemorrhagic hypotension requires blood transfusion; burnt patients require plasma; and patients suffering from salt-water depletion, as in cholera, require saline transfusion. Howard (1962), reporting on the U.S. Army Surgical Research Team results in Korea, drew attention to the danger of acute renal failure in wound shock. The kidney's function was sometimes irreversibly damaged by periods of haemorrhagic hypotension and general trauma lasting for 3 to 4 hours (see above).

Ancillary treatment has included the use of sympathomimetic agents or of sympatholytic drugs. There is little reliable evidence that *vasopressor* therapy employing the sympathomimetic agents has any favourable effect upon survival (Nickerson, 1962). On the contrary, it appears that the organisms's own resources in this respect are "optimal" in action, and any such attempts to bolster them, when they are failing, invites serious side effects.

Vasodilator therapy was introduced on the theory that blood flow through certain critical areas, rather than the blood pressure per se, was the main factor in determining survival. There is no question that sympathetic blockade will *hasten* death if used before haemorrhage (Chien, 1967). However, the use of sympatholytic drugs in animals that are suffering chronic haemorrhagic hypotension may, at certain stages of the shock, offset or remove the untoward effects of throttling of regional blood supply

(Nickerson, 1962; Kovách, 1961, 1971). Unfortunately, these agents do not only prevent the constriction of precapillary resistance vessels; they also eradicate the contraction of the venular and venous capacitance vessels. Thus, what may be gained by improving tissue blood flow for any given mean arterial pressure may well be lost by allowing a greater degree of venous pooling on the postcapillary side so that venous return falls. In addition, α-receptor blocking drugs, which are commonly used in this type of treatment, have several other effects besides that of blocking the constrictor fibre influence on the blood vessels (see Kovách, 1961, 1971). It is possible that these other effects are more important than those on the blood vessels.

References

Arturson, G., and S. Mellander (1964). "Acute changes in capillary filtration and diffusion in experimental burn injury," *Acta Physiol. Scand.* **62,** 457–63.

Bock, K. D., ed. (1962). *In Shock: pathogenesis and therapy.* Berlin: Springer.

Chien, S. (1967). "Role of the sympathetic nervous system in haemorrhage," *Physiol. Rev.* **47,** 214–88.

Epstein, A. N., J. T. Fitzsimons, and B. J. Simons (1969). "Drinking caused by the intracranial injection of angiotensin into the rat," *J. Physiol.* **200,** 98–100P.

Fine, J. (1965). "Shock and peripheral circulatory insufficiency," *Handbook of Physiology,* 2, Circulation **III,** 2037–70.

Fitzsimons, J. T., and B. J. Simons (1968). "The effect of angiotensin on drinking in the rat," *J. Physiol.* **196,** 39–41.

Grant, R. T., and E. B. Reeve (1951). "Observations on the general effects of injury in man," *MRC. Rep.* 227.

Gregg, D. E. (1962). "Haemorrhagic and post-haemorrhagic shock," in *Shock: pathogenesis and therapy* (ed. K. D. Bock), pp. 186–99. Berlin: Springer.

Hansson, L. O. (1965). "The influence of thrombocyte aggregation on renal circulation," *Acta Chir. Scand.,* Suppl., 345, 1–66.

Howard, J. M. (1962). "Haemorrhagic and posthaemorrhagic shock," in *Shock: pathogenesis and therapy* (ed. K. D. Bock), pp. 208–17. Berlin: Springer.

Knisely, M. H. (1965). "Intravascular erythrocyte aggregation (blood sludge)," *Handbook of Physiology*, 2, Circulation **III**, 2249–92.

Kovách, A. G. B. (1961). "Importance of nervous and metabolic changes in the development of irreversibility in experimental shock," *Fed. Proc.* **20,** Part 3, 122–37.

Kovách, A. G. B. (1971). "Shock," *Physiol. Rev.*, in press.

Lewis, D. H., and S. Mellander (1962). "Competitive effects of sympathetic control and tissue metabolites on resistance and capacitance vessels," *Acta Physiol. Scand.* **56,** 162–88.

Lillehei, R. C., J. K. Longerbeam, and J. C. Rosenberg (1962). "The nature of irreversible shock: its relationship to intestinal changes," in *Shock: pathogenesis and therapy* (ed. K. D. Bock), pp. 106–29. Berlin: Springer.

Mellander, S., and D. H. Lewis (1963). "Effect of haemorrhagic shock on the reactivity of resistance and capacitance vessels," *Circ. Res.* **13,** 105–18.

Nickerson, M. (1962). "Drug therapy of shock," in *Shock: pathogenesis and therapy* (ed. K. D. Bock), pp. 356–70. Berlin: Springer.

Seeley, S. F., and J. F. Weisiger, eds. (1961). "Recent progress and present problems in the field of shock," *Fed. Proc.* **20,** Suppl., 9, 1–268.

Wiggers, C. J. (1950). *Physiology of shock*. New York: Commonwealth Fund.

3 1

Physiological Aspects of Arterial Hypertension

General Considerations

Few disturbances of cardiovascular function are so common and at the
same time of such physiological interest as that of high blood pressure;
more than most pathophysiological conditions it is a "disease of regulation".

It is obvious from the preceding chapters that a raised systemic arterial
pressure can be accomplished in different ways: Cardiac output and/or
flow resistance can be increased, and the latter change can be due either
to an increased blood viscosity or to a narrowing of the resistance vessels
in the form of *structural* or *functional* changes. Again, in the latter case an
increased myogenic tone and/or extrinsic excitatory influences in the form
of neurogenic and blood-borne factors should be considered.

Thus, there are, theoretically, many ways in which the blood pressure
equilibrium can be raised, and this is true also for man's situation (see
below). For these reasons, high arterial pressure may be considered
rather as a symptomatic common denominator for a series of primarily
different disturbances. However, their long-term impact on the cardiovascular system implies the involvement of so many common secondary
changes that hypertension in man often gives the impression of a fairly
homogenous group of disorders.

Well-established hypertension—as it appears in the resting patient—is characterized primarily by a *raised systemic resistance to flow* due to a relatively uniform narrowing of the precapillary resistance vessels. This narrowing is *not* due to any sclerotic vascular "rigidity", because vasodilation readily occurs just as in normotensive subjects, when appropriate vasodilator factors are applied. Resting cardiac output and blood viscosity are—still considering a *well-established* hypertensive state—by and large normal.

The situation may, however, be a different one in the early gradual transformation from normotension to hypertension (see below), where the main difficulty is to draw a borderline between "normal" and "abnormal" as symptoms are few and the pressure level unstable, especially in the most common variant of high blood pressure, essential hypertension. It is usually agreed that diastolic pressure levels above 90 mm Hg imply that the borderline between normotension and hypertension is crossed, but, of course, this borderline is arbitrary. Thus, blood pressure—like all other biological entities—must show a fairly wide natural distribution. Theoretically, a person who normally has a resting diastolic pressure of 65 to 70 should perhaps be considered as abnormally hypertensive if his pressure were to increase to, say, 85 mm Hg. Clearly, the problems of definition—as long as the blood pressure alone forms the yardstick—must be considerable, and disagreements between authorities have often reached levels which cannot be good for their own blood pressure levels (see Pickering, 1968).

The presence of an increased, but not *rigidly* stabilized, systemic flow resistance suggests (1) a disturbance of precapillary smooth muscle function, and/or (2) a disturbance of vascular architecture, of such a nature as to set a higher equilibrium level for a range of luminal adjustments that is normal in itself.

The first alternative has by far attracted most attention throughout the years, being particularly directed towards *extrinsic* blood-borne and neurogenic vascular influences; far less interest has been devoted to *local* disturbances of myogenic activity, despite the fact that the "basal tone" of the resistance vessels is a consequence of such intrinsic mechanisms (Chapter 16). Still less attention has been paid to the possibility that an adaptive, per se "normal" change in vascular design, e.g. as a response to functionally imposed pressure loads, might be important, though recent findings strongly suggest that this is so (see below).

For authoritative reviews, and for contact with the enormous literature, the reader is referred to the penetrating survey of the physiology of hypertension by Page and McCubbin (1965) and the excellent monograph by Pickering (1968), as two examples. A symposium on the pathogenesis of essential hypertension (1960) is also recommended.

Among the true landmarks in the extensive search for the cause(s) of hypertension stands the classical Goldblatt discovery in the 1930's that most aspects of hypertensive disease in man could be mimicked in dogs if renal blood pressure, and flow, were lowered by means of clamps around the renal arteries (see Goldblatt, 1948). Another landmark in the 1930's was the independent discovery by Page and Braun-Menendez and their groups that renin—isolated from the kidneys as a "pressor substance" as early as 1898 by Tigerstedt and Bergman—is a *proteolytic enzyme*, splitting off from a *plasma globuline* (α-2-type) an extremely powerful vasoconstrictor polypeptide, now baptized *angiotensin* (earlier called hypertensin or angiotonin).

It is indeed understandable that these two findings greatly triggered research and, moreover, tended to focus the interest on the kidneys as the potential key to the problem of hypertensive disease in man. Further, until recently the safest way to produce high blood pressure in experimental animals—most species seldom acquire "spontaneous" hypertension—is to interfere with their renal blood supply. (A strain of genetically hypertensive rats has now been developed; Okamoto and Aoki, 1963.) It is therefore only natural that experimental studies of hypertension have until recently been primarily directed towards the *renal* variant of the disease which, however, is not necessarily an appropriate model for the initiation of the most common type of "spontaneously" occurring high blood pressure in man.

What greatly complicates the distinction between primary and secondary factors in such slowly developing disturbances as high blood pressure is the fact that the renal circuit appears to be especially vulnerable to a pressure load, with formation of degenerative-obstructive lesions. This may soon lead to the establishment of a "Goldblatt mechanism" in such variants of high blood pressure where there initially may have been no involvement of any renal mechanism. As a matter of fact, it appears evident that—no matter which might be *the* primary factor in any given case of hypertension—secondary factors of different nature (see below) are successively involved, so that by the time the patient sees his doctor,

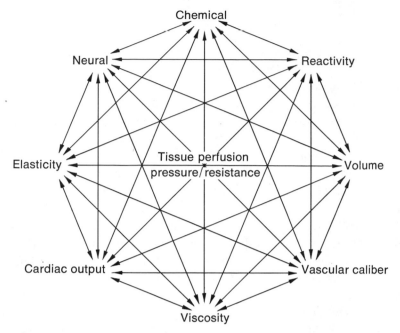

Fig. 31-1. The mosaic octagon illustrating the equilibrated system which controls tissue perfusion and how disturbance at one point will automatically lead to secondary changes of others. (From Page, 1949. By permission.)

several potentially causative factors may often be distinguished. To determine which one came *first* is by then usually impossible, but it is a natural inclination to direct the interest to the most obvious ones, and are renal changes detected, these are often considered as the chief villain. Considering the complexity of cardiovascular homeostasis—and the gradual development of high blood pressure with ample time for regulatory reset—it is not surprising that such problems arise, and the "mosaic theory", proposed by Page (1949), is certainly for such reasons justified (Fig. 31-1).

Different Types of Hypertension in Man

Before some especially important physiological interrelationships of potential etiological significance are dealt with, it may be justified to outline briefly the various types of hypertension in man.

Primary Hypertension

As matters stand today, it is clear that the *by far* most common type of high blood pressure (perhaps two-thirds) is *benign "essential" hypertension*, characterized by a strong hereditary element and an apparent lack of local or general signs of a specific causative mechanism; it is therefore often called *primary* hypertension. Thus, in early phases the subject is just hypertensive, and he appears in all other respects normal as far as cardiovascular control, kidney function, etc., are concerned. In fact, the impressive prefix "essential" simply means that we do not know with any certainty *why* there is a high blood pressure and what the nature of the hereditary element is.

In a sense, this diagnosis is, at present, one by *exclusion*, used where it is clear that none of the several types of "secondary" hypertension, where a distinct causative factor is identified, is involved. With refined diagnostic techniques, the frequency of essential hypertension will no doubt yield somewhat to the secondary ones, but it seems safe to state that it will always remain by far the most frequent type of high blood pressure. We will return to this important disturbance and its possible background, once the secondary types of hypertension have been outlined, as they are more clear-cut with respect to causative mechanisms. The "spontaneous", genetically linked hypertension in rats, referred to above ("Okamoto strain"), may be the best available "model" in experimental animals of essential hypertension in man.

Secondary Hypertension

Renal Hypertension

The most common among the secondary variants is renal hypertension, and here obvious disturbances of renal blood flow and/or other types of damage to the kidneys can be traced as the primary factor (see Page and McCubbin, 1968). In a way, therefore, the raised blood pressure should be considered more as one of several consequences, and symptoms, of a primary interference with renal function, even though the hypertensive state often dominates the clinical situation and may be the greatest threat to the patient.

A distinct renal element (nephritis, pyelonephritis, cystic kidneys, arterial obstructions, etc.) can be traced in perhaps 10 to 20% of hypertensive patients, depending on how penetrating the investigation is, but is it not necessarily true that in *all* these cases the renal factors came first. However, the cardinal position of the renal theory of hypertensive disease —historically, experimentally, and by its sheer attractiveness—has convinced many authorities that the kidney is the true villain of the plot also in essential hypertension and that only inadequate diagnostic techniques hinder the confirmation of this firm belief. Be this as it may, the kidney is a villain that sometimes dominates the scene in other types of high blood pressure also, once they have lasted long enough.

The sunny side of this—and most other types of secondary hypertension —is that a surgical correction of the primary disturbance may eliminate the hypertension, though quite often—especially in long-standing cases— the hypertensive state remains, at least in part. This fact again suggests that in most types of hypertension several factors become successively involved.

Phaeochromocytoma

In rare cases the adrenal medulla is the site of tumours, where the tumour cells produce mainly noradrenaline (NA). This pressor agent can sporadically, or more steadily, "spill over" into the bloodstream and later in the urine in surprisingly high concentrations. In fact, it is usually by the high NA content in the urine that a correct diagnosis is obtained. The excessively high NA concentrations in the blood lead to a hypertensive state that sporadically may reach dangerous levels. An *early* extirpation of the tumour usually implies elimination of the hypertensive stage.

Hypersecretion of Glucocorticoids (Cushing's disease)

In this serious syndrome, which involves gross disturbances in the hormonal control of intermediary metabolism, etc., a (usually) moderate degree of hypertension forms part of the syndrome, though it is quite overshadowed by other far more alarming symptoms and changes. Normalization of the underlying disturbance—be it a hypophyseal ACTH-producing tumour or a tumour in the zona fasciculata of the adrenals—usually relieves the hypertension as well.

Primary Aldosteronism

This interesting variant (Conn's disease) is due to hypersecretion in the zona glomerulosa of the adrenals, usually as a result of a tumour. On the surface, at least, it may exhibit most of the signs of essential hypertension with few other obvious expressions of the tumour, which is often very small. However, a correct diagnosis can be arrived at by a proper analysis of the [Na$^+$]-[K$^+$]-balance, which can reveal that excessive amounts of aldosterone must be secreted (Conn, 1961). It is also possible to measure aldosterone directly (Fig. 31-2). Exactly how the hypertensive stage is brought about is not fully understood, but it is known that any undue retention of sodium tends to raise the pressure equilibrium. It has been suggested that this "primary" disturbance of aldosterone secretion might be a fairly common variant of hypertensive disease, but probably it is not. It is quite another matter that a *secondary* increase of aldosterone secretion may occur in the course of other types of hypertension at least in their malignant phases (see below), in keeping with the "mosaic theory" (Fig. 31-2).

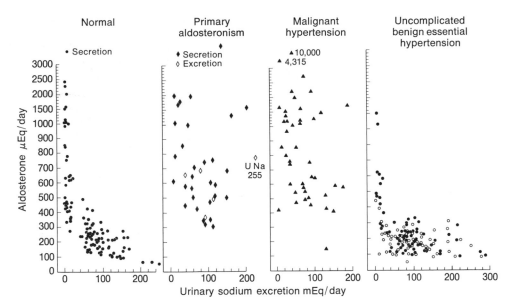

Fig. 31-2. Relation between aldosterone secretion and sodium excretion in normal subjects and in subjects with primary aldosteronism, malignant hypertension, and uncomplicated essential hypertension. Note the great rise in aldosterone secretion in primary aldosteronism and malignant hypertension, whereas that in uncomplicated essential hypertension is largely normal. (From Laragh *et al.*, 1966. By permission.)

Neurogenic Hypertension

It has been much debated whether a *primary* neurogenic hypertension—the term "neurogenic" is here used in the explicit sense that there should be a *steadily* increased sympathetic discharge—forms one of the entities, and there are no doubt cases where such a diagnosis is justified. Dickinson (1965) has with great skill and consequence argued for such a view. However, such cases are probably rather rare; it is an entirely different matter that the normal neurogenic control mechanisms, in the form of *intermittent* but perhaps frequent bouts of increased cardiovascular drive emanating from cortico-hypothalamic levels as a result of daily "stress", might form an important "trigger" element for the gradual development of essential hypertension (see below). Further, it appears that *resting* neurogenic discharge remains largely unchanged—instead of becoming reflexly damped as would be the case in acute hypertension by noradrenaline infusion, for example—because of the resetting of the baroreceptor control of the circulation (see Page and McCubbin, 1965; Kezdi, 1967).

Coarctation of the Aorta

This is one of nature's more interesting experiments, where the patient is hypertensive in the upper body parts that are supplied by aortic branches above the obstruction, but normotensive or even hypotensive, with greatly reduced pulse amplitude, in lower body parts. This abnormality illustrates the impact of pressure itself on vessels with respect to adaptive and degenerative changes, with the individual serving as his own control. No doubt the kidneys are often in a "Goldblatt situation", so that renal mechanisms are probably often involved early, with secondary involvement of other factors as well (see below). Nowadays it is common practice to correct the aortic obstruction surgically at an early age. Complications may arise, however, with obvious reactions of the vascular walls in lower body parts, when they suddenly become exposed to higher pressures than they are used to (see Pickering, 1968).

Malignant Hypertension

Any of the types of hypertension mentioned above, especially the primary but also the secondary variants, can occasionally escalate into a malignant phase with sharp rises in pressure, deteriorating cardiovascular control, and manifest vascular lesions, which will rapidly kill the patient if untreated. The diagnosis "malignant hypertension" is usually based not only on the over-all clinical picture, but on the eyeground changes as well. The retinal vascular bed serves as an excellent mirror of the systemic vessels, and the fourth grade changes with severe vascular lesions (see Pickering, 1968) are considered to be proof of a malignant state. Besides such types of malignant hypertension it has been suggested that there might also exist a "primary" malignant form, where severe and widespread vascular lesions rapidly develop in such a way that these lesions appear to be the primary disease which happens to lead to—among other things—high blood pressure. Probably most, or all, of such cases should be classified among the collagen diseases, such as polyarteritis nodosa (see Pickering, 1968). Most, and perhaps all, cases of truly malignant hypertension seem to be of a similar kind as the types described above, though escalating at a higher rate into very high pressure levels and severe complications.

Pathophysiological Aspects

Before possible *causative* elements in the most common and therefore most important type of high blood pressure—essential hypertension—are discussed, some key physiological mechanisms and their interrelationship will be outlined.

The Vasoconstrictor Effect of Angiotensin

Since the 1930's it has been well established that reductions of renal blood pressure and/or flow—whether due to gross arterial obstructions, to a regional narrowing of small preglomerular vessels, or to some other type of flow interference, including neurogenic flow reductions (Chapter 27)—lead to renin release and angiotensin formation (see Page and McCubbin, 1968). Angiotensin, being the most potent of known vasoconstrictor agents, almost selectively constricts the precapillary systemic vessels. Thus, when formed in high enough concentrations, it can produce, by this direct effect on the vascular effectors, a raised blood pressure, the haemodynamic pattern closely simulating that seen in well-established hypertensive disease: a raised systemic resistance to flow.

It is only natural that this straightforward mechanism has attracted wide interest; it was long considered as the only, or at least the main, "renal" mechanism for causing pressure rises. No doubt it may be of

considerable importance, especially in early phases of typically renal variants of hypertension where a major hindrance to blood flow has suddenly
been created. However, in most cases of essential hypertension, and in
other hypertensive states as well, it appears that the angiotensin concentrations in the blood are simply too low to produce any significant *direct*
vasoconstrictor effects. Important *indirect* effects of angiotensin will be
outlined below.

The Cardiovascular Impact of the Defence Reaction

This neuro-hormonal response of cortico-hypothalamic origin (Chapter
19) is not only displayed in moments of manifest threat to the individual:
it appears to become involved whenever alertness is raised, thus not only
by potentially harmful influences, but also by those which imply "stimulating" or even amusing challenges for the individual. From such a point
of view the term "defence reaction" may be somewhat misleading, as it
suggests an involvement only in troubled situations. It appears, in fact,
that this pattern in its milder or moderate forms plays repeatedly on the
cardiovascular system in normal daily life via its neuro-hormonal links.

With respect to the cardiovascular system, the defence reaction does
not only imply an acute rise in the pressure load, caused by an increased
cardiac output that is preferentially distributed to muscle, myocardium, and
brain with flow restrictions elsewhere, including the kidneys. A concomitant hormonal activation takes place, involving release of ADH, ACTH,
and glucocorticoids, adrenaline, and also aldosterone (see Charvat *et al.*,
1964; Folkow and Rubinstein, 1966). Several of these hormonal effects
are relatively slow in onset, but they are also long in duration, and they
may therefore in the long run have even more important effects on the
cardiovascular system than the direct neurogenic impact. It is clear that
this neuro-hormonal influence, which is perfectly normal in itself,
will considerably raise the *average* blood pressure over a long period of time
if repeated often enough. The consequences of this will be discussed below.
Compare the interesting "model" study on mice by Henry *et al.* (1967).
Further, Russian research has devoted much interest to central nervous
mechanisms of this general nature (see Simonson and Brožek, 1959;
"Symposium on the pathogenesis of essential hypertension," 1960).

Interrelationship between Angiotensin-aldosterone

The aldosterone release, causing retention of sodium and excretion of potassium, appears to be triggered at least in part by the neurogenic flow restriction in the kidneys, which restriction, incidentally, always forms part of the defence reaction. The consequent renin release is followed by a formation of angiotensin, and angiotensin proves to be the perhaps most potent of all stimuli for the zona glomerulosa of the adrenal cortex (see Davis *et al.*, 1962). These mechanisms imply an interesting and—especially in these connections—quite important link between everyday mental "stress" → neurogenic discharge to the cardiovascular system (with an *acute* rise in blood pressure) → restriction of renal cortical circulation → renin-angiotensin-aldosterone release → sodium chloride and water retention → *"chronically"* increased blood pressure. Thus, a primary neurogenic, and phasic, "pressor effect" may, via these hormonal interlinks, invite an important shift in the *milieu interieur* which, when pronounced enough, by itself tends to raise the systemic flow resistance in a more "chronic" fashion. Whether this is due to a secondary enhancement of myogenic activity, to an increased smooth muscle sensitivity to extrinsic stimuli, or to a mere water-salt logging of the vascular walls remains obscure. To this comes adaptive structural changes (see below).

Angiotensin Effects on Adrenergic Nerve Control

It has recently been shown that a continued renin-angiotensin release—subthreshold with respect to the direct precapillary constrictor effect of angiotensin (powerful in itself)—gradually *potentiates* the impact of the sympathetic nervous system on the cardiovascular system (Fig. 31-3; see also McCubbin *et al.*, 1965). It is not known to what extent this is due to a *local* effect of angiotensin on the NA release from the adrenergic nerve varicosities (an effect which has been experimentally demonstrated), to more centrally placed effects of angiotensin on the complex neurogenic machinery, or to angiotensin effects that are mediated by aldosterone and its effects on electrolyte balance (see above).

Whichever the case, current ideas about angiotensin effects have shifted from its direct vascular excitation to these *indirect* mechanisms, mediated via nervous and electrolyte changes and effective at decidedly lower angiotensin concentrations than those needed to produce direct vasoconstriction. Therefore, the mechanisms of the defence reaction, the angiotensin-aldosterone interrelationship, and the angiotensin effects discussed here *imply important mutual interactions between neurogenic and hormonal control factors*, so organized that whether the neurogenic or the

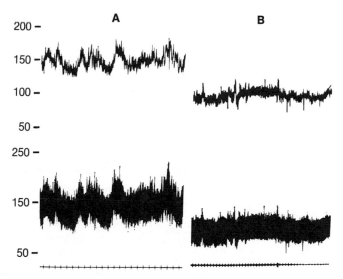

Fig. 31-3. Mean (top), systolic and diastolic (bottom) blood pressures in a resting dog after one week of infusion of initially subpressor amounts of angiotensin.
A. surrounded by normal laboratory activity.
B. laboratory completely quiet.
Note the marked lability and rise in pressure to trivial stimuli, which before the angiotensin infusion had only insignificant effects. (From McCubbin et al., 1965. By permission.)

hormonal factor is the initial one, they may together build up a gradually more sustained neuro-hormonal drive on the cardiovascular system.

It is, for example, possible that the trigger mechanism in such an interaction might simply be fairly mild but often repeated incidents of everyday mental "stress". In fact, often repeated but weak excitations of the hypothalamic defence area in rats can gradually produce a raised blood pressure level, present even during periods when no hypothalamic stimulation is performed (Fig. 31-4; see also Folkow and Rubinstein, 1966).

It may be because of this that mice, when exposed to environmental "social strain", tend to develop raised blood pressure (Henry et al., 1967).

Adaptive Changes of Vascular Structure

Last, but by no means least, there is another factor which may in itself be considered a *normal adaptive adjustment of vascular structure to increased load*. It

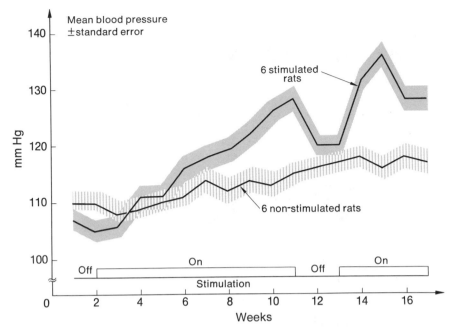

Fig. 31-4. Gradual change of resting mean blood pressure in rats, which for a prolonged period were exposed to intermittent but weak stimulations of the hypothalamic defence area. The resting mean pressure of control rats, identically treated with exception of the hypothalamic stimulations, is given for comparison. Note the gradual return towards normal upon a two-week cessation of stimulation with a prompt rise once the stimulations were resumed. (From Folkow and Rubinstein, 1966. By permission.)

is well-known that virtually all tissues, except the brain, rapidly adjust in structure to increases in load; this is particularly obvious in mesenchymal tissues. It is, for example, an everyday experience that skeletal muscles exposed to training increase in bulk. The *extent* to which this takes place seems to vary with the individual; those with a "mesomorphic" body build appear to respond more in this respect to the same degree of training than the "leptosomic" variants. Another common example: all the tissues of hands exposed to heavy use show the same type of change (compare hands of manual workers and desk workers).

The same holds true for visceral tissues as well. Thus, ureteral and intestinal walls become thickened proximal to a hindrance, an increased load on the heart leads to wall thickening, veins from the leg have thicker walls than those of equal size from the arm. Perhaps even more striking, veins used as surgical substitutes for damaged arteries rapidly display thickened walls. There are several reports (see Pickering, 1968) that arteriolar walls show "hypertrophy" in hypertensive subjects; exposure of part of the pulmonary vascular bed to the systemic pressure level rapidly produces thickened walls (Ferguson and Varco, 1955).

Strangely enough, the *haemodynamic* consequences of such adaptive changes of the vascular walls have been almost entirely neglected. To a large extent this may be due to the fact that the concept of a neurogenic and hormonal increase of arteriolar activity—especially when of renal origin—has so fascinated most investigators that other approaches seem to have been overlooked. However, it has been shown that regional flow resistance in well-established but uncomplicated essential hypertension is

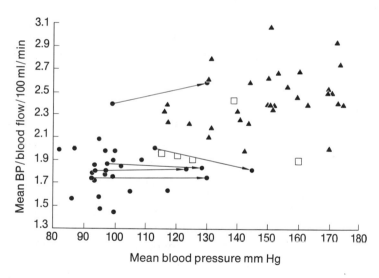

Fig. 31-5. The correlation between forearm blood flow resistance at *maximal* vasodilatation and mean blood pressure in normotensive individuals ●, individuals with essential hypertension ▲, and renal hypertension □. Note the largely proportional increase in mean blood pressure and resistance even at maximal vasodilatation in essential hypertension, with some change present also in renal hypertension. As a contrast, *acute* hypertension (noradrenaline infusion) in normotensive subjects (●———▶●) does *not* increase the **resistance. (From Folkow, 1956. By permission.)**

increased even at complete relaxation of the vascular smooth muscles, and, indeed, is increased largely to the *same* extent as resting over-all systemic resistance (Fig. 31-5) (Folkow, 1956; Folkow *et al.*, 1958). As "resting" regional flow resistance is largely increased to the same extent, it follows that the level of smooth muscle activity—best judged as the ratio between the resistances during "rest" and during maximal dilatation (Chapter 16)—is *not* raised. Hence, there is, in fact, nothing to indicate either increased amounts of constrictor agents in the blood or enhanced neurogenic activity in patients in this stage of their disease when they are kept in resting equilibrium. These results have been confirmed by Conway (1963) in an extensive study. Recently it has also been shown that in genetically hypertensive rats (Okamoto strain) the *entire* systemic vascular bed displays a raised resistance compared with that in normotensive controls, even at *maximal vasodilatation* (Folkow *et al.*, 1969).

The conclusion must be that the resistance vessels of hypertensive subjects (and of genetically hypertensive rats) have become *structurally* somewhat narrowed as compared with normotensive subjects. In other words, the very base from which the dynamic resistance control operates is reset to a higher level by adaptive morphological changes which are largely proportional to the increased pressure load.

To this come the effects of thickened vascular walls per se. It was theoretically predicted (see Folkow *et al.*, 1958)—and can be shown on models (e.g. Folkow and Sivertsson, 1964, 1968)—that for any given shortening of the contractile elements the flow resistance will increase *more* where the wall/lumen ratio is increased, as it is in hypertensive subjects (Fig. 31-6). This applies especially when vascular contractions originate from the *outermost* smooth muscle layer, as is the case with neurogenic effects (Chapter 16); such constrictions will push the entire wall mass towards the lumen. It follows that such vessels will appear more "reactive" to given stimuli, and so they are with respect to their *luminal* changes, but not necessarily with respect to their *smooth muscle* responses. The reason is simply that the thickened wall amplifies the luminal reduction produced by a given muscle excitation (see also Fig. 5-6, p. 98).

In later studies it has been illustrated in animal "model" experiments (Folkow and Sivertsson, 1968), and also on the hand blood vessels in man (Sivertsson and Olander, 1968), that an adaptive "reset" of vascular structure to the current level of pressure load leads to the theoretically predicted changes, i.e. to exaggerated luminal reduction in vessels where the wall/

lumen ratio is higher, though there is no shift in smooth muscle sensitivity as judged by threshold comparisons. Also the hand vessels of hypertensive subjects, like those of the forearm, *even at complete vascular relaxation*, exhibit a raised resistance which is largely proportional to the raised blood pressure level, but basal vascular *tone* is not raised. Results along these lines are summarized in Table 31-1, page 577. Furthermore, constant flow-perfusions of the hindquarters of "spontaneously" hypertensive rats and normotensive

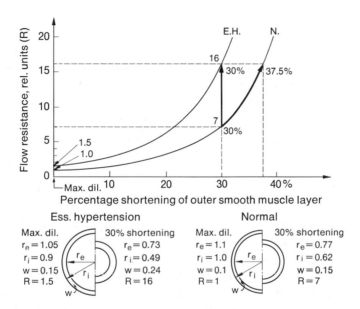

Fig. 31-6. Diagram illustrating in arbitrary figures the changed relationship between degree of vascular smooth muscle shortening and increase in flow resistance, once an adaptive structured change in wall/lumen ratio has occurred in essential hypertension (E.H.). Below is given the chosen figures for internal (r_i) external radius (r_e) and wall thickness (w), where at maximal dilatation r_i and w in hypertension are set at 90% and 150%, respectively, of those in normotension (N). Note the increased resistance already at maximal dilatation and the exaggerated resistance increases in E.H., compared with N for a given smooth muscle shortening. If the raised flow resistance in hypertension were *only* due to increased smooth muscle activity, this change would occur along curve N (arrow) and maximal dilatation would yield the same low resistance value as in normals. (Modified from Folkow *et al.*, 1958. By permission.)

controls show that both groups display the *same* responsiveness to vasopressor agents in terms of threshold sensitivity. However, when given higher (up to supramaximal) doses of pressor agents (noradrenaline, vasopressin, barium ions), the hypertensive animals display *exaggerated* luminal reductions and are able to maintain *higher* pressure levels, largely in proportion to their higher resting blood pressure and the higher flow resistance displayed already at maximal vasodilatation (Folkow *et al.*, 1970). All these changes suggest an increased wall/lumen ratio as the main difference (see also Sivertsson, 1970).

Now, if such presumably adaptive vascular changes are generalized throughout the systemic circuits—and they are in hypertensive rats and there is no reason to believe that they are *not* in man, because the underlying type of structural response to load appears to be a general feature— the following conclusions can hardly be sidestepped:

In essential hypertension (and in "spontaneous" hypertension in rats), there is an adaptive re-build of the resistance vessels, which implies that flow resistance is raised largely in proportion to the arterial pressure, even at *complete* vascular relaxation.

This re-build, expressing itself also as an increased wall/lumen ratio, *enhances* the luminal reduction produced by a given effector shortening; it results in an increased vascular "reactivity".

These factors have the consequence that there is usually little or no increased *effector activity* behind the raised "*resting*" resistance in well established essential hypertension.

If generalized, these structural changes of arteries-arterioles would reduce wall distensibility also at the baroreceptor sites, explaining the well known "resetting" of these receptors to the raised pressure level.

This structural "reset" of arteries-arterioles still allows for a completely *normal*, or even increased, range of luminal adjustments, though operating from a "raised baseline".

Figure 31-6 summarizes schematically some of these differences between normotension and essential hypertension and also the difference between this disease and such types of hypertension that may be *solely* due to an increased vascular smooth muscle activity.

The question arises whether a morphological "reset" of the mentioned type is slow or rapid in onset. It should then be stressed that adaptive tissue changes of this nature can usually be traced within weeks. In the mentioned "model" study on cats (Folkow and Sivertsson, 1968) this was certainly the case. It may be in line with this that Aars (1968) was able to show a reduced wall distensibility in the aortic baroreceptor area within a week after a hypertensive stage had been enforced upon rabbits. These are short periods in the course of development of essential hypertension and may imply that functional and structural elements go largely hand in hand. Such problems are summarized in a recent survey (Sivertsson, 1970).

	Normotensives	Hypertensives	Significance
Mean arterial blood pressure	100% (82 mm Hg)	141% (116 mm Hg)	$p < 0.001$
Resistance at max. dilatation	100% (1.6 PRU_{100})	163% (2.5 PRU_{100})	$p < 0.001$
Basal resistance	100% (3.8 PRU_{100})	156% (5.9 PRU_{100})	$0.02 > p > 0.01$
Basal tone	100%	96%	$p > 0.9$
NA threshold dose ($\mu g/min \times 100$ g)	100% (0.032)	94% (0.030)	$0.9 > p > 0.5$
NA dose producing resistance of 30 PRU_{100}	100% (0.14)	43% (0.06)	$0.02 > p > 0.01$
NA dose producing resistance of 50 PRU_{100}	100% (0.20)	39% (0.078)	$0.01 > p > 0.001$
Steepness of NA dose-response curve	100%	178%	$0.05 > p > 0.02$

Table 31-1. Hand blood flow resistance in normotensives and hypertensives (mainly essential hypertension) at maximal vasodilatation, at "basal tone," and when the vessels are exposed to increasing noradrenaline (NA) amounts (i.a. infusion). Note that resistance at maximal dilatation is raised about as much as is mean blood pressure: basal tone is not changed, nor is the threshold to NA, but the luminal reductions to suprathreshold doses of NA are stronger in the hypertensives. (From Sivertsson and Olander, 1968. By permission.)

Etiological Aspects of Essential Hypertension

With the hypertension types and pathophysiological aspects as a general background it may be justifiable to consider possible primary and secondary factors in the development of essential hypertension. This means a shift from facts to hypothesis: little is known, and discussing the topic raises as much ire as disturbing a hornet's nest. Some general considerations may still be justified. Antidotes against the views given here will, no doubt, be found in other surveys of this controversial topic.

There are, indeed, many reasons why the etiology of essential hypertensions contains more theory than facts. Early phases of essential hypertension give no symptoms: when and how does it start, and where, on the whole, should the borderline between health and disease be drawn? To base that borderline only on such a flexible and shifting parameter as the blood pressure has its problems, as continuous pressure recordings on perfectly "normotensive" subjects have revealed surprising pressure tops in moments of even trivial mental strain (Fig. 31-7) (Hinman *et al.*, 1962; Bevan *et al.*, 1969).

Suppose that an important "trigger" element *is* constituted simply by normal central neuro-hormonal influences, if only these are repeated often enough. No doubt such reiterated influences can, in otherwise perfectly "normotensive" rats, produce a raised blood pressure level (Folkow and Rubinstein, 1966), so why not in man as well? This would then constitute an "environmental factor" because the true pressure load on man's cardiovascular system is not the *resting* blood pressure, as recorded in the doctor's office, but the *average* pressure in daily life over months and years. Fig. 31-7 suggests that these two pressure levels may be entirely different in many situations and subjects.

It is clear that in most subjects accidental neurogenic episodes of raised

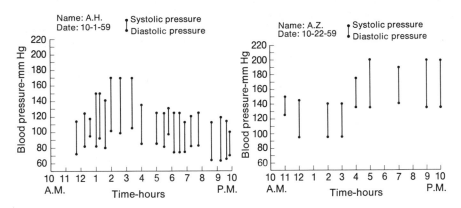

Fig. 31-7. Levels of arterial blood pressure during the day (portable recorder). Subject A.H. drove in traffic 1:00 p.m. and spoke at meeting 2:00–3:30 p.m. Subject A.Z. had a heated discussion about his work at 4–5 p.m. and cared for his children from 7–10 p.m. (From Hinman *et al.*, 1962. By permission.)

pressure will hardly affect the resting blood pressure level; otherwise we would all have hypertension. However, if such episodes are repeated often enough in particularly susceptible persons, the situation may be a different one, and it may be here that the hereditary element of essential hypertension comes in. There appears to be a prevalence of mesomorphic body build in subjects with essential hypertension (Robinson and Brucer, 1940). It is possible that the hereditary element—the common "inherent" denominator for this type of hypertension—is simply an especially pronounced tendency of tissues to react with hypertrophy as a response to increased load (Folkow, 1956). If so, manifest essential hypertension might occur only where intermittent bouts of centrally elicited neuro-hormonal discharge happen to affect a vascular bed which by inheritance has an especially pronounced tendency to respond with adaptive increases in arteriolar wall/lumen ratio. The balance between the two elements— environmental and inherent—can no doubt vary considerably, but their *sum* or *product* would determine the outcome. The situation in the "spontaneously" hypertensive rats, discussed earlier as perhaps the best animal "model" of essential hypertension in man, may be largely the same.

Thus, there is no need to presuppose either any abnormal "emotional lability" or "undue emotional strain" in predisposed subjects or any definitely *pathological* inheritance to get the ball slowly rolling from normotension via a labile to a more stable hypertensive state. This is not a revolutionary thought; it is in many ways more surprising that most people *remain* normotensive, considering the many functional disturbances that a so-called civilized lifespan exposes them to. It should in this context be stressed that in *early* stages of essential hypertension, the pressure is relatively labile, and Brod's group has shown in excellent studies that the haemodynamic situation seems to be characterized by an increased cardiac output, increased muscle but reduced renal blood flows (e.g. Fejfar and Widimsky, 1960), and hardly by any over-all increase in flow resistance (as appears to be the case in *late* stages). In fact, this cardiovascular pattern suggests the presence of a neuro-hormonal drive, identical or closely similar to that of the defence reaction; moreover, acute mental stress in man is known to produce this type of response (Brod, 1963), just as it does in rats, cats, and other animals (Chapter 19).

Such an approach to the etiology of essential hypertension thus takes into account both the hereditary element and such changes in cardiovascular control and in vascular structure that seem to characterize this type of hypertension in its uncomplicated stages. As the neuro-hormonal influences mentioned above are so closely interlinked with the mechanisms of the angiotensin-aldosterone interrelationship and angiotensin effects on adrenergic nerve control, either of them may—depending on circumstances and subjects—dominate vascular tone, but towards a background of gradual vascular re-build. Therefore, this latter structural factor serves by its very nature as a *stabilizing element*, slowly resetting upwards the "baseline" from which the dynamic influences on smooth muscle activity operate, and the ball rolls slowly on if the chain of events is not broken somewhere.

It should be stressed that no truly *pathological* factor has so far been invoked—it is rather a matter of a gradual shift in balance between elements that are in themselves normal. For these reasons such a theory has much in common with the view held by Pickering, based mainly on his interesting clinical-epidemiological approach. According to Pickering essential hypertension is a disease characterized by a *quantitative* rather than a qualitative deviation from the norm, thus differing from other types of hypertension which take their origin from a renal artery obstruction, an adrenal tumour, etc. Pickering has met violent criticism—though not seldom off the point—but he stands firm and defends his view with great vigour and brilliance; the reader should consult his succinct text on this matter (Pickering, 1968).

However, many other authorities look to the kidney as the potential key to essential hypertension, though there seems to be no real evidence for any distinct renal "trigger" mechanism, apart from such types of renal involvement as outlined above. This by no means denies that a "Goldblatt mechanism" may soon develop in essential hypertension because of the vulnerability of the renal vessels to increased pressure loads and that then, indeed, such a mechanism may even dominate the situation. As patients often come to investigation and treatment relatively late in their disease, both primary and secondary factors are apt to be present. It is then easiest to pick the most palpable one and blame everything on this, and a renal artery narrowing is no doubt more palpable than, for example, diffuse neuro-hormonal mechanisms. It is tantalizing that it is so difficult to gain full insight into the *early* development of essential hypertension. The approach by Sokolow, Harris, and their collaborators (see Pickering, 1968), performing long-term studies of blood pressure changes on normotensives and hypertensives in daily routine life by means of portable automatized recorders, may here reveal important secrets.

Even in typically *renal* hypertension, with distinct and primary lesions in the kidneys, it is clear from what has been outlined above that neurogenic elements may soon become engaged via the angiotensin effects on sympathetic vascular control. It is probably unavoidable that adaptive structural changes of the vascular walls come in as well; also subjects with renal hypertension show signs of a raised flow resistance in maximal vasodilatation (Folkow *et al.*, 1958, Conway, 1963). In *late* stages, therefore, cases with renal and essential hypertension may look rather similar, thanks to the mixture of primary and secondary factors, of which several are common for both but where the primary factors differ. The problem is often: Which came first? This may in part explain why authorities disagree so violently in debates about the relationship between these two diseases. Lastly, even in such types of hypertension as primary aldosteronism, phaeochromocytoma, etc., secondary factors of a structural, renal, or neurogenic nature may come in, probably explaining why surgical removal of the primary cause sometimes leaves the hypertension behind.

References

Aars, H. (1968). "Static load-length characteristics of aortic strips from hypertensive rabbits," *Acta Physiol. Scand.* **73,** 101–10.

Bevan, A. T., A. J. Honour, and F. H. Stott (1969). "Direct arterial pressure recording in unrestricted man," *Clin. Sci.* **18,** 543–51.

Brod, J. (1963). "Haemodynamic basis of acute pressor reactions and hypertension," *Brit. Heart J.*, Vol. XXV, 227–45.

Charvat, J., P. Dell, and B. Folkow (1964). "Mental factors and cardiovascular disease," *Cardiologica*, **44,** 121–41.

Conn, J. W. (1961). "Aldosteronism and hypertension," *Arch. Intern. Med.* **107,** 813–28.

Conway, J. (1963). "A vascular abnormality in hypertension: a study of blood flow in the forearm," *Circ.* **27,** 520–29.

Davis, J. O., C. C. J. Carpenter, and C. R. Ayers (1962). "Relation of renin and angiotensin II to the control of aldosterone secretion," *Circ. Res.* **11,** 171–81.

Dickinson, C. J. (1965). *Neurogenic hypertension.* Oxford: Blackwell.

Fejfar, Z., and J. Widimsky (1960). "Juvenile hypertension," *Proc. of joint WHO-Czechoslovak Cardiological Society Symposium on the Pathogenesis of Essential Hypertension*, pp. 33–42. Prague: State Medical Publ. House.

Ferguson, D. J., and R. L. Varco (1955). "The relation of blood pressure and flow to the development and regression of experimentally induced pulmonary arteriosclerosis," *Circ. Res.* **3**, 152–58.

Folkow, B. (1956). "Structural, myogenic, humoral and nervous factors controlling peripheral resistance," *Hypotensive drugs*, pp. 163–74. London: Pergamon.

Folkow, B., and E. H. Rubinstein (1966). "Cardiovascular effects of acute and chronic stimulations of the hypothalamic defence area in the rat," *Acta Physiol. Scand.* **68**, 48–57.

Folkow, B., and R. Sivertsson (1964). "Aspects of the difference in vascular 'reactivity' between cutaneous resistance vessels and A-V anastomoses," *Angiologica*, **I**, 338–45.

Folkow, B., and R. Sivertsson (1968). "Adaptive changes in 'reactivity' and wall/lumen ratio in cat blood vessels exposed to prolonged transmural pressure difference," *Life Sci.* **7**, Part I, 1283–89.

Folkow, B., G. Grimby, and O. Thulesius (1958). "Adaptive structural changes of the vascular walls in hypertension and their relation to the control of the peripheral resistance," *Acta Physiol. Scand.* **44**, 255–72.

Folkow, B., M. Hallbäck, Y. Lundgren, and L. Weiss (1969). "Structurally based increase of flow resistance in spontaneously hypertensive rats. XIII Scandinavian Congress of Physiology," *Acta Physiol. Scand.*, Suppl., 330, 94.

Folkow, B., M. Hallbäck, Y. Lundgren, and L. Weiss (1970). "Background of increased flow resistance and vascular 'reactivity' in spontaneously hypertensive rats," *Acta Physiol. Scand.*, **80**, 93–106.

Goldblatt, H. (1948). *The renal origin of hypertension.* Springfield, Ill.: Charles C. Thomas.

Henry, J. P., J. P. Meehan, and P. M. Stephens (1967). "The use of psychosocial stimuli to induce prolonged hypertension in mice," *Psychosomatic Medicine*, **27**, 408–32.

Hinman, A. T., B. T. Engel, and A. F. Bickford (1962). "Portable blood pressure recorder accuracy and preliminary use in evaluating intradaily variations in pressure," *Am. Heart J.* **63**, 663–68.

Kezdi, P., ed. (1967) "Baroreceptors and hypertension," Pergamon Press.

McCubbin, J. W., R. Soares DeMoura, I. H. Page, and F. Olmsted (1965). "Arterial hypertension elicited by subpressor amounts of angiotensin," *Science*, **149**, 1394–95.

Okamoto, K., and K. Aoki (1963). "Development of a strain of spontaneously hypertensive rats," *Jap. Circulat. J.* **27**, 282–93.

Page, I. H. (1949). "Pathogenesis of arterial hypertension," *J. Am. Med. Assoc.* **140**, 451–60.

Page, I. H., and J. W. McCubbin (1965). "The physiology of arterial hypertension," *Handbook of Physiology*, 2, Circulation **III**, 2163–208.

Page, I. H., and J. W. McCubbin (1968). *Renal hypertension*. Chicago: Year Book Med. Publ.

Pickering, G. (1968). *High blood pressure*. London: Churchill.

Proceedings of the Joint WHO-Czechoslovak Cardiological Society Symposium on the Pathogenesis of Essential Hypertension (1960). Prague: State Medical Publ. House.

Robinson, S. C., and M. Brucer (1940). *Arch. Int. Med.* **66**, 393–417.

Simonson, E., and J. Brozek (1959). "Russian research on arterial hypertension," *Ann. Int. Med.* **50**, 129–93.

Sivertsson, R. (1970). "The hemodynamic importance of structural vascular changes in essential hypertension," *Acta Physiol. Scand.* **79**, suppl. 343.

Sivertsson, R., and R. Olander (1968). "Aspects of the nature of the increased vascular resistance and increased 'reactivity' to noradrenaline in hypertensive subjects," *Life Sci.* **7**, 1291–97.

Index